MASTER TECHNIQUES IN ORTHOPAEDIC SURGERY

■

KNEE ARTHROPLASTY

MASTER TECHNIQUES IN ORTHOPAEDIC SURGERY

■

Series Editor
Roby C. Thompson, Jr., M.D.

Volume Editors

THE FOOT AND ANKLE
Kenneth A. Johnson, M.D.

RECONSTRUCTIVE KNEE SURGERY
Douglas W. Jackson, M.D.

KNEE ARTHROPLASTY
Paul A. Lotke, M.D.

THE HIP
Clement B. Sledge, M.D.

THE SPINE
David S. Bradford, M.D.

THE SHOULDER
Edward V. Craig, M.D.

THE ELBOW
Bernard F. Morrey, M.D.

THE WRIST
Richard H. Gelberman, M.D.

THE HAND
James W. Strickland, M.D.

KNEE ARTHROPLASTY

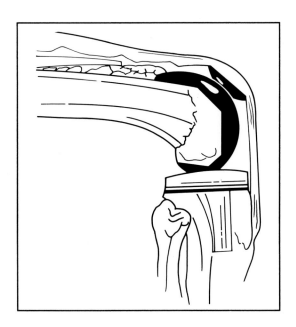

Editor

PAUL A. LOTKE, M.D.
Professor
Department of Orthopaedics
Hospital of the University of Pennsylvania
Philadelphia, Pennsylvania

Illustrator

Caspar Henselmann
New York, New York

Raven Press ✎ New York

Raven Press, Ltd., 1185 Avenue of the Americas, New York, New York 10036

Made in the United States of America

Library of Congress Cataloging-in-Publication Data

Knee arthroplasty / editor, Paul A. Lotke ; illustrator, Caspar
   Henselmann.
      p. cm.—(Master techniques in orthopaedic surgery)
   Includes bibliographical references and index.
   ISBN 0-7817-0032-9
   1. Knee—Surgery. 2. Total knee replacement. 3. Knee—
Reoperation. I. Lotke, Paul A. II. Series.
   [DNLM: 1. Arthroplasty—methods—atlases. 2. Knee—surgery—
atlases. WE 168 M423 1995]
RD561.K573 1995
617.5'82059—dc20
DNLM/DLC
for Library of Congress   93-42856

The material contained in this volume was submitted as previously unpublished material, except in the instances in which credit has been given to the source from which some of the illustrative material was derived.

Great care has been taken to maintain the accuracy of the information contained in the volume. However, neither Raven Press nor the editor can be held responsible for errors or of any consequences arising from the use of the information contained herein.

Materials appearing in this book prepared by individuals as part of their official duties as U.S. Government employees are not covered by the above-mentioned copyright.

9 8 7 6 5 4 3 2 1

To my wife, Dorothy-Sue,
and my children, Michael, Eric, and Pam,
who have accepted and supported the time-consuming
lifestyle of an orthopaedic surgeon.

■

CONTENTS

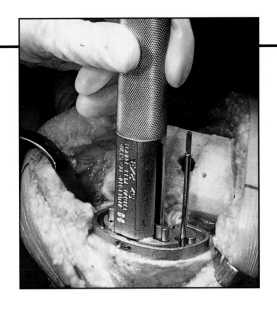

CONTRIBUTORS

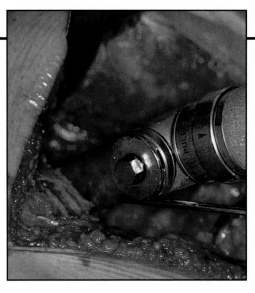

Frederick F. Buechel, M.D.
Clinical Professor, Department of Orthopaedic Surgery, South Mountain Orthopaedics, P.A., 61 First Street, South Orange, New Jersey 07079

Clifford W. Colwell, Jr., M.D.
Clinical Professor, Department of Orthopaedics and Rehabilitation, University of California San Diego; Head, Division of Orthopaedic Surgery, Scripps Clinic and Research Foundation, 10666 North Torrey Pines Road, La Jolla, California 92037

Lawrence D. Dorr, M.D.
Director and Professor, The Center for Arthritis & Joint Implant Surgery, USC University Hospital, 1510 San Pablo Street, Suite 634, Los Angeles, California 90033-4634

William F. Flynn, Jr.
Fellow, Adult Reconstructive Service, The Hospital for Special Surgery, 535 East 70th Street, New York, New York 10021

Mark L. Harlow, M.D.
Attending Surgeon, Department of Orthopedic Surgery, Rapid City Regional Hospital, and Black Hills Orthopaedic Clinic, 2805 Fifth Street, Suite 120, Rapid City, South Dakota 57701

Aaron A. Hofmann, M.D.
Professor, Division of Orthopedic Surgery, University of Utah School of Medicine, 50 N. Medical Drive, Salt Lake City, Utah 84132

David S. Hungerford, M.D.
Professor, Department of Orthopaedic Surgery, Johns Hopkins University School of Medicine, 5601 Loch Raven Boulevard, Baltimore, Maryland 21239

John N. Insall, M.D.
Clinical Professor, Department of Orthopaedic Surgery, Mt. Sinai School of Medicine; Attending Orthopaedic Surgeon, Beth Israel Medical Center—North, New York, New York; and Director, Insall Scott Kelly Institute for Orthopaedic and Sports Medicine, 170 East End Avenue, New York, New York 10128

Kurt J. Kitziger, M.D.
Clinical Professor, Department of Orthopaedics, Louisiana State University Medical Center, New Orleans, Louisiana, Orthopaedic Associates, 3525 Prytania, Suite 402, New Orleans, Louisiana 70115

Norman A. Johanson, M.D.
Associate Professor of Orthopaedic Surgery, Temple University School of Medicine, Broad and Ontario Streets, Philadelphia, Pennsylvania 19140

Brian P. Johnson, M.D.
Orthopaedic Surgery Service, Brooke Army Medical Center, HSHE-SBR, Building 2376, Fort Van Huston, Texas 78234-6353

Don LaRossa, M.D.
Professor, Department of Surgery, Hospital University of Pennsylvania, 10 Penn Tower, 3400 Spruce Street, Philadelphia, Pennsylvania 19104

Paul A. Lotke, M.D.
Professor, Department of Orthopaedic Surgery, Hospital University of Pennsylvania, 3400 Spruce Street, Philadelphia, Pennsylvania 19104

John B. Meding, M.D.
Kendrick Memorial Hospital, and Sports Medicine & Joint Reconstructive Surgery, P.C., Center for Hip and Knee Surgery, 1199 Hadley Road, Mooresville, Indiana 46158

Bernard F. Morrey, M.D.
Chair, Department of Orthopedic Surgery, Mayo Clinic and Mayo Foundation, Professor of Orthopedics, Mayo Medical School, 200 First Street, SW, Rochester, Minnesota 55905

Chitranjan S. Ranawat, M.D.
Professor, Department of Orthopaedic Surgery, Cornell University Medical College, Chief, Combined Arthritis Service, The Hospital for Special Surgery, 535 East 70th Street, New York, New York 10021

James A. Rand, M.D.
Consultant, Division of Orthopedic Surgery, Mayo Clinic Scottsdale, 13400 East Shea Boulevard, Scottsdale, Arizona 85259, and Professor of Orthopedics, Mayo Medical School, Rochester, Minnesota

Merrill A. Ritter, M.D.
Professor, Department of Orthopaedic Surgery, Indiana University Medical Center, Kendrick Memorial Hospital and, Sports Medicine & Joint Reconstructive Surgery, P.C., Center for Hip and Knee Surgery, 1199 Hadley Road, Mooresville, Indiana 46158

Alexander A. Sapega, M.D.
Assistant Professor, Department of Orthopaedic Surgery, University of Pennsylvania Sports Medicine Center, 235 South 33rd Street, Philadelphia, PA 19104

Richard D. Scott, M.D.
Associate Clinical Professor, Department of Orthopedic Surgery, Harvard Medical School, 125 Parker Hill Avenue, Boston, Massachusetts 02120

Giles R. Scuderi, M.D.
Attending Orthopaedic Surgeon, Insall Scott Kelly Institute for Orthopaedic and Sports Medicine, Beth Israel Medical Center—North Division, 170 East End Ave, New York, New York 10128

Thomas P. Sculco, M.D.
Professor of Orthopaedic Surgery, Cornell University Medical College, New York, New York; Director of Orthopaedic Surgery, The Hospital for Special Surgery, 535 East 70th Street, New York, New York 10021

Roby C. Thompson, Jr., M.D.
Professor and Head, Department of Orthopaedic Surgery, University of Minnesota Hospital and Clinic, 420 Delaware Street, SE, Minneapolis, Minnesota 55455

Thomas S. Thornhill, M.D.
Associate Clinical Professor of Orthopaedics, Harvard Medical School, Brigham and Women's Hospital, New England Baptist Hospital, 75 Francis Street, Boston, Massachusetts 02115

Russell E. Windsor, M.D.
Associate Professor, Department of Orthopaedic Surgery, Cornell University Medical College, and Associate Chief of the Knee Service, The Hospital for Special Surgery, 535 East 70th Street, New York, New York 10021

ACKNOWLEDGMENTS

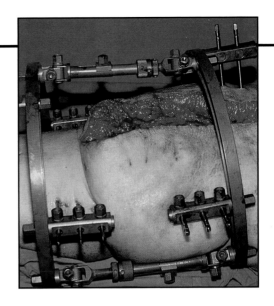

I gratefully acknowledge the authors who contributed their time and expertise to this textbook. Without exception, they are leaders in their field and have learned the hard way how to perfect their surgical techniques. They are true masters and have dedicated their time and energy to help us become better knee surgeons.

In addition, I acknowledge the fine support given by the publishers and their staff, particularly Kathey Alexander, Danette Knopp, and Joyce-Rachel John. Their long hours and dedication to making this textbook successful is a credit to them and the publisher.

SERIES PREFACE

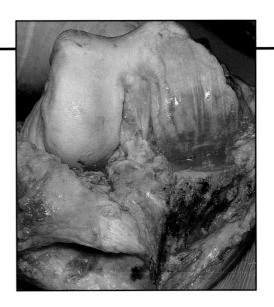

Master Techniques in Orthopaedic Surgery is a series of nine volumes designed to provide direct, detailed access to techniques preferred by orthopaedic surgeons who are recognized by their colleagues as "masters" in their specialty. The volume editors are leaders who, through their research and educational efforts, have earned the respect of their peers. The chapter authors, selected for their experience and skills, present the techniques in a personal manner bringing their unique perspectives and observations to the reader.

These atlases are designed to help the practitioner deal with the difficult but common problems encountered in daily practice. Experimental techniques and technology that are so sophisticated that most cases are referred to a treatment center are avoided, as are straightforward surgical techniques that seldom cause difficulty.

These books take you into the operating room and let you peer over the shoulder of the surgeon at work. The color photographs and accompanying drawings guide you step-by-step through a procedure. The commentary, organized in a standardized format throughout the series, offers you specific technical advice, as well as tips and pearls gained through the surgeons' years of experience.

The shared knowledge and expertise found in these pages are presented to enable the surgeon to undertake surgical procedures with greater confidence and improved proficiency.

Roby C. Thompson, Jr. M.D.
Series Editor

PREFACE

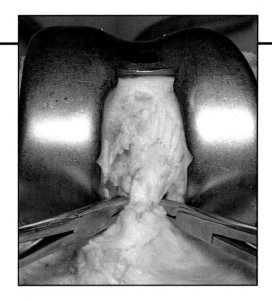

Orthopaedic surgery is a craft. It requires the surgical skills that allow us to accomplish the goals of any given procedure. Although good clinical judgment and the wisdom regarding a particular surgical treatment precede any exposure in the operating theater, the product of the orthopaedic surgeon's experience and clinical skills depends on the ability to master the techniques of surgery. The teaching of these skills is an art in itself and, ideally, is best accomplished through listening and watching an experienced surgeon. This book attempts to accomplish that educational goal. It is a personalized surgical technique book written by experienced masters that is designed to help solve a series of orthopaedic problems concerning the knee. These master technicians explain to the reader their own approach to a particular problem and how they solve it. We all recognize that there are many ways to accomplish the same objective; this text teaches the reader individual preferences in orthopaedic surgical technique.

The book is organized so that the first five sections outline methods of surgical exposure. These are generalized approaches to the knee that can be used in a variety of knee problems. They are not meant to solve a specific case but to give a broad approach to most common problems related to adult reconstructive surgery.

The second section is devoted principally to total knee arthroplasty. This procedure has demonstrated excellent longevity and function, and it has become the procedure of choice for many problems related to the adult knee. This section has been divided into three subsections starting from a standard approach towards a primary total knee with minimal or moderate deformities to unusual problems not encountered in a routine arthroplasty (i.e., loss of bone, limited motion, or significant preoperative patella problems).

The third section reviews methods of approach to a revision total knee. With over 200,000 joints being replaced each year with a 95 percent success rate, we still have 10,000 joints each year requiring some form of revision. The management of this problem is outlined in detail and includes not only the routine approach to revision surgery but also the management of unusual problems, such as skin necrosis, extensor mechanism problems, and the septic knee.

A number of other important reconstructive procedures that address specific knee problems are discussed in the fourth section. These include unicompartmental arthroplasty, tibial and femoral osteotomies, patellectomy, arthrodesis, and joint debridement. All these techniques are explained in detail and the personal approach of the masters is carefully outlined.

The focus of this book is to teach the surgical skills necessary to complete the immediate tasks at hand. It is not designed to be an all-inclusive textbook but, rather, a learning session with the surgeons along with discussions and illustrations as guides.

As editor, I have learned a great deal from the masters who have put forth their efforts in explaining their approaches to the knee. Their efforts will be equally rewarding to you.

Paul A. Lotke, M.D.

MASTER TECHNIQUES IN ORTHOPAEDIC SURGERY

■

KNEE ARTHROPLASTY

PART I

Surgical Exposures

Master Techniques in Orthopaedic Surgery,
KNEE ARTHROPLASTY, edited by P. A. Lotke,
Raven Press, Ltd., New York © 1995.

1

Anterior Medial Exposures

Paul A. Lotke

INDICATIONS/CONTRAINDICATIONS

The anterior medial incision is the classic approach to the knee joint (Fig. 1). It has very few drawbacks and offers many advantages. It is extensile, follows anatomic planes, gives excellent access to the intraarticular and periarticular structure, and allows large exposure with relatively short incision and minimal soft-tissue dissection. In addition, this approach is safe and avoids the neurovascular structures.

The specific indications for a *short* anterior medial arthrotomy (Fig. 1A) incision would include such procedures as removal of loose bodies, open meniscectomies, retrieval of broken arthroscopy instruments, tibial tubercle surgery, and patellar tendon realignments, quadriceps tendon repair or reconstruction, and drainage of sepsis.

The moderate length anterior medial arthrotomy (Fig. 1B) incision would be useful for such surgical procedures as open synovectomy or joint debridement, patellectomy, unicompartmental arthroplasty, and medial tibial plateau fracture.

The *long* exposure (Fig. 1C), which is extensile both proximally and distally, can be used classically for total knee arthroplasty. It may also be extended proximally to provide exposure for the internal fixation of distal femur fractures, and extended distally for tibial plateau fractures.

The contraindications to the anterior medial incision are relatively few. It allows no exposure posteriorly and is not recommended for anterior lateral procedures such as proximal tibial osteotomies, or other isolated procedures to the lateral side of the knee. A relative contraindication to this incision is a previous long parallel lateral incision. Care should be taken to avoid parallel incision to every practical extent; if possible, one may use a previous longitudinal skin incision, and dissect under a skin flap to the anterior medial aspect of the knee for the

P. A. Lotke, M.D.: Department of Orthopedic Surgery, Hospital University of Pennsylvania, Philadelphia, PA 19104.

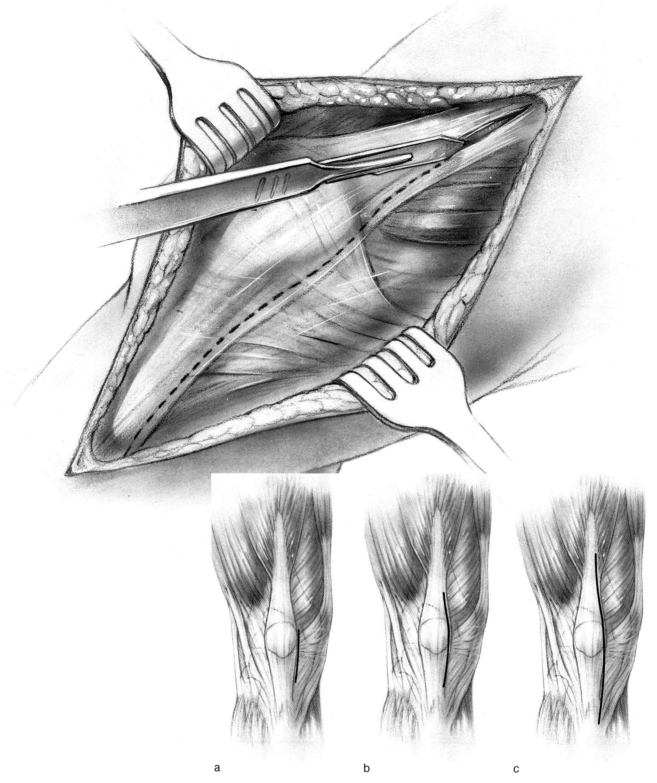

a   b   c

Figure 1. The anterior incision is extensile and gives excellent access to the intraarticular and periarticular structures, depending on the length of the incision. **a:** The short anterior medial arthrotomy incision is placed parallel to the patellar tendon, 4 cm proximal and distal to the joint line. **b:** The midlength anterior medial incision extends from a few centimeters above the patella to a few centimeters below and medial to the tibial tubercle. **c:** The long anterior incision starts 7 cm proximal to the midline of the superior pole of the patella and extends down over the patella and distally along the medial border of the patellar tendon and tibial tubercle to 7 cm below the lower pole of the patella.

capsular incision. Transverse skin incisions do not appear to affect the healing of the vertical anterior medial approach, and short previous medial or lateral incisions may be disregarded. However, when possible, the anterior incision should incorporate other previous longitudinal incisions about the knee.

PREOPERATIVE PLANNING

The most important aspect of the preoperative planning for the anterior medial incision involves recognition of the importance of previous incisions, as mentioned above. If there are two preexisting longitudinal incisions about the knee, I will generally choose the longer of the two. In addition, if there is a preoperative incision that seems impossible to incorporate within the anterior medial incision, then one should move as far away from that previous incision as practical. The length of the anterior incision will vary somewhat according to body type (i.e., excellent exposure can be obtained in thinner, more frail patients with shorter incisions, in contrast to very muscular or obese patients.

SURGERY

The patient is placed supine on the operating table. A protective belt should always be applied across the upper body to allow tilting of the table as needed. A tourniquet is applied to the upper thigh (Fig. 2). The tourniquet should be applied snugly and as far proximally as practical. In the very obese patient, the fat may be pulled distally from beneath the tourniquet, causing it to bulge from the distal edge of the tourniquet. This prevents it from migrating and ensures that the tourniquet is placed as far proximal as practical. A sandbag is taped to the table at a level just distal to the joint line. When the knee is fully flexed, the foot engages the sandbag and can be maintained in the flexed position without the use of an assistant.

There are many ways to prep and drape a patient for the anterior medial incision, but I have found that suspending the heel in a leg holder gives excellent access to the knee and allows surgical personnel to be available for other purposes. We use an organic iodine solution which we partly remove to enable an adhesive plastic drape to adhere more tightly to the skin. An impermeable, waterproof stockinette is placed over the unprepped foot (Fig. 3), after which a double-knit stockinette is placed over the entire leg and over the tourniquet. A limb extremity

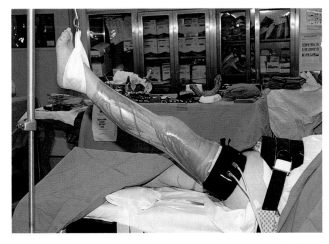

Figure 2. Leg suspended and completely prepped. Tourniquet is placed on the thigh as proximal as possible.

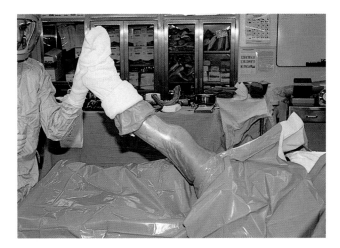

Figure 3. Draping is done in stages, using a plastic sheet to drape away the tourniquet.

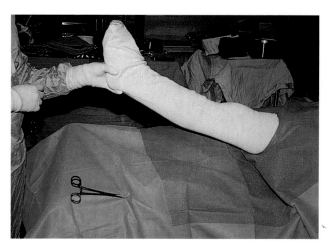

Figure 4. A "limb" sheet is used to cover the upper body and table. A large cuff under the thigh allows motion of the leg without moving the drapes. A clamp prevents the drapes from migrating during the procedure.

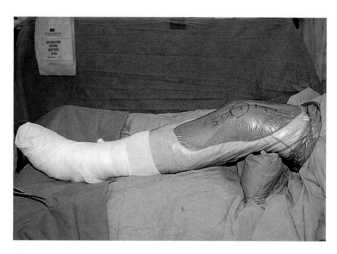

Figure 5. A plastic sheet can be used to keep the skin sterile.

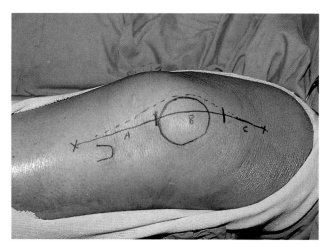

Figure 6. The incision is marked on the front of the knee from the midportion of the quadriceps tendon to the medial aspect of the tibial tubercle.

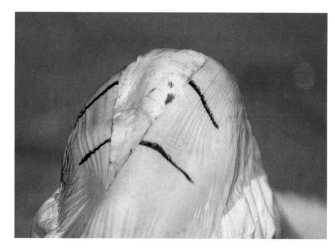

Figure 7. As the deep fascia is split, the quadriceps tendon and patellar retinaculum are readily exposed.

sheet with a rubberized central portion having a hole in it is then slipped over the stockinette and pulled proximally to the tourniquet level (Fig. 4). A folded cuff is tucked under the most proximal portion of the thigh in order to prevent the drape sheets from migrating when the knee is flexed. The cuff allows full, unrestricted motion of the lower extremity, which is a valuable benefit of this draping technique. With paper drapes, there is a tendency for the drapes to move on each other, and I clip these drapes to the foot of the mattress in order to prevent this migration. The front of the stockinette is removed over the anterior aspect of the knee, and transverse lines are drawn with an ink pen in order to reapproximate the skin anatomically. An adhesive plastic drape is applied to encircle the leg (Fig. 5). A folded sheet is placed under the knee in order to slightly flex the knee.

Prior to making the incision I check to be sure there is enough area exposed to incorporate the entire incision, that the cuff is large enough to prevent pulling of the drapes, and that the covering over the extremity is thin enough so that I can appreciate the alignment and bone landmarks in the lower leg.

Technique

Any part of the anterior medial incision may be used to approach the knee (Fig. 6). The incision may be extended as far proximally and distally as necessary in order to obtain adequate exposure. The long anterior incision starts 7 cm proximal to the midline of the superior pole of the patella, and extends down over the patella and distally along the medial border of the patellar tendon and tibial tubercle to 7 cm below the lower pole of the patella. Any segment of this incision may be utilized for a variety of reasons, and the incisions may be extended more proximally and distally for fracture or tumor surgery (Fig. 1).

Long Anterior Medial Incision. The long anterior medial incision may be considered the standard full-exposure approach to the knee for such procedures as total knee arthroplasty.

The incision is taken through the skin, fat, and Scarpa's fascia to the anterior border of the quadriceps tendon, patella, (Figs. 7 and 8), and medial border of the patellar tendon. The quadriceps tendon is incised in the line of its fibers, 1

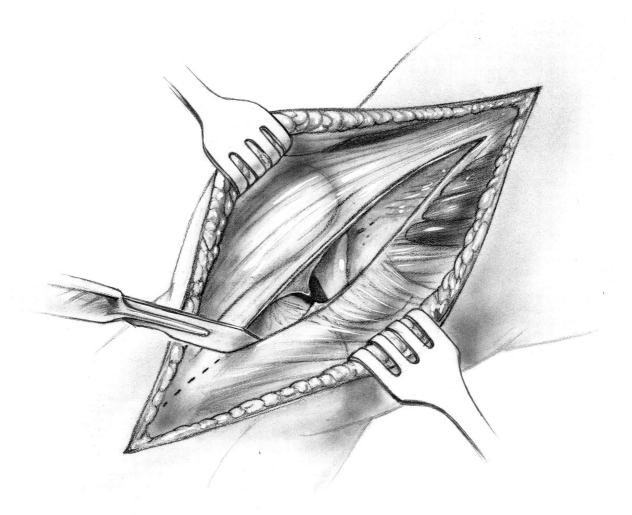

Figure 8. The anterior incision is taken straight vertically in front of the knee joint, with a slight medial orientation. It begins at the midportion of the quadriceps tendon and ends parallel to the tibial tubercle along the anterior tibial spine. The deep incision splits the quadriceps tendon in the line of its fibers, approximately 1 cm from the insertion of the vastus medialis. It curves gently along the medial edge of the patella, leaving a 5-mm rim of retinaculum attached to the patella, and then extending distally parallel to the patellar tendon. The synovium is incised parallel to the deep incision.

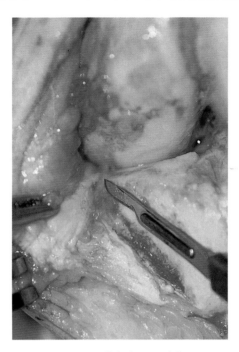

Figure 9. The medial sleeve of the exposure can be readily developed with a retractor on the meniscus and a scalpel incising the coronary ligaments and entering into the pes anserinus bursa.

cm from the vastus medialis. It curves gently in the line of the quadriceps muscle insertion along the medial edge of the patella, and gently back along the medial border of the patella (Fig. 1). It extends distally to the rim of the meniscus and distally onto the proximal tibial, medial and parallel to the tibial tubercle.

The arthrotomy incision is made through the medial retinaculum, capsule, and synovium; just medial to the patella, 5 mm of retinaculum and capsule remain to the patella in order to facilitate repair. The incision is taken distally, parallel to the patellar tendon. The joint space is entered and if the meniscus is to be excised, such as for an arthroplasty, the meniscus is incised vertically just medial to its anterior horn attachment. With a sharp rake placed on the cut edge of the medial segment of the meniscus, it is folded medially and the coronary ligaments are exposed. These can be incised sharply with a knife (Fig. 9). Using the principle of the acute or stripping angle of Henry (1), the knife incises the coronary ligament and is advanced distally under the medial retinaculum within the bursa of the pes anserinus (Fig. 10). With mild knee flexion, the supraperiosteal plane is readily developed with the edge of a small scalpel held on top of the periosteum. The blade is advanced distally and posteriorly. The posterior segment of this dissection is completed with a periosteal elevator. The bursa lies beneath the pes tendons and medial collateral ligaments, and superficial to the periosteum. Working within this bursa leaves the periosteal blood vessels intact, and the dissection may be readily carried as far posterior as the semimembranosus tendon. A Z-retractor is placed at the posterior margin of the dissection to maintain exposure. With this dissection, the entire media sleeve, which includes the medial collateral ligament, the pes anserinus tendons, and the medial retinaculum remain as one unit and can be readily resutured into their anatomic positions at closure.

The proximal extension of the long anterior medial incision follows the line of fibers within the quadriceps tendon. If the extension is placed properly, the

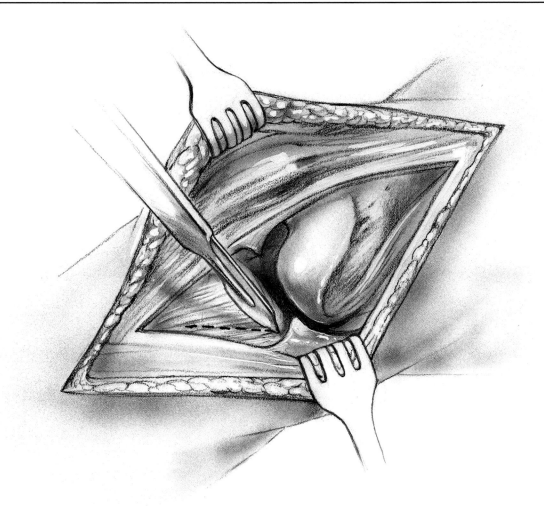

Figure 10. The medial segment of this incision is developed as one continuous sleeve, including the medial retinaculum, the meniscal attachment, the medial collateral ligament, and the pes anserinus tendons. The coronary ligament is incised and a scalpel is advanced distally under the medial retinaculum within the pes anserinus bursa. With mild knee flexion and varus positioning, the supraperiosteal plane is readily developed as one advances distally and posteriorly. The most posterior segment of this dissection is completed with a periosteal elevator. The bursa lies between the pes tendons and the medial collateral ligament, and superficial to the periosteum. Remaining within this bursa leaves the periosteal blood vessels intact. This dissection can be readily carried posteriorly to the semimembranosus tendon.

quadriceps tendon is split without cutting the fibers. The incision is extended approximately 6 cm above the patella. The patella may then be everted and the knee flexed. If a total knee arthroplasty is contemplated and wide exposure laterally is indicated, the anterior capsule behind the fat pad is incised. Prior to flexing the knee, a right-angle retractor is placed into the bursa posterior to the patellar fat pad. With minimal dissection, the entire anterior lateral aspect of the knee is exposed through this bursa (Figs. 11 and 12). Sharp dissection detaches the fat pad from the lateral meniscus. This allows the patella to be readily mobilized for eversion. The ligamentum mucosa should also be sectioned. With the patella everted, the knee is gradually flexed to ensure that there is adequate exposure without too much tension on the soft-tissue structures. If the quadriceps tendon is too tight, the incision may be extended proximally in the line of the fibers by

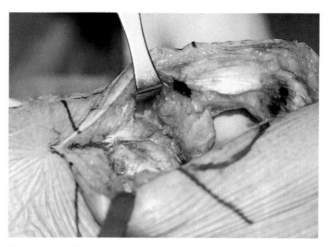

Figure 11. The bursa behind the patellar fat pad gives ready access to the anterior and lateral aspects of the joint. A right-angle retractor exposes this bursa.

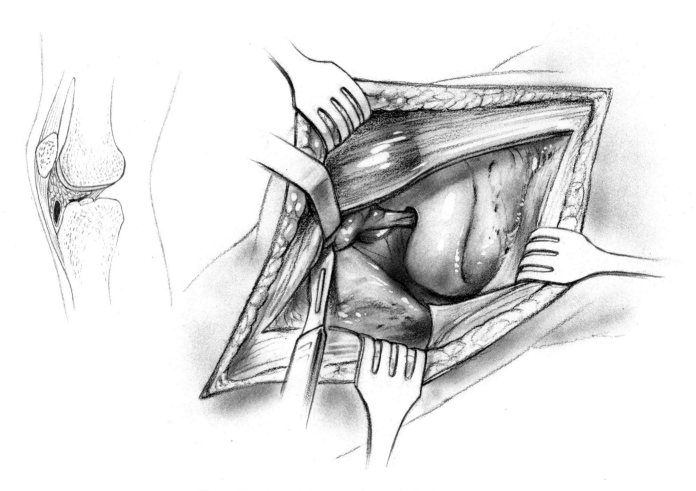

Figure 12. The anterior capsule can be incised behind the fat pad of the retropatellar tendon. A right-angle retractor is placed into the bursa posterior to the fat pad. With minimal dissection the entire anterior lateral aspect of the knee is exposed through this bursa. Sharp dissection detaches the fat pad from the lateral meniscus and the anterior capsular attachments. This allows the patella to be readily mobilized for eversion.

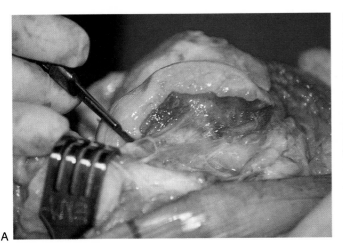
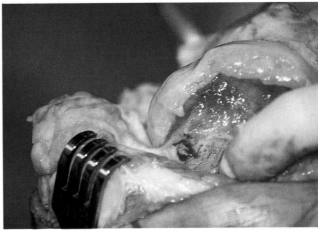

Figure 13. A,B: On the lateral side of the joint, the patellar femoral ligament serves to tether the patellar tendon, and its release gives excellent access to the lateral side of the tibial plateau.

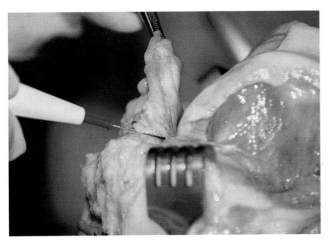
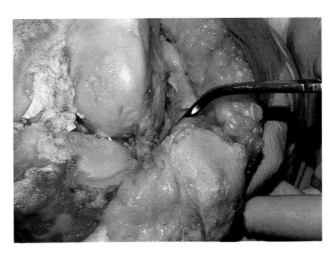

Figure 14. The posterior portion of the fat pad and its attachment to the lateral meniscus may be excised to give better exposure to the lateral corner of the knee.

Figure 15. A Homan retractor placed over the lateral edge of the tibial plateau retracts the soft tissues from the lateral side of the knee.

gently dissecting and separating the fibers longitudinally. The patella is then reflected laterally with a sharp rake or Homan retractor, and the patella femoral ligament is identified and incised (Fig. 13 A,B). This ligament is sometimes a very dense structure that prevents adequate access to the lateral aspect of the knee during an arthroplasty. For a total knee arthroplasty, the posterior aspect of the fat pad may be excised. The extent of fat-pad removal depends on the type of prosthesis and size of the patient (Fig. 14). In order to obtain better exposure along the lateral aspect of the knee, especially for total knee arthroplasty, the lateral meniscus should be detached at its anterior horn and incised along the lateral margin of the tibial plateau; the incision may be continued into the meniscal popliteal hiatus. The inferior lateral geniculate artery is encountered in this location and should be identified and cauterized (Fig. 15). For most total knee arthroplasties, the anterior cruciate ligament is sacrificed, permitting the entire tibia to be subluxed forward (Fig. 12), thus allowing complete exposure to the tibial platea. The details for obtaining maximal exposure and ligamentous balance for a total joint arthroplasty are further elucidated in the chapters devoted to that procedure.

Pearls   I would like to emphasize a few of my personal practices that facilitate exposure of the knee and make the surgery on it flow efficiently. The anterior medial retinacular incision leaves a 5-mm remnant of tissue attached to the patella and expedites closure. I like to utilize the bursae that exist about the knee and thereby minimize surgical dissection. The two principal bursae into which I enter are the bursa behind the fat pad of the patella and the pes anserinus bursa. The former allows extension over the entire anterior lateral aspect of the knee without disrupting a blood vessel on the periosteum. The pes bursa beneath the medial collateral ligament and pes anserinus tendons is entered from above and through the coronary ligament attachment. This approach allows very rapid and minimally traumatic exposure of the medial and posterior aspects of the tibial metaphysis. A Homan retractor, bent in its midportion to a right angle, is a handy instrument to place on the edges of the lateral tibial plateau; it effectively holds back the patellar tendon and gives excellent exposure to the lateral side of the knee (Fig. 16).

Exposure of the knee with this anterior medial approach can become very efficient and offer several other advantages to the knee surgeon. If care is taken to make a single incision through the medial retinacular structures, without multiple small defects, the repair is quite simple, with smooth borders clearly defined. With flexion and external rotation, the dissection along the proximal medial tibia allows good access to the posterior medial aspect of the tibia, where the semimembranosus tendon can be exposed or incised. With increasing external rotation and flexion, the entire posterior medial corner of the knee can be approached. This is further described in the chapters on ligament release and balance for total knee arthroplasty.

Extra Long Incision. The anterior medial incision may be extended proximally and distally in order to assist in the treatment of supracondylar fractures, femoral osteotomies, or fractures and tumors of the tibial plateau.

Proximally, the skin and quadriceps tendon incisions are extended and the anterior aspect of the distal femur may be well visualized.

Distally, after the anterior incision is made in the prepatellar bursa, the skin is reflected from the deep fascia, permitting ready exposure of both the medial and lateral retinaculum. Entry into the joint on either side of the patella can be completed if necessary. As the knee is flexed, the skin is separated from deep fascia and reflected posteriorly for excellent exposure of both sides of the proximal tibia (Fig. 7). This is an excellent incision for bicondylar plateau fractures, medial or lateral plateau fractures, and proximal tibial tumor surgery.

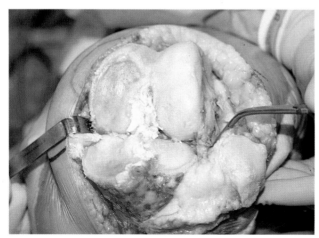

Figure 16. After the exposure has been completed, the entire knee is widely exposed for any surgical procedure.

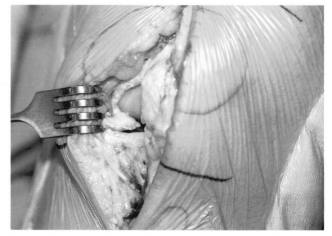

Figure 17. A small arthrotomy can be completed on the medial side of the knee by using the midportion of the wound. This centers over the joint line and allows ready access to the menisci and joint-line structures.

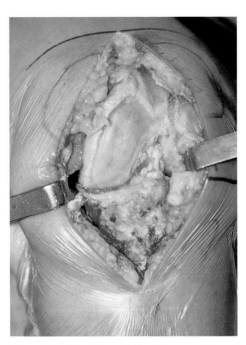

Figure 18. A midlength incision may be utilized to allow exposure of and surgical intervention in the medial compartment of the knee.

Short Arthrotomy Incision. A short arthrotomy incision utilizes the distal segment of the approach to the knee described above. The incision is placed anteriorly, 4 cm proximal and distal to the joint line (Figs. 12 and 17). It is taken through the skin and subcutaneous tissue, and down through the deep fascia. The wound edges are retracted medially and the medial retinaculum is incised medial to the skin incision, 5 mm from the medial border of the patella. The arthrotomy is taken through the medial capsule and synovium. Upon entering the joint, a right-angle retractor may be placed anteriorly to retract the patellar tendon and fat pad (Fig. 17). A Z-retractor is placed under the medial collateral ligament just above the meniscus. Through this small arthrotomy incision the joint may be well inspected, loose bodies removed, the medial meniscus excised, and other pathology identified and removed from the medial side of the knee.

The midlength anterior medial incision extends from 3 cm above the superior pole of the patella to 3 cm below the medial aspect of the tibial tubercle (Fig. 12). This incision is appropriate for unicompartmental arthroplasty, allografts to articular defects, the treatment of osteochondritis dissecans, and other purposes. The arthrotomy is made through the medial retinaculum, capsule, and synovium just medial to the patella, as noted above, leaving the 5 mm of retinaculum attached to the patella. The joint space is entered and if the meniscus is to be excised, such as for unicompartmental arthroplasty, the medial supraperiosteal dissection is performed as described above. By extending the incision proximally as far as necessary, usually 2 to 3 cm above the proximal pole, the patella is allowed to slide off the lateral femoral condyle as the knee is flexed (Fig. 18). This midlength approach gives excellent visualization of the medial condyle and medial proximal tibia without complete patellar eversion.

POSTOPERATIVE MANAGEMENT

The postoperative management of the anterior medial arthrotomy depends on the underlying procedure for which the arthrotomy was completed. With a short anterior medial incision, the recovery time is very brief. Patients can usually bear weight immediately, start motion within the first 24 hours, and expect to be returning to usual activities within 4 to 6 weeks. On the other hand, with long arthrotomies, including total joint procedures, the course is more prolonged and is individualized for such procedures, as noted in the succeeding chapters.

COMPLICATIONS

The most common complications of anterior medial arthrotomy are those associated with wound healing. Unless adequate soft-tissue closure is achieved, areas of wound separation or drainage can occur. The combination of swelling, long incision, and early mobilization can contribute to the retardation of healing. Therefore, careful management of the closure is important, and there is no substitution for good surgical technique.

Lesser complications include the sacrifice of the infrapatellar branch of the saphenous nerve. Depending on the individual size of this nerve, there will be an area of numbness or dysesthesia on the skin anterolateral to the proximal tibia. This gradually becomes less noticeable. It is noteworthy because some patients confuse the associated dysesthesia and numbness with a problem resulting from the intraarticular procedure.

An uncommon but potentially devastating complication results from overzealous eversion of the patella and flexion of the knee, which can avulse the patellar tendon from the tibial tubercle. This can be an extremely disabling problem and every effort should be made to avoid it. Techniques to avoid this complication are described in Chapter 6 on difficult exposures. Recognition of a partial avulsion of the patellar tendon will help prevent this problem. The more difficult the exposure, the greater is the risk of avulsion of the patellar tendon from the tibial tubercle.

In general, the anterior medial incision into the knee is a versatile, safe, and extensile approach that can be utilized for a variety of clinical problems, with relatively few complications.

RECOMMENDED READING

1. Henry, A. K.: *Extensile Exposure*, 2nd ed. pp. 4–5. E. S. Livingston Ltd., Edinborough, 1962.

Master Techniques in Orthopaedic Surgery,
Knee Arthroplasty, edited by P. A. Lotke,
Raven Press, Ltd., New York © 1995.

2

Submedialis Approach

Aaron A. Hofmann and Mark L. Harlow

INDICATIONS/CONTRAINDICATIONS

The submedialis (subvastus) approach is becoming increasingly popular in total knee arthroplasty. Although first described in the German literature in 1929, it has only recently been advocated for exposure of the knee joint for unicompartmental or total condylar replacements (1–5). The essential feature of the submedialis approach, which distinguishes it from the standard medial parapatellar approach, is that it does not divide the quadriceps tendon, but instead passes medially through the tendinous attachment of the vastus medialis to the patella and medial retinaculum (Fig. 1). When done properly, this technique provides excellent exposure of the articular surfaces of the knee, and offers the advantages of maintaining the integrity of the extensor mechanism and minimizing the disruption of the vascular supply to the patella.

It has been shown that the patellar blood supply comprises six major vessels (Fig. 2) (6). The medial parapatellar approach, of necessity, disrupts the medial circulation, and if combined with a lateral release may significantly deplete the anastomotic plexus. The submedialis approach spares the supreme geniculate vessel, which is contained within the belly of the vastus medialis.

The ideal candidate for the use of the submedialis approach is one who meets the following criteria: (i) primary arthroplasty, (ii) primary distal femoral osteotomy, (iii) no prior arthrotomies, and (iv) non-obese.

These guidelines provide a general framework for decision-making that must be individualized for each patient. As the surgeon becomes more facile with the submedialis approach, the indications may expand.

M.L. Harlow, m.d.: Department of Orthopedic Surgery, Rapid City Regional Hospital, and Black Hills Orthopaedic Clinic, Rapid City, South Dakota 57701.

A. A. Hofmann, m.d.: Division of Orthopedic Surgery, University of Utah School of Medicine, Salt Lake City, Utah 84132.

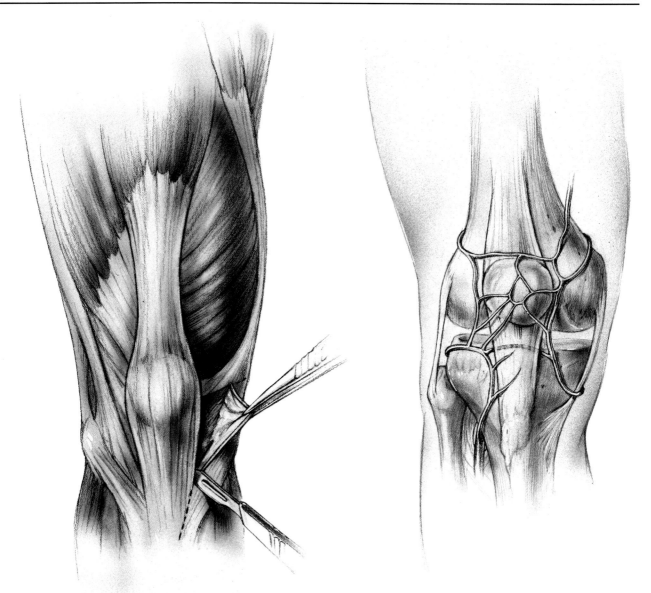

Figure 1. The inverted L capsular incision used in the submedialis approach.

Figure 2. Vascular supply of the patella. (Redrawn with permission from ref. 7.)

Relative contraindications to this surgical exposure include: (i) revision arthroplasty, (ii) prior major arthrotomy, (iii) prior proximal tibial osteotomy, (iv) prior arthrotomies, and (v) obesity.

Previous surgical procedures about the knee may have led to the formation of significant scar tissue, which may make patellar eversion more difficult. This may compromise the exposure of the joint surfaces and potentially jeopardize the insertion of the patellar ligament. Obesity, especially when combined with short stature, is associated with excessive soft-tissue impingement and difficult visualization.

SURGERY

A general or spinal anesthetic with complete motor paralysis is recommended. When the tourniquet is inflated, the knee should be in a flexed posture so as not to limit the excursion of the extensor mechanism.

Technique

The incision is made with the knee flexed to approximately 90 degrees, which facilitates the identification and separation of the tissue planes. The midline incision begins at a point approximately four finger-breadths proximal to the patella and extends distally to the level of the tibial tubercle (Fig. 3). The distal extent of the incision curves slightly medially to avoid placing the scar over the bony prominence of the tibial tubercle.

The first key structure to identify is fascial layer I, which is the continuation of the deep fascia of the thigh, found immediately deep to the subcutaneous adipose layer (Fig. 4) (7). Fascial layer I is incised in line with the skin incision. Blunt dissection is then used to separate layer I from the underlying perimuscular fascia of the vastus medialis. This should proceed in a proximal-to-distal fashion until the tendinous portion of the vastus medialis is visualized (Fig. 5). Occasionally these two fascial planes are adherent distally as they become confluent with the medial retinaculum. With layer I under tension, gentle dissection with a scalpel allows their separation.

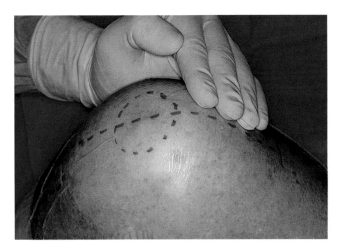

Figure 3. The skin incision is made with the knee flexed, and begins approximately four finger-breadths proximal to the superior pole of the patella.

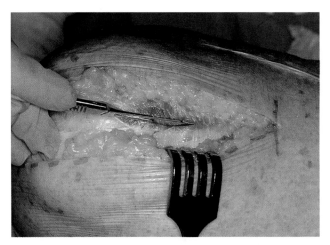

Figure 4. Fascial layer I is encountered immediately deep to the subcutaneous adipose layer.

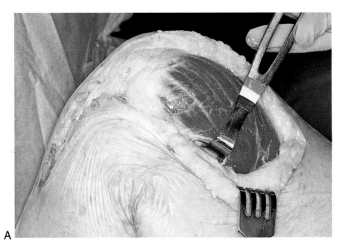

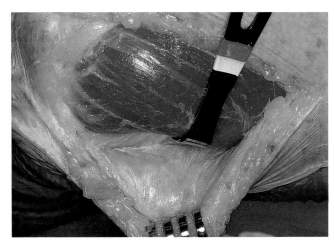

A   B

Figure 5. A: Layer I and the perimuscular fascia are separated to the point where the tendinous portion of the vastus medialis is identified. B: Layer I remains attached to the subcutaneous tissue.

The posterior margin of the muscle belly is now identified and bluntly elevated from the medial intermuscular septum (Fig. 6). This should proceed in a distal-to-proximal direction with the knee in a position of approximately 45 degrees of flexion. This diminishes the tension on the muscle belly, which allows it to be more easily mobilized. The muscle belly should be freed to a point approximately 10 cm proximal to the adductor tubercle. Occasionally, a small perforating vein passes through the medial septum into the muscle belly, and should be ligated or coagulated when encountered.

With the knee still flexed to approximately 45 degrees, the muscle belly is elevated anteriorly off the suprapatellar pouch (Fig. 7). This serves to put the tendi-

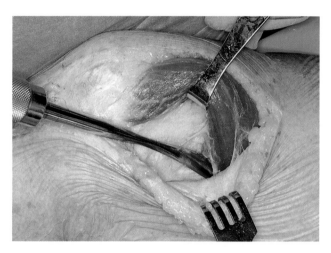

Figure 6. The vastus medialis muscle belly is elevated from the medial intramuscular septum with the knee in approximately 45 degrees of flexion.

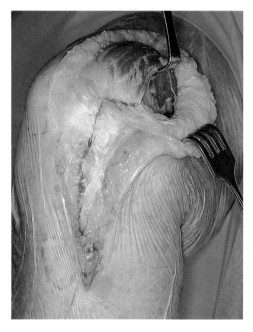

Figure 7. The muscle belly is now separated from the underlying suprapatellar pouch. The path of the inverted L capsular incision is seen outlined with methylene blue.

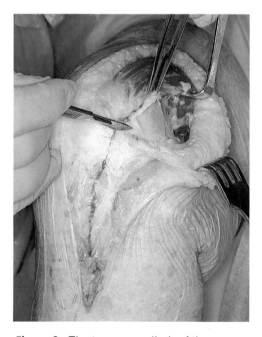

Figure 8. The transverse limb of the capsular incision is completed through the tendinous attachment of the vastus medialis to the medial retinaculum.

nous attachment of the vastus medialis under tension and facilitates its identification. The transverse limb of this inverted L incision is then completed through this tendinous attachment by lightly touching the scalpel to its fibers (Fig. 8). Care should be taken to ensure that a bridge of tendon stays attached to the muscle belly to ensure stable closure at the end of the procedure. Care should also be taken to avoid incising the underlying synovium when making the transverse limb of the incision.

The vertical limb of the incision is now completed. With the extensor mechanism retracted laterally, a curvilinear longitudinal arthrotomy is made through the suprapatellar pouch and continued distally through the medial retinaculum to the medial aspect of the tibial tubercle (Fig. 9). With the retinaculum released, the extensor mechanism can be retracted even further laterally, which will allow the fat pad incision to be made on its most medial border, which minimizes bleeding, maximizes local vascularity, and decreases postoperative adhesions (Fig. 10).

The knee is now taken to full extension and the patella everted (Fig. 11). If the patella is not easily everted, a more extensive release of the suprapatellar pouch

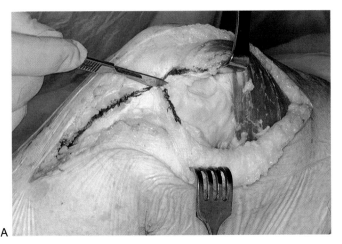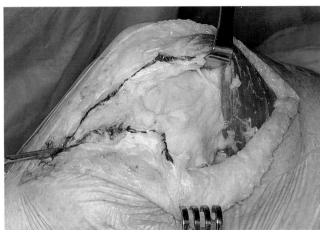
A   B

Figure 9. A,B: The vertical limb of the arthrotomy is now made through the suprapatellar pouch and the medial retinaculum.

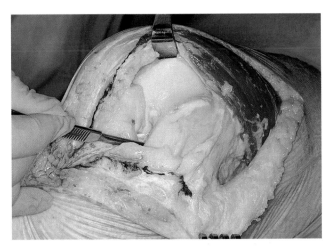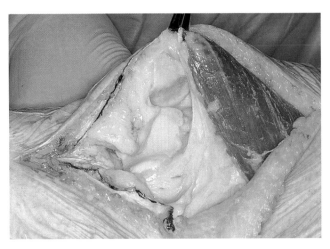

Figure 10. With the retinaculum released, the extensor mechanism may be retracted more laterally to allow for incision of the fat pad at its most medial aspect.

Figure 11. Patellar eversion is now attempted. For demonstration purposes, the suprapatellar pouch has been incompletely incised.

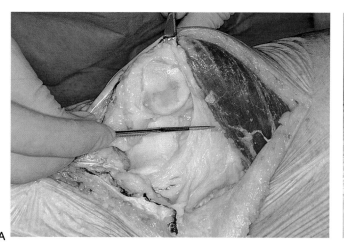
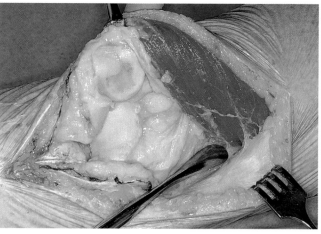

A   B

Figure 12. If patellar eversion is difficult, then **A:** a more extensive release of the suprapatellar pouch may be required or, **B:** more of the vastus medialis muscle belly may be mobilized from the medial intramuscular septum.

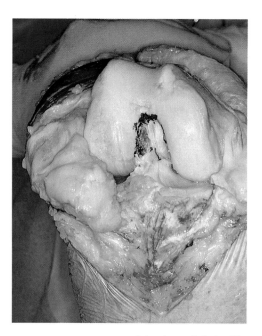

Figure 13. Exposure of the knee joint with the submedialis approach.

or a more proximal release of the muscle belly from the medial intermuscular septum may be required (Fig. 12). In severely arthritic knees, the removal of osteophytes or release of the lateral patellofemoral ligament may be required. In the rare case in which these maneuvers are not effective in achieving patellar eversion, the patella may be laterally dislocated and the knee maximally flexed. Over several minutes, while other steps of the procedure are being attended to, the soft tissues should gradually stretch enough to allow eversion of the patella.

Once the patella has been successfully everted, the knee is slowly and carefully flexed while visualizing the attachment of the patellar ligament to the tibial tubercle. If this appears to be jeopardized, then further release maneuvers should be undertaken, as described above. With proper technique, the visualization of the knee joint is equivalent to that achieved with a medial parapatellar arthrotomy (Fig. 13).

Lateral Release

Following insertion of the components, the final element of soft-tissue balancing is the assessment of patellar tracking. With this approach, visualization of the patellofemoral articulation is easily accomplished through the inferomedial window (Fig. 14A). With the extensor mechanism intact, the surgeon has the distinct advantage of being able to reliably assess patellar tracking and to accurately titrate a lateral release. If a lateral release is required, it is performed with the knee flexed. Fascial layer I is bluntly separated from the lateral retinaculum. The incision is

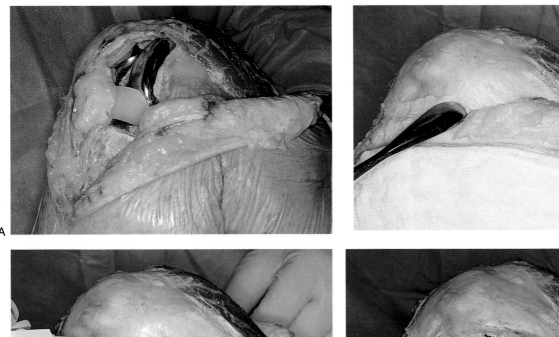

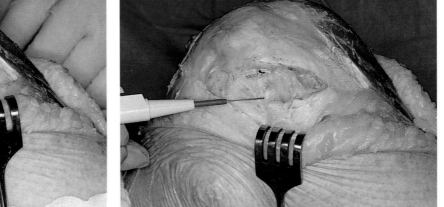

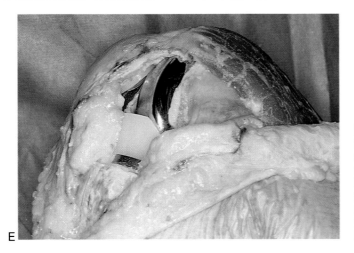

Figure 14. A: Visualization of the patellofemoral articulation through the inferomedial window of the submedialis approach. The patella is seen riding on the lateral femoral condyle. View of the knee from the lateral side showing **B:** blunt dissection of layer I from the underlying lateral retinaculum, **C:** lateral release 1.5 cm lateral to patellar margin, and **D:** preservation of underlying synovial tissue. **E:** Proper patellofemoral relationship following lateral release.

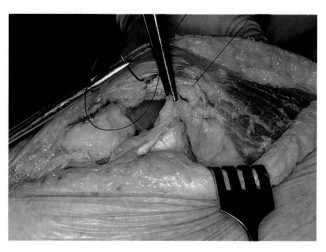

Figure 15. The synovial tissue is reapproximated with a running absorbable suture.

made approximately 1.5 cm lateral to the lateral margin of the patella, which should allow for avoidance of the lateral inferior geniculate and recurrent anterior tibial vessels (5). The release is titrated by direct visualization of the patellofemoral articulation through the inferomedial window (Fig. 14 B–E). If possible, the synovium should be preserved.

Following release of the tourniquet, hemostasis should be meticulously obtained. Particular attention should be paid to the medial intermuscular septum. The synovial tissue is closed with a running absorbable suture (Fig. 15). The key to capsular closure is the reapproximation of the apex of the "L" to its point of origin (Fig. 16). The transverse limb of the capsular incision is then closed by reapproximating the tendon of the vastus medialis to the medial retinaculum with interrupted sutures. The vertical limb is then closed by reapproximating the medial retinaculum, as would be done for a medial parapatellar approach. No reattachment of the muscle belly to the intra-muscular septum is necessary. Fascial layer I is then closed with interrupted absorbable sutures, and the skin is closed according to the surgeon's preference. The authors favor the application of a bulky compressive Jones' dressing.

COMPLICATIONS

The major complications related to the subvastus medialis approach are the same as with any surgical approach to the knee joint. However, two complications are unique to this particular surgery. The first is a subvastus hematoma, and the second is traumatization of the muscles from stretching and ischemia.

A subvastus hematoma may occur during the dissection of the vastus medialis from the septum of the inner musculature. A series of vessels run parallel to the posterior insertion of this septum and branch into the muscles in the posterior aspect of the vastus medialis. They can be visualized and coagulated during the surgical dissection. However, this dissection creates a space that does not readily compress, and proper attention to the potential for bleeding in this area is necessary.

The second complication related to the subvastus medialis approach is the overstretching and ischemia that may occur within the vastus medialis. This is most

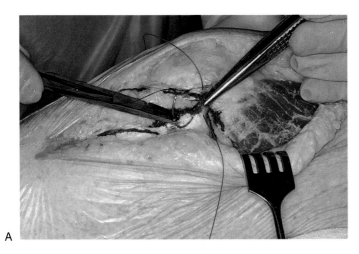

A

Figure 16. A: The key to anatomic closure is reapproximation of the apex of the L. **B:** Approximation of two corners with a suture.

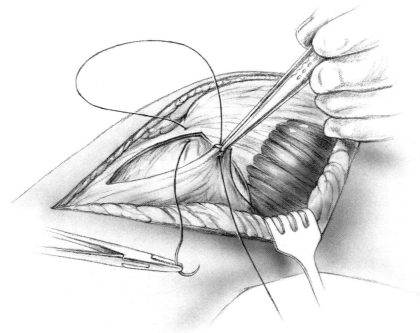

B

likely to occur in individuals with either bulky muscles or obese thighs, in whom greater exposure is necessary. When the vastus medialis is mobilized from the septum of the inner musculature, the patella is everted and the knee is flexed, there can be considerable stretching of the medialis muscle. This can be eliminated by further proximal dissection. However, if the muscle is very bulky or the thigh very obese, the stretching and tension on the vastus medialis will be notably uncomfortable to the patient in the postoperative period. This does not appear to be associated with a long-term muscular deficit, but does make rehabilitation more difficult. Attention to these observations will help avoid such complications.

RECOMMENDED READING

1. Bechtol, C. O.: *Richards Patello-Femoral Replacement Surgical Technique Brochure.* pp. 2, 14, 26, 1976, 1978.

2. Erkes, F.: Weitere Erfahrungen mit physiologischer Schnitt fuhrung zue Eroffnung des Kneige-lenks. *Bruns. Beitr. Klin. Chir.*, 147: 221, 1929.
3. Gustke, K. D.: Southern approach for total knee replacement. Florida *Orthop. Trans.*, 1989.
4. Hofmann, A. A., Plaster, R. L., and Murdock, L. E.: Subvastus (southern) approach for primary total knee arthroplasty. *Clin. Orthop.*, 269: 70, 1991.
5. Kayler, D. E., and Lyttle, D.: Surgical interruption of patellar blood supply by total knee arthroplasty. *Clin. Orthop.*, 229: 221, 1988.
6. Mullen, M. T.: A VMO approach to total knee surgery—A modified technique. AAOS Video Library, 1989.
7. Scapinelli, R.: Blood supply of the human patella. *J. Bone Joint Surg.*, 49: 563, 1967.
8. Warren, L. F., and Marshall, J. L.: The supporting structures and layers on the medial side of the knee. *J. Bone Joint Surg.*, 61: 56, 1979.

Master Techniques in Orthopaedic Surgery,
KNEE ARTHROPLASTY, edited by P. A. Lotke,
Raven Press, Ltd., New York © 1995.

3

Lateral Approach

Frederick F. Buechel

INDICATIONS/CONTRAINDICATIONS

The lateral parapatellar approach should be considered in fixed valgus knee deformities that are isolated or combined with flexion contractures or external tibial rotation contractures. Severe valgus deformities of up to 90° with combined flexion contractures and external tibial rotation deformities have been corrected using this approach. Such knees have remained stable in extension and flexion for 8 years without the need for constrained knee replacement implants, and have functioned well with the use of unconstrained, mobile-bearing knee replacements.

The severe fixed varus knee deformity represents the only relative contraindication to the lateral approach, since the medial contractures that require release are not well visualized from the lateral side without undermining the medial skin and subcutaneous tissue sleeve. Varus knee deformities are best approached by the medial parapatellar deep incision.

PREOPERATIVE PLANNING

Evaluation of the Valgus Deformity

The varus stress test in full extension is the standard clinical test used to evaluate the amount of fixed valgus deformity. If the knee can be brought to a neutral or 5-degree overall valgus position on varus stress, the condition is considered to be passively correctable and may then be approached either medially or laterally, since a lateral bone-stock deformity is the reason for valgus, rather than contracture of the lateral knee-stabilizing structures.

F. F. Buechel, M.D.: Department of Orthopaedic Surgery, New Jersey Medical School, Newark, New Jersey 07079.

A fixed valgus deformity exists when a varus stress in extension does not bring the knee into a neutral alignment of 5°, but rather maintains a valgus alignment of more than 8° or causes the mechanical axis line to be lateral to the center of the knee joint.

Mild fixed valgus deformities are malaligned by less than 10 degrees and usually require release of only the iliotibial tract (ITT) for correction (step 1). Moderate fixed valgus deformities are malaligned by 10 to 20 degrees and usually require release of the ITT, the lateral collateral ligament (LCL), and the popliteus tendon (PT) for correction (step 2). Severe fixed valgus deformities are more than 20 degrees out of alignment and may require the additional procedure of fibular head resection for complete correction and decompression of the peroneal nerve (step 3).

Evaluation of the Flexion Contracture

Fixed flexion contractures are present when full extension cannot be achieved under anesthesia. These contractures may be of a bony or soft tissue nature, and require surgical release of bony, capsular, or other soft-tissue structures to gain terminal extension.

Evaluation of the External Tibial Rotation Contracture

External tibial rotation contractures are those deformities in which the leg and foot lie externally rotated in the frontal plane, causing the axis of the second metatarsal bone to extend outward from the tibial axis. These deformities result from progressive contractures of the ITT and the posterior cruciate ligament (PCL), requiring release of these structures to restore frontal-plane alignment in the flexed-knee position. Frontal-plane alignment in the extended-knee position requires external rotational alignment of the femoral component to compensate for this external tibial rotation position as long as the hip joint can rotate internally to a sufficient degree to accommodate this rotational position and place the knee and foot into the frontal plane for a normal forward translational gait. In the absence of sufficient internal hip rotation it is preferable to leave the tibia in an externally rotated position and correct only the valgus deformity.

Radiologic Evaluation of the Valgus Knee

Passively correctable and fixed valgus knees without associated flexion or external tibial rotation contractures are best evaluated by standing anteroposterior (AP) radiographs to determine the amount of valgus and the bone loss involved. Varus and valgus stress radiographs are useful to document the deformities and their ability to be corrected passively.

Fixed flexion and external tibial rotation contractures tend to confuse the radiographic picture in the AP view because of distortion, thus limiting the usefulness of radiographic evaluation for determining the degree of valgus contracture. In such cases, bone loss can be appreciated on AP, lateral, and "skyline" patellar radiographs, but contractures must be assessed clinically.

Preoperative radiographic templates may give an erroneous picture in the AP plane because of the distortion and increased magnification caused by fixed flexion and external tibial rotation contractures. Thus, the use of lateral radiographs to determine the size range for total knee components is more predictable and useful. Final sizing of components, however, must be done by direct intraoperative measurements of the exposed femur, tibia, and patella.

Figure 1. Midline curved skin incision.

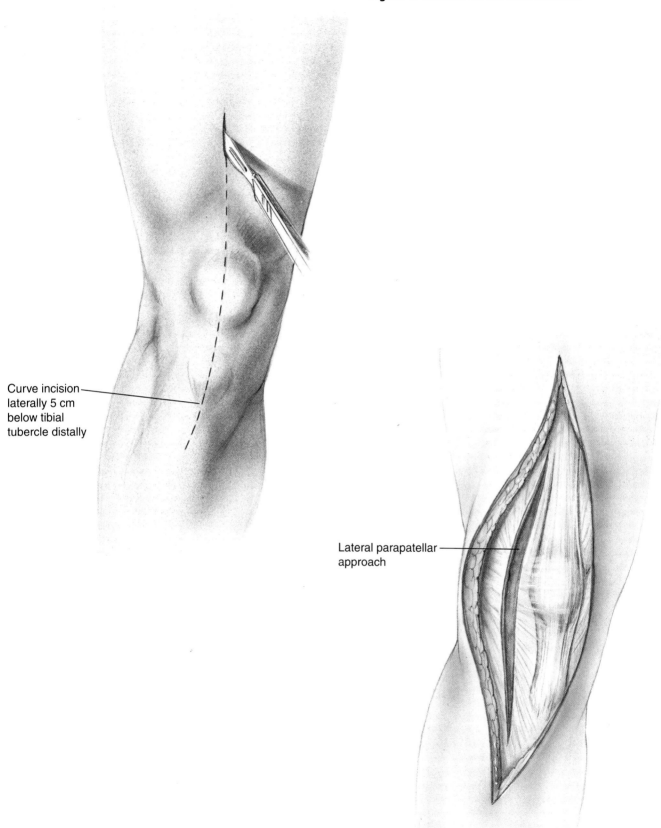

Curve incision laterally 5 cm below tibial tubercle distally

Lateral parapatellar approach

Figure 2. Deep lateral parapatellar incision.

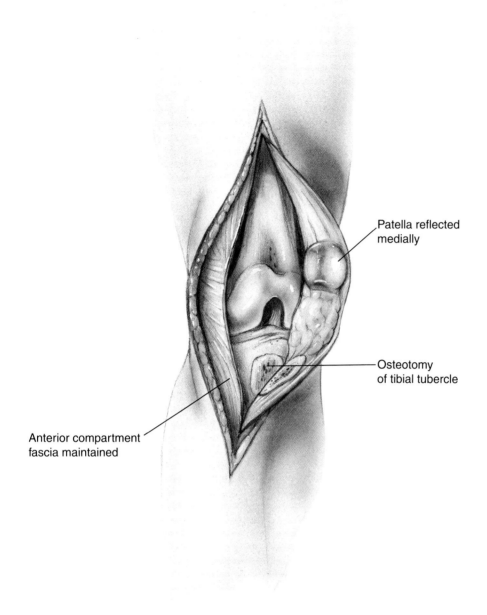

Patella reflected
medially

Osteotomy
of tibial tubercle

Anterior compartment
fascia maintained

Figure 3. Elevation of the tibial tubercle
and medial displacement of the patella.

SURGERY

Technique

A midline curved skin incision is made for primary total knee arthroplasty, or
a lateralmost incision in total knee arthroplasty for knees that have undergone
multiple operations (Fig. 1). The incision is finished distally over the lateral portion
of the tibial tubercle. Combined incisions may be necessary to avoid less than a
45-degree angle between previously healed scars.

Next, a deep lateral parapatellar incision is made into the joint (Fig. 2). The
distal portion of the incision is continued into the anterior compartment fascia,
1.5 cm from the tibial tubercle for a distance of 3 cm distal to the tubercle.

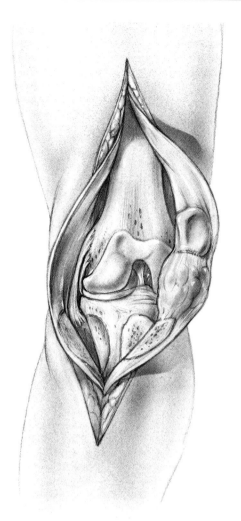

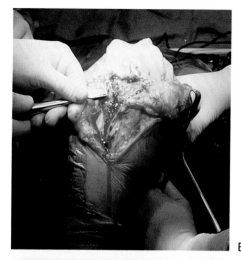

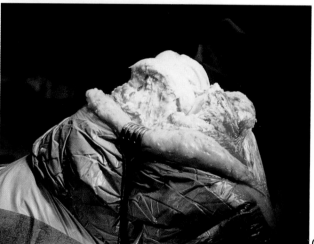

A

B

C

Figure 4. A: Step 1, the anterior compartment muscle and the ITT from Gerdy's tubercle are elevated. **B:** The ITT is elevated from Gerdy's tubercle in the frontal plane. **C:** Lateral view of the elevated ITT and anterior compartment musculature completing step 1. Step 2 incision is marked on the lateral femoral condyle.

For elevation of the tibial tubercle (Fig. 3), a thin segment of the tubercle is osteotomized with the attached patellar tendon. The patella is reflected medially while the sleeve of the anterior compartment fascia is retained laterally, and a periosteal hinge of the tibia is retained medially. The infrapatellar fat pad is maintained on the patellar tendon for later use in closing the lateral retinacular defect.

The three-step lateral release to correct fixed valgus (1) is used in mild fixed valgus deformities of less than 10° (usually only step 1), moderate fixed valgus deformities of 10° to 20° (usually steps 1 and 2), and severe fixed valgus deformities of more than 20° (steps 1, 2, and occasionally step 3). The steps include elevating (a) the ITT from Gerdy's tubercle, (b) the LCL and PT, and (c) the entire periosteum of the fibular head, followed by resection of the fibular head.

In step 1, the musculature of the anterior compartment and the ITT from Gerdy's tubercle are elevated subperiosteally back to the level of the fibular head (Fig. 4). This will remove the deforming force of the ITT and derotate the tibia in cases of fixed external rotation contractures. The knee is brought to full extension and the overall correction is checked using alignment rods or osteotomes on the femur and tibia. Under varus stress, the knee should reach 0° and spring back to 5° to 8° of valgus to be considered released. If further fixed valgus continues to exist, the LCL and PT should be elevated as described in step 2.

In step 2, the knee is flexed to 90°, and the LCL and PT are elevated (Fig. 5) as a subperiosteal flap, based proximally on the lateral femoral shaft. The knee is then brought into extension, and the alignment is checked by applying a varus stress. If the knee does not correct to 0° and spring back to 5° to 8° of valgus, the subperiosteal flap should be released more proximally on the femur. If the release at this point remains uncorrected, as in some moderate (10–20° fixed valgus) and severe (more than 20° fixed valgus) deformities, then the entire lateral femoral periosteum should be elevated. Additionally, if the peroneal nerve begins to sublux after release of the LCL and PT, the fibular head should be resected, as explained in step 3.

In step 3, knee flexion should be maintained at 90° and the entire periosteum of the fibular head elevated while protecting the peroneal nerve in the region of the fibular neck (Fig. 6). Next, the fibular head at the neck is resected. The knee is brought into full extension and the alignment and extension position of the peroneal nerve are checked to be sure the nerve falls into the space provided by

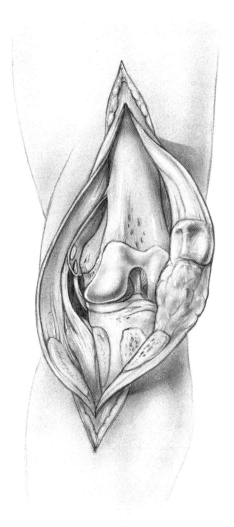

A

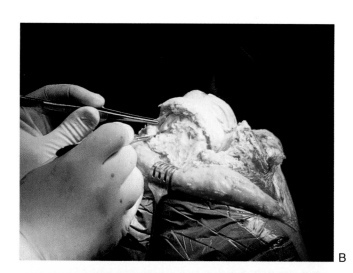

B

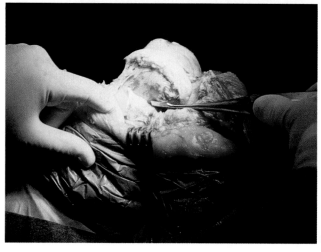

C

Figure 5. A: Step 2, the LCL and PT are elevated. **B:** The periosteum is incised to outline the area to be elevated on the lateral femoral condyle. **C:** The LCL, PT, and periosteum are elevated from the lateral femoral condyle, sumpleting step 2.

the resected fibular head. At this stage all fixed valgus components of even the most severe deformities should be corrected.

If after these last three procedures the tibia translates forward into neutral from an externally rotated position, and cannot be displaced posteriorly beneath the femur at 90° of flexion, then the PCL should be released to allow the tibia to reduce beneath the femur in the neutral position (Fig. 7). The PCL contributes to the external rotational deformity and resists attempts at correction. The use of a PCL-sacrificing implant is indicated in these conditions.

The amount of leg–foot external rotation (Fig. 8) should be assessed with the knee in full extension after release of the PCL, and should be compared with the normal extremity. The degree of excess external rotational deformity in full extension should be recorded and used to rotate the AP cuts externally on the distal femur. This is done to eliminate the deformity by internally rotating the hip and knee to realign the leg–foot position. This step requires at least normal internal rotation of the hip, so that after femoral resection the knee can be rotated into a

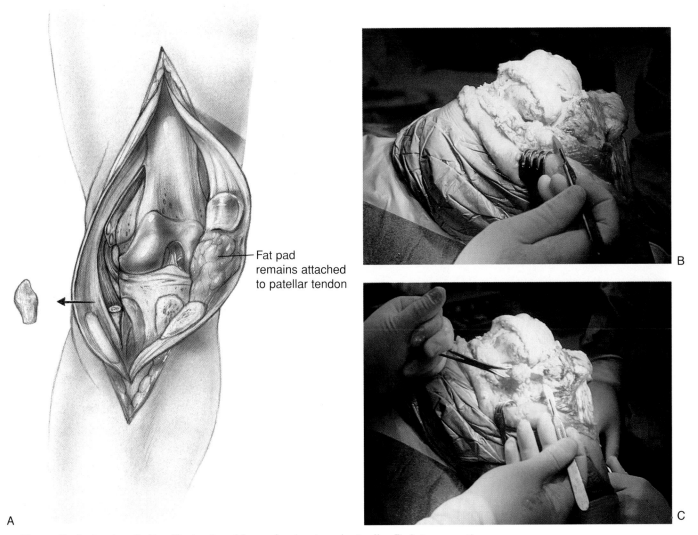

Fat pad remains attached to patellar tendon

A

B

C

Figure 6. A: In step 3, the fibular head is excised subperiosteally. **B:** Intraoperative view shows the fibular head exposed subperiosteally. **C:** The fibular head is resected at the level of the neck to complete step 3.

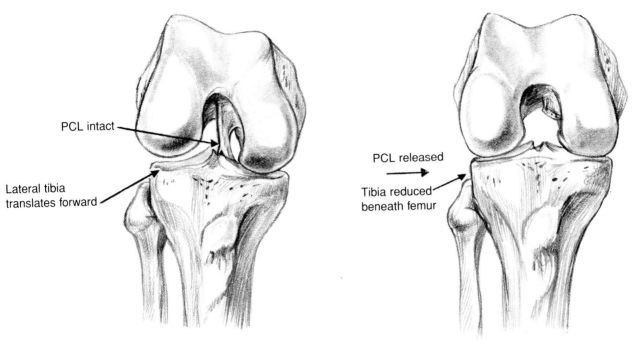

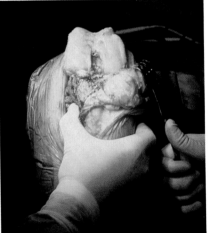

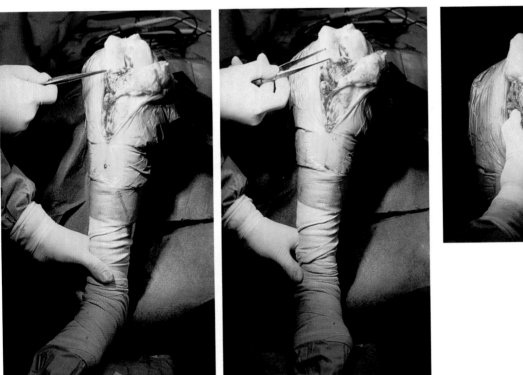

Figure 7. A,B: Correction of external tibial rotation deformity following lateral release. **C:** External rotation deformity of the leg can be seen with the tibia reduced beneath the femur. **D:** Correction of the tibial external rotation contracture to neutral subluxes the tibia forward from the femur because of a contracted PCL, which needs to be resected to allow correction. **E:** Resected PCL allows tibia to reduce beneath lateral femoral condyle and maintains correction of the external tibial rotation contracture.

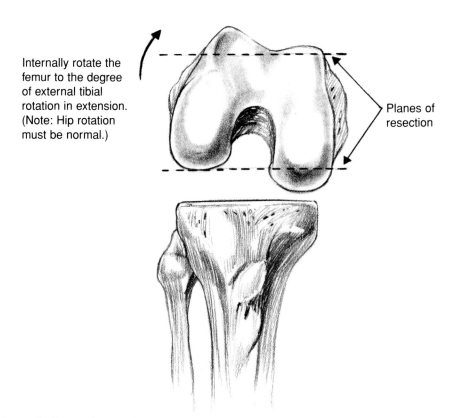

Internally rotate the
femur to the degree
of external tibial
rotation in extension.
(Note: Hip rotation
must be normal.)

Planes of
resection

Figure 8. Derotational alignment cuts on the femur for external tibial rotation contracture.

neutral position with respect to the opposite extremity. To accomplish this, an axial positioner is used on the tibial cut to orient the AP femoral resection guide into the desired amount of external rotation. A lamina spreader is used to distract the lateral compartment and internally rotate the femur with respect to the guide positioner; this provides a stable tension on the lateral compartment while allowing the desired rotation as determined in full extension. Once the exact external rotational position of the guide has been determined, the guide is pinned into place and the guide positioner can be removed. Usually, a significant amount of the posterior medial femur and a small amount if any of the posterior lateral femur will be removed.

If there is insufficient internal rotation at the hip to rotate the knee internally after external AP femoral resections, the knee will remain in external rotation and inhibit a normal forward transitional gait. In this case it is preferable to leave the external tibial rotational deformity alone and correct only the valgus deformity.

For alignment of a total knee arthroplasty, alignment of the mechanical axis should be maintained in extension (Fig. 9). Generally, more of the distal medial femoral condyle will be removed than of the distal lateral femoral condyle. Distal femoral and chamfer cuts should parallel the anterior and posterior femoral cuts. The position of the tibial component should be perpendicular to the ankle axis in the AP plane and have 5° to 10° of posterior inclination, matching the anatomic inclination in the lateral plane.

Closure is done by expanding the fat pad (Fig. 10 A–D). A lateral patellar tendon attachment is maintained, and the midsubstance is incised and unfolded superiorly and inferiorly to cover the lateral retinacular defect over the knee implants (Fig. 10 E–H).

The quadriceps tendon is closed, patellar tracking is assessed, and the lateral retinacular closure that maintains central patellar tracking is continued.

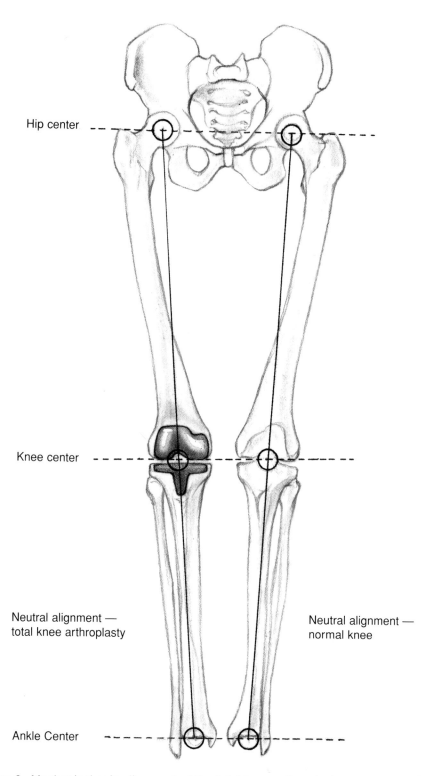

Hip center

Knee center

Neutral alignment —
total knee arthroplasty

Neutral alignment —
normal knee

Ankle Center

Figure 9. Mechanical axis alignment of the total knee arthroplasty versus normal.

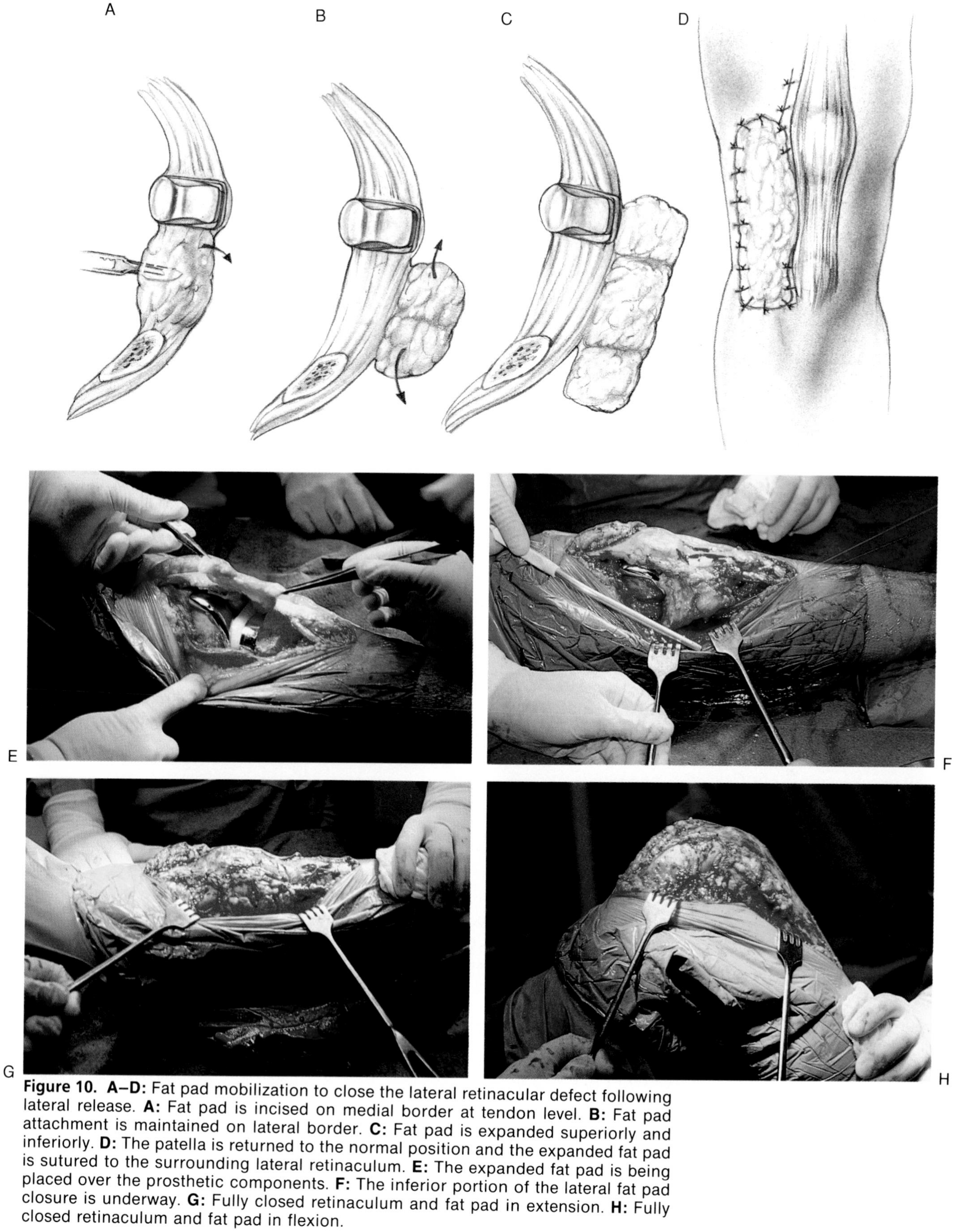

Figure 10. A–D: Fat pad mobilization to close the lateral retinacular defect following lateral release. **A:** Fat pad is incised on medial border at tendon level. **B:** Fat pad attachment is maintained on lateral border. **C:** Fat pad is expanded superiorly and inferiorly. **D:** The patella is returned to the normal position and the expanded fat pad is sutured to the surrounding lateral retinaculum. **E:** The expanded fat pad is being placed over the prosthetic components. **F:** The inferior portion of the lateral fat pad closure is underway. **G:** Fully closed retinaculum and fat pad in extension. **H:** Fully closed retinaculum and fat pad in flexion.

POSTOPERATIVE MANAGEMENT

Immediate Postoperative Management

Patients who have undergone total knee arthroplasty through a lateral approach are placed in a knee immobilizer for 2 days in full extension, after which any drains are removed. Isometric quadriceps setting is begun on the first postoperative day and continued daily to gain active terminal extension and the ability for straight leg raising. Immediate weight bearing to tolerance is also begun on the first postoperative day regardless of whether the patient has cemented or cementless component fixation.

Gravity-assisted flexion is begun on the second postoperative day and continued in conjunction with active-assistive range-of-motion (ROM) exercises in physical therapy. The use of continuous passive motion (CPM) or manipulation to gain flexion has been unnecessary with this approach.

Wound healing has been complete in all patients having arthroplasty by the lateral approach, and no infections have yet been encountered in more than 40 patients with valgus deformities of up to 90°. Normal ROM occurs earlier and wound healing appears to be less painful with the lateral approach than with the medial approach (1,3–6). Central patellar tracking without disruption of the medial blood supply is automatic when the lateral approach is used (7). No patellar subluxations, dislocations, or fractures have been observed in this group of patients, despite the complexity of their treatment. Correction of valgus, flexion, and external tibial rotation contractures has been maintained over the long term even in patients with the most severe deformities. Unconstrained mobile-bearing implants have been used in all of these cases of fixed valgus deformity, and remain clinically and radiographically stable, thus providing a significant, wear-resistant alternative to the more constrained implants previously advocated for these conditions.

Patients generally regain flexion of more than 100° in the first 7 days following surgery and then progress to approximately 120° of flexion over the next 5 weeks. Knee stability is maintained and instability has been rare, even though both cruciate ligaments have been resected and an unconstrained rotating-platform device is used in most cases. A painless, functional knee joint is the typical result with the lateral approach to arthroplasty with either cemented or cementless implants.

REHABILITATION

Knees with lateral-soft tissue sleeve releases in which periosteal attachments are maintained may be mobilized immediately without fear of sudden detachment. Early passive or active ROM does not appear to affect the long-term outcome of stability as long as proper soft-tissue closure is done to cover the prosthesis at the end of the procedure. Thus, unconstrained mobile-bearing implants can be successfully used in these patients without fear of the problems of late instability associated with complete sectioning of the lateral stabilizing structures of the knee (8).

COMPLICATIONS

Because the lateral parapatellar approach was developed to eliminate many of the complications seen with the medial parapatellar approach, it is gratifying to see that it has been quite successful. The lateral approach has virtually eliminated wound-healing problems often associated with medial approaches (1,3–6). Patellar maltracking problems have also been virtually eliminated. Early or late instability has not been a problem when subperiosteal sleeve releases have been performed in conjunction with the lateral approach.

Peroneal palsy remains a potential complication in the fixed valgus knee, especially in the presence of a fixed flexion or external tibial rotation deformity. Resection of the fibular head as described will minimize this problem, but nerve palsy must be considered and described to the patient preoperatively. The sudden onset of a foot drop in the recovery room should alert the surgeon to flex the knee for 24 to 48 hours to remove pressure on the peroneal nerve.

Complete peroneal palsies generally resolve within 6 months unless an intraoperative misadventure caused disruption of the nerve fibers. It is important to protect the peroneal nerve during resection of the fibular head so as to avoid this complication. Postoperative drop-foot braces should be prescribed, along with muscle stimulation via the peroneal nerve, until functional recovery of the leg and foot has been achieved.

ILLUSTRATIVE CASE FOR TECHNIQUE

A 67-year-old clergyman developed osteoarthritis and a progressive 18-degree fixed valgus deformity of the right knee over a 10-year period. His pain became refractory to pain medications, walking aids, and physical therapeutic modalities during the year prior to his presentation. Examination of his right knee revealed a mild effusion and clinical valgus of 20 degrees on weight bearing, which could be passively corrected to 10°. His range of motion was from 0 to 110°, actively and passively. An external rotation contracture of 20° was observed compared to the unaffected extremity. A 2+ anterior instability was appreciated at 90° of flexion. Extension and flexion muscle strength were rated at 5/5, or excellent. The patient's preoperative knee score (11) was 53 points out of 100, a poor score.

The patient underwent a cementless, New Jersey LCS Rotating Platform total knee arthroplasty using a lateral parapatellar approach and a three-step lateral release (1). He was allowed immediate weight bearing to tolerance, with crutches, combined with isometric quadriceps setting exercises and an active-assistive ROM program in physical therapy. A mild but painless knee effusion persisted for 6

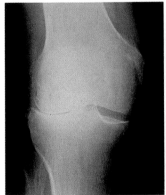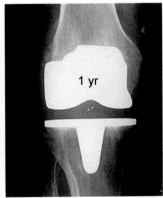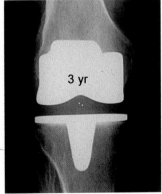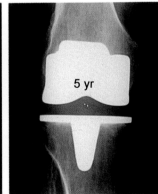

Figure 11. Sequential AP radiographs of the right knee of 67-year-old, 85 kg active osteoarthritic male with a preoperative fixed valgus deformity of 18°. Postoperative radiographs of his cementless LCS rotating platform total knee arthroplasty are shown at 1, 3, and 5 years, respectively.

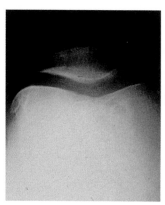 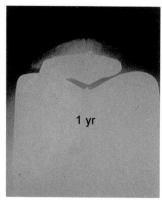 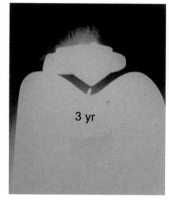 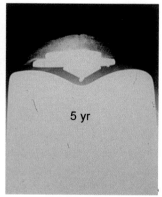

Figure 12. Sequential skyline radiographs of right knee of patient in Figure 9. Postoperative radiographs of his cementless LCS rotating-bearing patellar replacement are shown at 1, 3, and 5 years, respectively.

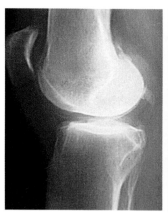 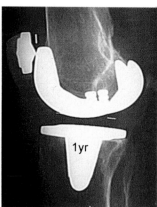 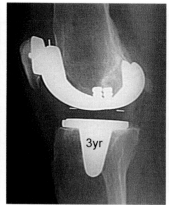 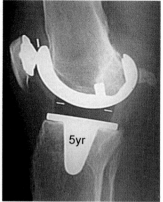

Figure 13. Sequential lateral radiographs of the right knee of the same patient following total knee arthroplasty with a cementless LCS rotating platform.

months because of overactivity with his clerical duties. Extension and flexion stability in the medial–lateral plane have remained excellent during his postoperative period. His AP flexion stability at 90° remains 1+ to 2+ with no instability sensation noted by the patient. His range of motion at 3 months was 0 to 105°; at 1 to 4 years, 0 to 121°; and at 5 years, 0 to 130°. His knee score improved from 53 points (poor) preoperatively to 95 points (excellent) at one year postoperatively to 97 points at 2 to 5 years postoperatively. He remains an active weekend golfer and walks 2 miles per day at work without pain or instability.

Postoperative radiographs demonstrated stable bone–prosthesis interfaces of the tibial, femoral and rotating patellar components at 1, 3, and 5 years following surgery (see Figs. 11, 12, 13).

Acknowledgment   The author thanks Linda A. Carter for her excellent technical assistance in the research and preparation of this manuscript.

RECOMMENDED READING

1. Buechel, F. F.: A sequential three-step lateral release for correcting fixed valgus knee deformities during total knee arthroplasty. *Clin. Orthop.*, 260: 170, 1990.

2. Buechel, F. F.: A simplified evaluation system for the rating of knee function. *Orthop. Rev.,* 11: 9, 1982.

3. Buechel, F. F.: How to correct valgus and lateral approaches. AAOS Course: Techniques of Total Knee Arthroplasty. Philadelphia, Pennsylvania, May 7, 1988.

4. Keblish, P. A.: The lateral approach to the valgus knee: Surgical technique and analysis of 53 cases with over two-year follow-up evaluation. *Clin. Orthop.,* 271: 52–62, 1991.

5. Keblish, P. A.: Valgus deformity in TKR: The lateral retinacular approach. *Orthop. Trans.,* 9: 28, 1985.

6. Keblish, P. A.: Valgus deformity in TKR: The lateral retinacular approach. Proc. AAOS 53rd Annual Meeting, New Orleans, Louisiana, February 20–25, 1986.

7. Scapinelli, R.: Blood supply of the human patella. *J. Bone Joint Surg.,* 49B:563, 1967.

8. Sharkey, P. F., Hozack, W. J., and Booth, R. E.: Posterior dislocation of total knee arthroplasty. *Clin. Orthop.,* 278: 128–133, 1992.

Master Techniques in Orthopaedic Surgery,
Knee Arthroplasty, edited by P. A. Lotke,
Raven Press, Ltd., New York © 1995.

4

Popliteal Approach

Kurt J. Kitziger

INDICATIONS/CONTRAINDICATIONS

The popliteal approach is seldom required in orthopedic surgery; when indicated, however, its execution requires extensive knowledge of the posterior anatomy of the knee. Numerous authors have described the popliteal approach, but Henry's description of it remains the classic one and will be referred to in the following discussion.

The popliteal fossa is a diamond-shaped area bounded above by the biceps femoris laterally and the semimembranosus medially, and below by the two heads of the gastrocnemius. The fossa contains the common peroneal and tibial branches of the sciatic nerve as well as the popliteal artery and its numerous collateral branches. For most orthopaedic surgeons, surgical approach through the popliteal fossa is similar to tying a bowtie: it is not commonly performed, and therefore schematic diagrams are of indispensable assistance.

The indications for the popliteal approach are limited. Removal of a Baker's cyst, which usually can be treated by addressing intraarticular pathology anteriorly, has become a less common procedure today. Repair of a tibial avulsion of the posterior cruciate ligament usually requires this approach. Release of fixed flexion contractures of the knee is another important use of the posterior approach. Total synovectomy, such as that required in the treatment of pigmented villonodular synovitis (PVNS) and synovial chondromatosis, often mandates the use of combined popliteal and anterior approaches. Finally, access to the neurovascular structures of the popliteal fossa may be gained by the posterior route.

The popliteal approach is obviously contraindicated when another means of access to the knee would suffice. This includes treatment of isolated damage to either the posteromedial or posterolateral corner ligaments. Each of these injuries is best addressed through a more direct approach either medially or laterally, as indicated.

K. J. Kitziger, M.D.: Department of Orthopaedics, Louisiana State University Medical Center, New Orleans, LA; Orthopaedic Associates, Suite 402, New Orleans, LA 70115.

PREOPERATIVE PLANNING

A meticulous physical examination and standard radiographs are usually all that are required during the stage of preoperative planning for knee surgery using the popliteal approach. This includes a thorough examination and documentation of the neurovascular status of the limb. Angiography is necessary when distal pulses are not palpable or when vascular pathology is suspected. To preoperatively define the extent of synovial pathology for conditions such as PVNS, magnetic resonance imaging (MRI) can be invaluable.

SURGERY

The patient is placed in the prone position with careful placement of chest rolls. A small bolster across the foot of the operating table will prevent excessive prolonged plantar flexion of the ankles. A proximal thigh tourniquet is placed. A stout assistant is required to hold the extremity during the surgical preparation, owing to the lack of extension at the hip and the tendency of the knee to buckle into flexion (Fig. 1). After placement of an impervious stockinette over the foot and ankle, the extremity is draped free (Fig. 2). This facilitates movement of the knee during surgery. The limb is exsanguinated and the tourniquet inflated, except for cases of vascular repair.

Technique

In order to maximize exposure and minimize scar formation, a long S-shaped incision is used (Fig. 3). A pen is used to mark cross-hatches on the skin to assist later in wound closure. I prefer to begin over the medial hamstrings, about 7 to

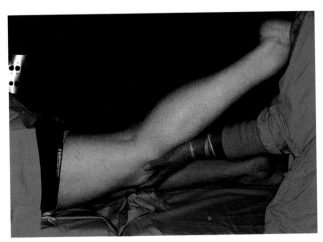

Figure 1. An assistant must support the knee during the surgical preparation.

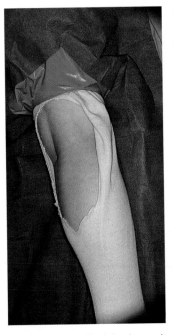

Figure 2. The limb is draped free.

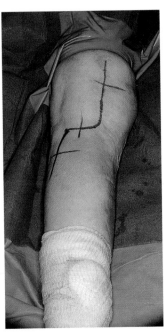

Figure 3. The incision starts over the medial hamstrings of this left knee, crosses below the popliteal crease, and extends laterally over the gastrocnemius.

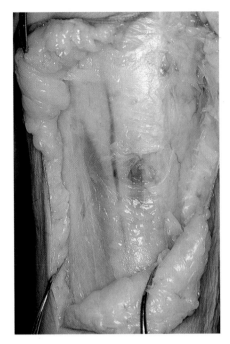

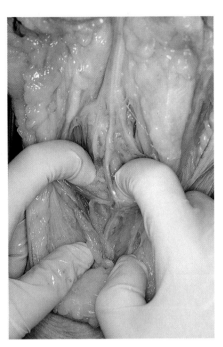

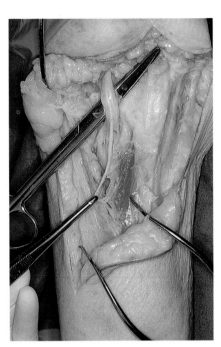

Figure 4. The blue guide, or small saphenous vein, is more easily found in this fresh cadaver specimen than in the live patient. The fascial incision is medial to the vein.

Figure 5. Using the white guide as a midline marker, the heads of the gastrocnemius are bluntly separated.

Figure 6. The white guide, or medial sural cutaneous nerve, seen here in the forceps, leads proximally to the tibial nerve, which is seen overlying the Mayo scissors.

10 cm above the joint line. The semitendinosus tendon is a good landmark. The incision is then gently curved transversely for about 5 cm at the level of the joint. The joint line may be palpated medially and laterally in the thin patient; however, in obese patients, it is important to be aware that the joint line is just distal to the skin-flexion crease. The incision is carried distally over the lateral gastrocnemius and deepened down to the popliteal fascia, and the skin flaps containing the subcutaneous tissue are reflected medially and laterally. Self-retaining retractors placed above and below offer wide exposure of the roof of the popliteal fossa.

As an alternative skin incision, the S of the incision may be reversed by starting the proximal incision over the biceps femoris laterally and ending distally over the medial gastrocnemius. This method, however, limits the ability to extend the incision toward the vascular structures proximally and toward the peroneal nerve distally, should either maneuver become necessary.

The next segment of the procedure involves identifying the large nerves, a step made easier with the help of Henry's "guides." The small saphenous vein, or blue guide, usually lies superficial to the fascia and is lateral to the medial sural cutaneous nerve, or white guide (Fig. 4). In the distal portion of the wound, the popliteal fascia is incised medial to the veins and the medial sural cutaneous nerve is identified in the grove between the conjoined heads of the gastrocnemius. The white guide is traced proximally through the popliteal fat to identify the tibial nerve. It is helpful to bluntly separate the heads of the gastrocnemius with one's fingers in order to open the fossa (Fig. 5). The tibial nerve is followed toward the proximal apex formed by the medial and lateral hamstrings. Here the tibial nerve joins the common peroneal nerve, which is then dissected back distally under the belly of the biceps femoris (Fig. 6). A large Penrose drain is looped around the common peroneal nerve (Fig. 7).

The vascular structures lie deep to the tibial nerve. For cyst removal, the cystic mass can usually be identified and traced to its origin in the posterior capsule.

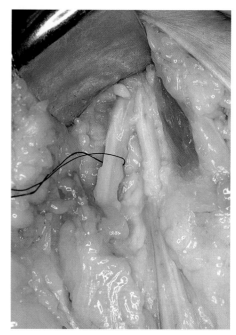

Figure 7. The common peroneal nerve, marked with a black suture, joins the tibial nerve in the apex of the popliteal fossa.

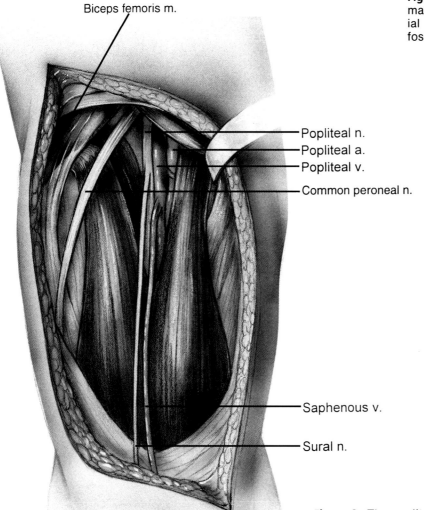

Biceps femoris m.

Popliteal n.
Popliteal a.
Popliteal v.
Common peroneal n.

Saphenous v.

Sural n.

Figure 8. The popliteal vein lies medial to the artery as it enters the fossa, and then comes to lie posterior to the artery.

With luck, the tibial nerve and its popliteal vessels may be bluntly retracted as a bundle medially and laterally to provide adequate exposure. Slight flexion of the knee will relax the muscles and improve visualization. When wider exposure of the capsule is required, further dissection is necessary to protect the vessels.

Knowledge of the vascular relationships in the popliteal fossa is essential, especially in the enveloping mass of popliteal fat. The popliteal vein lies superficial or posterior to the artery, in the middle of the wound. In the distal aspect, the vein is medial and superficial to the artery (Fig. 8). The popliteal artery is tethered to the back of the knee by five collateral branches; the medial and lateral superior geniculate arteries, the medial and lateral inferior geniculate arteries, and the middle geniculate artery (Fig. 9). The superior geniculate arteries arise just above the medial and lateral epicondyles, and these vessels pass just proximal to the heads

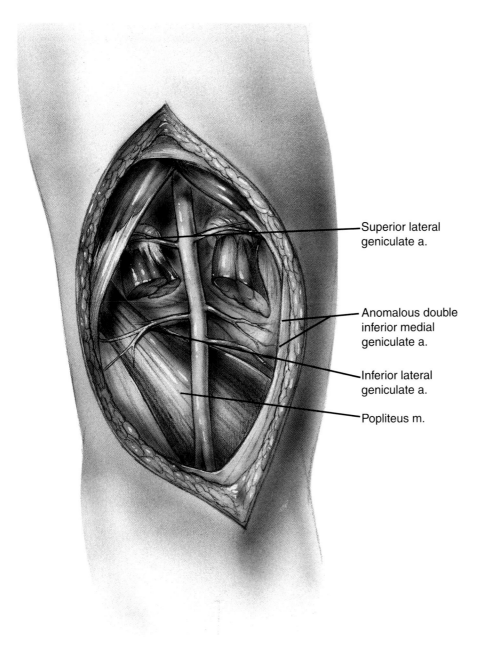

Superior lateral
geniculate a.

Anomalous double
inferior medial
geniculate a.

Inferior lateral
geniculate a.

Popliteus m.

Figure 9. Drawing depicting the relationships of the geniculate arteries.

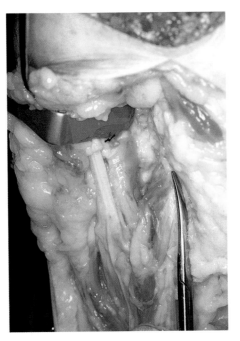

Figure 10. The superior medial geniculate artery has been ligated with a silk suture, and the tibial artery, vein, and nerve are being retracted laterally as a bundle. The scissors marks where the medial head of the gastrocnemius will be taken down.

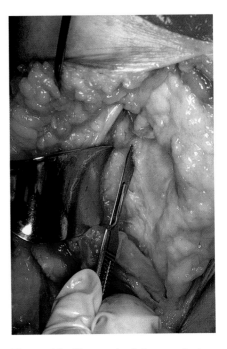

Figure 11. The scalpel demonstrates the arthrotomy through the posterior oblique ligament.

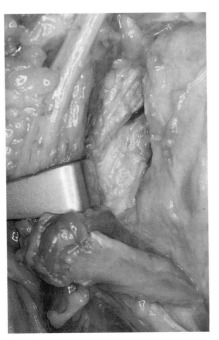

Figure 12. With the bundle retracted laterally, the posterior cruciate ligament is readily visualized. Repair of a tibial avulsion can be directly accomplished.

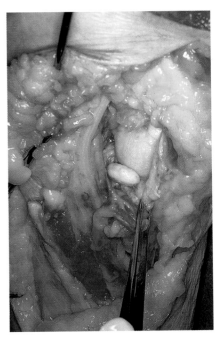

Figure 13. To obtain better visualization of the medial compartment, the posterior capsule can be reflected off the back of the medial condyle, in this case revealing a loose body.

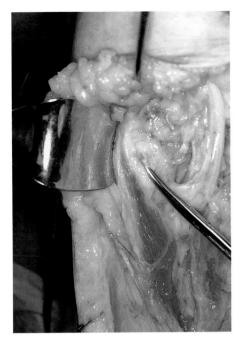

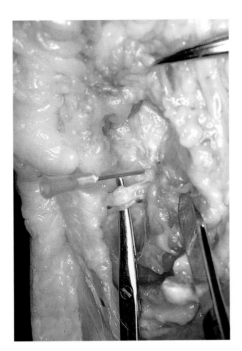

Figure 14. The common peroneal nerve is being retracted laterally. The scissors marks the origin of the lateral head of the gastrocnemius.

Figure 15. The hemostat in the upper portion of the wound clamps the lateral superior geniculate artery; the lateral head of the gastrocnemius has been taken down and reflected medially with the bundle. The needle in the arcuate ligament marks the joint level, and the scissors demonstrates the lateral inferior geniculate artery.

of origin of the gastrocnemius against the bone. The inferior geniculate arteries arise near the joint line and pass along the capsule medially and laterally. The middle geniculate artery passes through the oblique popliteal ligament to enter the posterior cruciate ligament. The medial and lateral sural arteries are the muscular branches that supply the respective heads of the gastrocnemius, and should be protected. Those geniculate vessels impeding exposure of the posterior capsule can safely be ligated during the procedure.

To obtain the best exposure of the posterior capsule, one or both heads of the gastrocnemius must be taken down. To approach an avulsion of the posterior cruciate ligament, the medial head is taken down (Fig. 10). The origin of the medial head lies more proximal than that of the lateral head. The thumb and index finger are used to palpate the muscle belly and bluntly dissect it up to its broad origin on the femur. The superior medial geniculate vessel is ligated if necessary, so as to improve access. The tendinous origin of the muscle belly is released sharply, leaving a stump on the femur for repair. Because the neurovascular supply to each of the bellies of the gastrocnemius comes from the midline, the released muscle will be reflected toward the center of the wound. Usually, the middle geniculate artery will have to be ligated to approach the posterior cruciate ligament. A vertical incision is made through the posterior oblique ligament near the midline to readily visualize the PCL (Fig. 11). The PCL courses to its insertion distally on the back of the tibia (Figs. 12 and 13).

When approaching the knee through release of the lateral gastrocnemius, the common peroneal nerve must be protected (Figs. 14 and 15). When both bellies of the gastrocnemius have been taken down, the entire posterior capsule can be thus exposed (Fig. 16). In cases requiring synovectomy, the capsule is usually distended. Appropriate vertical arthrotomies may be made on either side of the cruciate ligament. The heads of the gastrocnemius are repaired with heavy, nonabsorbable suture. The remainder of the wound is closed in routine fashion.

Careful identification and protection of the neurovascular structures are essential in this operation. One can confidently proceed with the dissection by mastering the popliteal anatomy. There should be no hesitation in taking down the gastrocnemius to improve exposure, because the morbidity from this procedure is small and the benefit great.

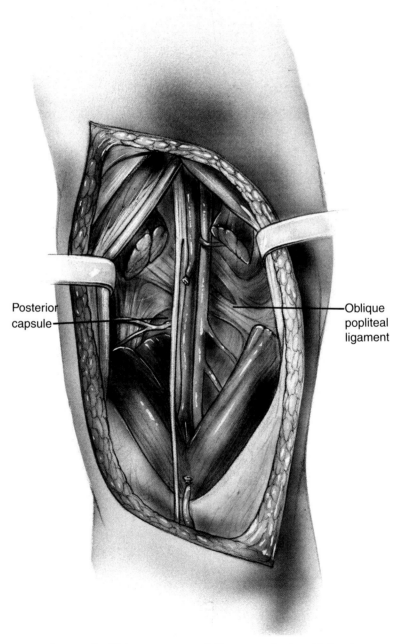

Posterior
capsule

Oblique
popliteal
ligament

Figure 16. Wide exposure of the capsule is obtained when both heads of the gastrocnemius are taken down.

POSTOPERATIVE MANAGEMENT

Postoperative care is dictated by the type of procedure performed. A well-padded dressing is applied in the operating room, followed by splints with the knee in slight flexion. A careful neurovascular examination is documented postoperatively. With sturdy repair of the gastrocnemius origins, I allow range-of-motion exercises to begin on the second postoperative day when pain has begun to subside. I delay weight bearing for 4 to 6 weeks to protect the gastrocnemius repair.

COMPLICATIONS

The complications of the popliteal approach are neurovascular. Damage to the medial sural cutaneous nerve can cause a painful neuroma, and injury to the major nerves will cause significant disability. In the posterior approach, skin problems occur much less commonly than with anterior incisions.

The popliteal approach to the knee, although not commonly performed, is an important procedure for the orthopaedic surgeon.

ILLUSTRATIVE CASES FOR TECHNIQUE

Case 1

A 26-year-old woman with a history of recurrent PVNS presented with effusion, pain, increased swelling, and nodular masses in the popliteal area of the knee. Three years previously, she had had an open anterior arthrotomy and synovectomy, followed by intraarticular radiation therapy.

An MRI scan showed nodular masses in the posterior aspect of the knee, corresponding to the findings in the physical examination. Very few areas of low signal intensity, representing the patient's PVNS, remain anteriorly (Figs. 17 and 18).

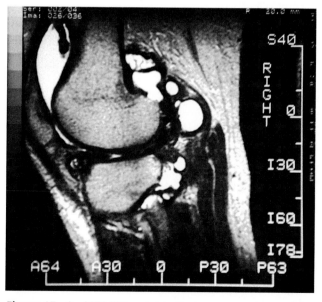

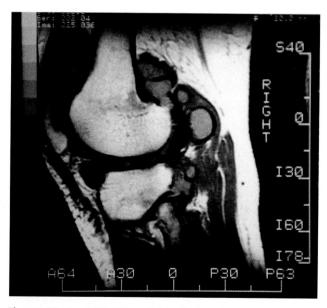

Figure 17. An MRI (T2 weighted) shows massive nodular lesions of high signal intensity in the posterior aspect of the knee, proximally and distally and extending into the tissues.

Figure 18. An MRI (T1 weighted) also demonstrates the recurrent tumors in the posterior aspect of the knee.

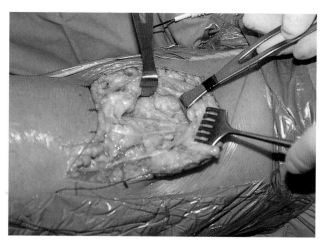

Figure 19. A curvilinear popliteal incision is taken through the flexor crease in the posterior aspect of the knee, and the deep fascia is incised, allowing wide retraction in the area.

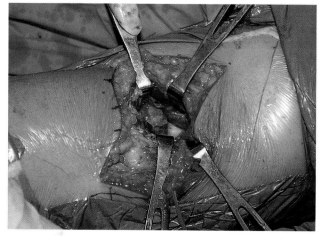

Figure 20. The gastrocnemius muscles are separated and exposure to the posterior capsule reveals PVNS bulging from the posterior aspect of the joint.

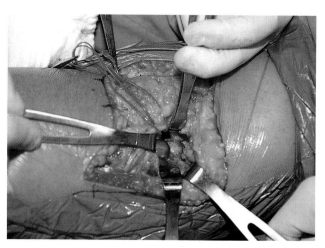

Figure 21. With resection of the pigmented synovial masses, the posterior aspect of the joint can be entered and visualized, and removal of remaining synovium can be expedited.

A posterior approach was utilized to remove the recurrent masses in the posterior aspect of the patient's knee (Figs. 19 through 21).

Case 2

A 42-year-old woman, the wife of an orthopaedic surgeon, noted increasing pain, effusions, and limitation of motion of her knee over a 2-year period, which she and her spouse disregarded. She denied previous injury or symptoms within the knee. Examination showed a mild synovitis, a small effusion, and significant limitation of motion from 3 to 90 degrees of flexion. There was no tenderness,

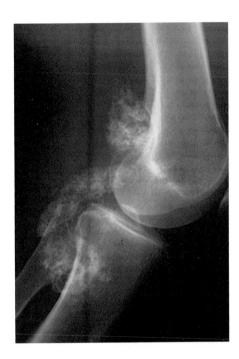

Figure 22. Radiograph demonstrating large synovial masses of osteochondromatosis, which have begun to ossify in the posterior aspect of the knee, extending distally and proximally.

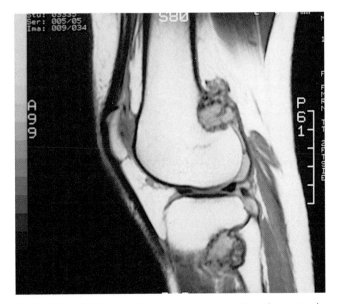

Figure 23. MRI scan showing that osteochondromatosis has begun to erode into the posterior femur as well as into the proximal tibiofibular joint.

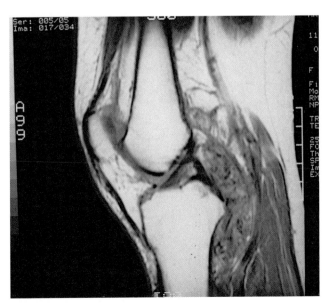

Figure 24. Mass of synovial chondromatosis lies beneath the gastrocnemius tendon and extends well distal to the joint.

and the ligaments were intact. A radiograph and MRI showed large synovial osteo-chondromatosis involving the posterior aspect of the knee. Prior to removal of the masses in the posterior aspect of the knee, an arthroscopic examination was done which showed small osteochondromatous foci within the joint. A synovec-tomy was completed arthroscopically (Fig. 25). The patient was then placed in the prone position and the posterior approach to the knee was utilized to remove the osteochondromatous masses from behind the knee (Figs. 26 and 27).

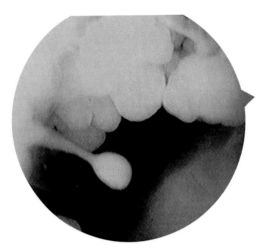

Figure 25. Intraarticular arthroscopic photo-graph of lesions of synovial chondromatosis embedded within the synovium, prior to syno-vectomy.

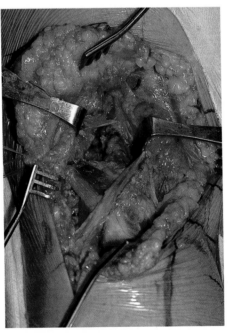

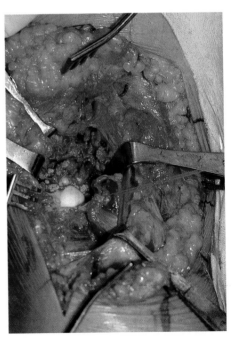

Figure 26. Popliteal dissection carefully retracts the gastrocnemius muscles and isolates the popliteal artery, nerve, and vein, as well as their medial and lateral branches.

Figure 27. The gastrocnemius muscle is partially reflected from its attachment, and the posterior aspect of the joint can be entered and debrided. The peroneal nerve is carefully protected.

RECOMMENDED READING

1. Abbott, L. C., and Carpenter, W. F.: Surgical approaches to the knee joints and bone joint. *Surgery,* 27B: 277–310, 1945.
2. Brackett, E. G., and Osgood, R. B.: The popliteal incision for the removal of joint mice. *Boston Med. Surg. J.,* 165: 975–977, 1911.
3. Henry, A. D.: *Extensile Exposure,* 2nd ed. pp. 241–255. Churchill Livingstone, New York, 1973.
4. Hoppenfeld, S., and DeBoer, P.: *Surgical Exposures in Orthopaedics.* pp. 427–436. J. B. Lippincott, Philadelphia, 1984.
5. Kelikian, H.: Posterior approach to the knee. *Surg. Clin. North Am.,* 27: 157–181, 1947.
6. Knight, R. A.: Surgical approaches. In: *Campbell's Operative Orthopaedics,* 3rd ed., edited by J. S. Speed. pp. 213, 217, C. V. Mosby, St. Louis, 1956.
7. Trickey, E. L.: Rupture of the posterior cruciate ligament of the knee. *J. Bone Joint Surg.,* 50B: 334–341, 1968.

Master Techniques in Orthopaedic Surgery,
KNEE ARTHROPLASTY, edited by P. A. Lotke,
Raven Press, Ltd., New York © 1995.

5

Biopsy Techniques Around the Knee

Roby C. Thompson, Jr.

INDICATIONS/CONTRAINDICATIONS

The goal of biopsy is to obtain a diagnosis with minimal compromise of subsequent definitive surgery. Whenever a malignant tumor is suspected in the vicinity of the knee joint, placement of the biopsy incision is critical in the determination of potential limb-sparing surgery. Even though the general indication for biopsy is to obtain a diagnosis, the biopsy incision may in some circumstances require further extension for primary treatment. For example, infection or certain benign tumors, diagnosed on frozen section, may best be treated at the time of biopsy. Postsurgical function will rest on the ability of the surgeon to reconstruct the knee with optimum soft tissue and bone reconstruction, and both of these may be compromised by an inappropriate biopsy incision.

The principles of biopsy as they refer to the knee include: (i) A longitudinal incision that can be excised in continuity with underlying structures. (ii) Avoidance of contamination of the femoral or popliteal vessels or sciatic nerve or its branches. (iii) A biopsy procedure should not violate the synovium, nor contaminate the joint, unless the pathology is intraarticular and arthrotomy is unavoidable.

When possible, the posterior compartment of the distal thigh should be avoided for biopsy, since the femoral artery and vein as well as the posterior tibial and peroneal division of the sciatic nerve may be contaminated.

R. C. Thompson, Jr., M.D.: Department of Orthopaedic Surgery, University of Minnesota Hospital and Clinic, Minneapolis, MN 55455.

PREOPERATIVE PLANNING

When approaching an intraosseous lesion, minimum preoperative planning must include an AP radiograph (Fig. 1), a bone scan (Fig. 2), and an axial image made either by computerized axial tomography or magnetic resonance imaging (Fig. 3), in order to plan the biopsy incision. This is particularly important in lesions of the deep posterior compartment or lesions that are not palpable on physical examination, in which it is difficult to determine whether a medial or lateral incision would be best.

SURGERY

The limb is prepared circumferentially and elevated for exsanguination before the tourniquet is inflated. Depending upon the location and presentation of the mass, I prefer to place the biopsy incision medially or laterally to avoid disruption of the rectus and intermedius divisions of the quadriceps. Using these approaches, I can obtain an adequate specimen. If the diagnosis is suitable for a limb-sparing surgical procedure, a small cuff of vastus medialis or lateralis can be excised at the time of resection, with the biopsy site and the remaining quadriceps reflected from the femur for resection and then reapproximated over the reconstruction (Figs. 4–7).

Biopsies of the proximal tibia should be done either anteromedially or anterolaterally in order to avoid contamination of the posterior neurovascular structures. When placing these incisions, I avoid the patellar tendon, so that when limb-sparing surgery is appropriate, the tendon is not contaminated by the biopsy.

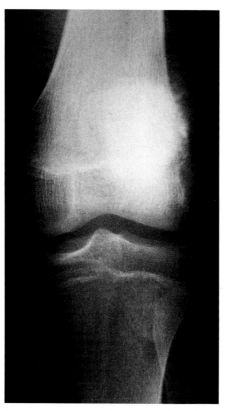

Figure 1. An AP radiograph of the knee showing an expansile mass involving the lateral aspect of the distal femur.

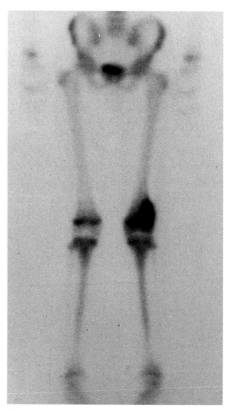

Figure 2. Nuclear image of the same limb showing increased activity in the lateral aspect of the distal femur.

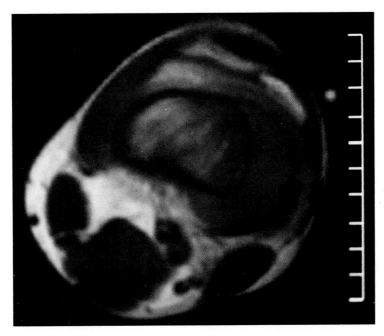

Figure 3. Magnetic resonance image showing the extracortical mass on the lateral aspect of the distal femur, with the preferred biopsy approach in line with the arrows.

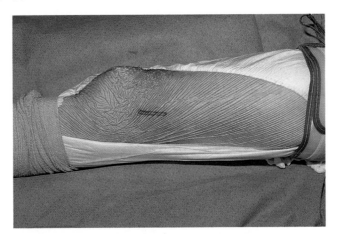

Figure 4. Placement of biopsy at time of resection.

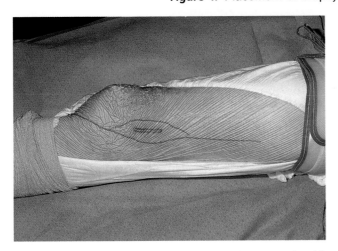

Figure 5. Opportunity for elipsing the biopsy track with the primary incision.

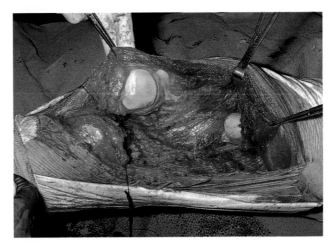

Figure 6. The distal femur can be excised by reflecting the entire quadriceps muscle medially.

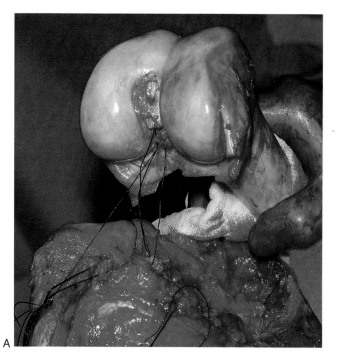

A

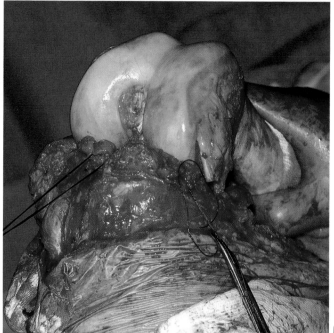

B

Figure 7. Reconstruction of the joint. **A:** Distal femoral allograft in place with ligamentous repair; sutures positioned for tightening. **B:** Posterior, capsular, and medial ligament sutures have been placed and secured. **C:** With the osteoarticular structures of the joint reduced, the quadriceps mechanism can now be repositioned over the allograft with minimum surgical disruption of quadriceps function.

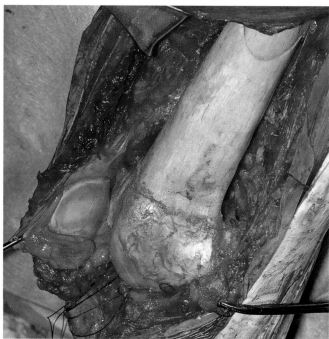

C

Masses in the popliteal region are treated much like those in the posterior compartment of the thigh, with incisional biopsies when the mass is subcutaneous, avoiding the neurovascular structures.

In cases of osseous lesions that are not palpable, intraoperative radiographs should be made prior to the incision, in order to accurately locate the defect to be biopsied.

POSTOPERATIVE MANAGEMENT

It is essential to have meticulous hemostasis in the biopsy wound. Particularly in those osseous lesions that require biopsy, it is critical to have the limb elevated and rested for at least 24 hours in order to avoid unnecessary hemorrhage and dissection of hematoma into soft-tissue planes that can potentially spread the tumor. Mobilization of the limb is permitted between 24 and 48 hours, depending on the underlying diagnosis and the treatment that is necessary.

COMPLICATIONS

When the incision is placed appropriately, the most troublesome complication of biopsy surgery is hemorrhage. Careful preoperative planning and evaluation to avoid entering a highly vascular tumor mass can minimize this complication. When physical findings such as erythema, warmth, and venous engorgement suggest an increased blood flow to the area of the lesion, it may be important to undertake further diagnostic studies, including nuclear imaging and/or angiography. Fortunately, in the region of the distal femur and the proximal tibia, most intraoperative hemorrhage can be controlled by the use of a tourniquet on the proximal thigh. However, when the tourniquet is released, intraosseous bleeding into the biopsy wound may be a problem and can disseminate neoplastic cells. I recommend releasing the tourniquet prior to wound closure, and if hemostasis cannot be obtained, I leave the wound open with a sterile dressing to allow spontaneous coagulation and hemostasis, and perform a delayed secondary closure. Other authors have suggested using a methacrylate plug in the bone to control hemostasis, and this is occasionally appropriate. Another troubling complication is a nondiagnostic biopsy. This can usually be avoided by obtaining a frozen-section evaluation, asking the pathologist to identify ''pathologic tissue consistent with clinical findings.'' In the absence of pathologic tissue considered to be eventually diagnostic, additional tissue must be obtained. A culture for microbial identification should be obtained in all biopsies.

ILLUSTRATIVE CASE FOR TECHNIQUE

Figures 1 through 7 illustrate a typical approach to a previously biopsied lesion in the distal femur, and show how the biopsy incision has allowed optimum reconstruction of the distal femur and knee joint.

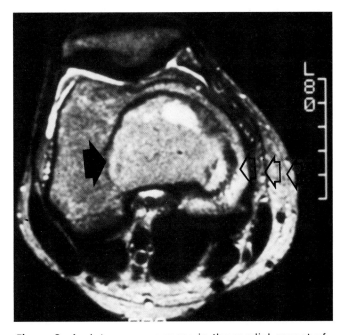

Figure 8. An intraosseous mass in the medial aspect of the femoral condyle (black arrow), which was approached for biopsy through the medial incision outlined by the open arrows.

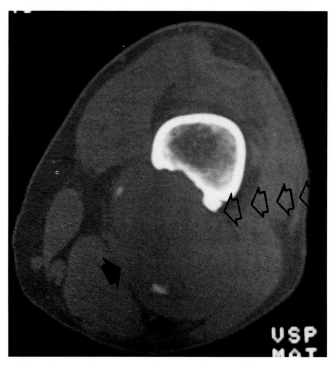

Figure 9. Large posterior mass in the distal femur, with the posterior extent identified by the solid black arrows and my preferred biopsy approach identified with the open arrows coming from the lateral side through the vastus lateralis and back to the region of the linea aspera.

Other examples of biopsy with less obvious site selection include Figure 8, in which the mass was intraosseous and there was no palpable lesion outside of the bone, yet proved optimum for a posterior medial approach. Figure 9 illustrates a soft-tissue mass in the posterior aspect of the distal femur just above the popliteal space, which represents a more difficult choice for biopsy-site selection, but one in which the optimum biopsy track is outlined in the posterior lateral aspect of the thigh through the vastus lateralis to the linea aspera.

RECOMMENDED READING

1. Lawrence, W.: Concepts in limb-sparing treatment of adult soft tissue sarcomas. *Semin. Surg. Oncol.*, 4–1: 73–77, 1988.
2. Mankin, H. J., Lange, T. A., and Spanier, S. S.: The hazards of biopsy in patients with malignant primary bone and soft tissue tumors. *J. Bone Joint Surg.*, 64A: 1121–1127, 1982.
3. Rydholm, A., Berg, N. O., Persson, B. M., and Akerman, M.: Treatment of soft tissue sarcoma should be centralized. *Acta Orthop. Scand.*, 54-3: 333–339, 1983.
4. Shives, T. C.: Biopsy of soft-tissue tumors. *Clin. Orthop.*, 289: 32–35, 1993.

PART II

Total Knee Arthroplasty

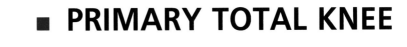

■ PRIMARY TOTAL KNEE

Master Techniques in Orthopaedic Surgery,
KNEE ARTHROPLASTY, edited by P. A. Lotke,
Raven Press, Ltd., New York © 1995.

6

Primary Total Knees
Standard Principles and Techniques

Paul A. Lotke

INDICATIONS/CONTRAINDICATIONS

A total knee arthroplasty is indicated for severe disability resulting from pain, deformity, and limited function as a result of rheumatoid arthritis, osteoarthritis, or other arthritides about the joint. Surgery should be considered only after an adequate trial of conservative therapy, including physical therapy, antiinflammatory medication, and modification of daily activities. In addition, both pain and deformity should be present. Pain alone should lead the physician to look for other diagnoses and treatment alternatives. Structural deformity without significant pain or disability is very well tolerated, especially in the elderly, and should not alone be an indication for surgery. The patient should also have realistic goals. Even a well-placed total knee will neither feel nor function like a normal knee. Younger patients must be carefully advised about abuse and overactivity leading to a failure. Older patients should recognize that reconstruction of a single joint alone may not alter their overall functional abilities.

When the disease involves a single compartment, other surgical alternatives should be considered. A high tibial osteotomy or unicompartmental arthroplasty can offer excellent results with less bone loss and morbidity than total knee arthroplasty. These procedures are especially useful for younger people with unicompartmental disease who want to engage in high-level activities.

When there is deformity in both knees, arthroplastic surgery can be performed in either one or two stages. One-stage surgery may be considered for younger, more vigorous patients because they are at lower risk of fat-embolization syndrome and are more capable of handling the inconvenience of simultaneous knee

P. A. Lotke, M.D.: Department of Orthopaedic Surgery, Hospital University of Pennsylvania, Philadelphia, PA 19104.

rehabilitation. In general, it is safer to stage arthroplastic surgical procedures in the elderly, or to monitor these patients very carefully for sequelae of the fat-embolization syndrome, which often occurs in one-state bilateral procedures.

The contraindications to total knee replacement are relatively few and include inactive or latent infection. The relative contraindications include Charcot's joint, poor skin coverage, ankylosis of a joint in a good position, lack of muscle control, and inability to cooperate in the postoperative period with realistic activity modifications.

PREOPERATIVE PLANNING

Although it sounds simplistic, a good history and examination of the patient are the most effective ways to ensure that the patient meets the indications and criteria for a total knee replacement. Once it is established that the patient is a satisfactory candidate for knee arthroplasty, the specific details of the procedure can be addressed.

The standing anteroposterior (AP) radiograph is usually the most important study for evaluating the preoperative status of the knee. However, lateral and patellar views are also relevant in assessing the preoperative knee. Some surgeons consider it essential to obtain a full-length radiograph from the hip to the ankle. However, I do not routinely obtain such a film, and feel that most of the necessary information can be obtained on a 17-inch cassette. If a patient has a history of surgical procedures or trauma to the hip or lower leg, these areas should have

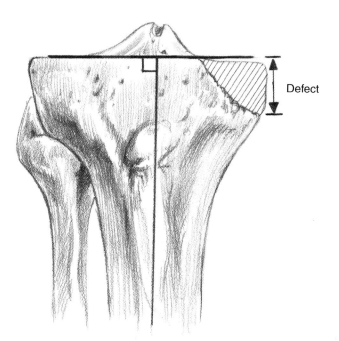

Figure 1. The standing AP radiograph will allow determination of whether there is significant bone loss at the time of surgery. A horizontal line drawn perpendicular to the long axis of the tibia at the level of the uninvolved plateau will allow measurement of the depth of the defect. In general, no specific consideration will be necessary when the maximum bone loss reduces the height of the plateau by less than 15 mm below the height of the normal plateau.

radiographs to rule out unrecognized bone pathology. The standing AP radiograph will allow a determination of whether there will be significant bone loss at the time of surgery, and whether augmentation for this loss will be necessary during surgery (see Chapter 9). A horizontal line is drawn perpendicular to the long axis of the tibia at the level of the uninvolved plateau (Fig. 1). In general, no specific considerations will be necessary if the maximal bone loss is no more than 15 mm from the height of the normal plateau. The standing radiograph also permits assessment of the amount of subluxation and ligamentous laxity that may exist on the medial or lateral side of the knee. In addition, observations are made of the size and position of osteophytes that should be removed during surgery when reconstructing the anatomic contours of the knee.

The lateral and patellar views are also important for preoperative planning. The patellar view will show whether there are erosive changes and thinning of the patella, which are commonly seen in valgus deformities. The lateral radiograph is important to assess if there is patella baja from a previous osteotomy or arthroscopic procedure, and more importantly whether the posterior compartment of the knee contains large osteophytes that will require removal during the surgical procedure.

The preoperative examination should document the condition of the skin and location of previous scars. Psoriasis is not a contraindication to surgery, but the condition of the skin should be optimized prior to surgery. Previous incisions and scars are very important. Every effort should be made to incorporate old incisions into the surgery through careful planning of the new incision. In general, I choose the longest scar and extend it as necessary. Parallel incisions should be assiduously avoided.

SURGERY

The patient is placed in the supine position and carefully prepped and draped. I utilize a long anterior medial incision (described in Chapter 1). A tourniquet is applied on the most proximal portion of the thigh. The incision starts approximately 3 inches above the superior pole of the patella and extends approximately 5 inches to the inferior pole of the patella (Fig. 2). The skin, subcutaneous tissue, and deep fascia are incised. The quadriceps mechanism is cut along its medial border in line with its fibers, and then medially along the border of the patella and patellar tendon (Fig. 3). The knee joint is entered and the soft tissue is dissected from the proximal medial metaphysis within the pes anserinus bursa and

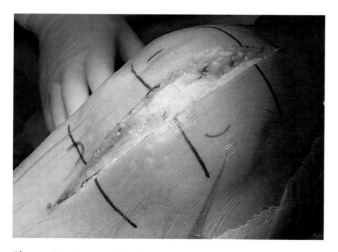

Figure 2. An anterior incision is taken from 3 inches above the patella to 3 inches below the patella.

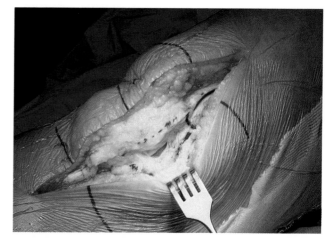

Figure 3. The knee joint is entered through a median parapatellar arthrotomy.

extending back to the posterior medial corner of the knee (Fig. 4). The medial soft-tissue sleeve is carefully kept intact. The bursa beneath the retropatellar fat pad is entered and the anterior lateral capsule incised. The patella is everted, the knee flexed, and the incision extended, if necessary, in order to be sure that there is no undue tension on the soft tissues about the knee. A bent, narrow Homan retractor is inserted laterally to the lateral meniscus and the patellofemoral ligament is incised. Removing the posterior half of the infrapatellar fat pad offers good exposure and reduces the bulkiness of this fat pad, which may bulge out after surgery (Fig. 5). The fat pad is removed with the lateral meniscus. The lateral inferior geniculate vessels are usually identified and coagulated (Fig. 6). They run along the lateral border of the meniscus and are best visualized in the midlateral position of the tibial plateau. The anterior cruciate ligament is incised, as are the posterior horn attachments of the menisci. With external rotation and anterior displacement of the tibia, complete exposure of the tibial plateau and femoral condyles can be obtained (Fig. 7).

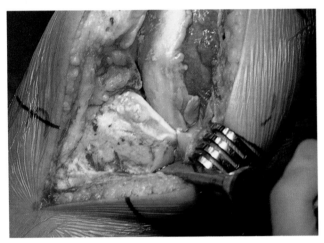

Figure 4. The medial soft-tissue sleeve is dissected within the pes anserinus bursa, and extends back to the posterior medial corner of the knee.

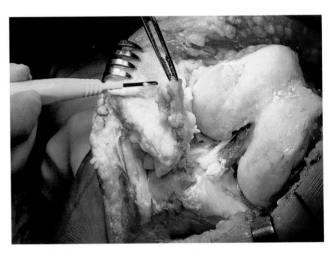

Figure 5. The posterior aspect of the fat pad is resected for better exposure of the lateral compartment of the knee.

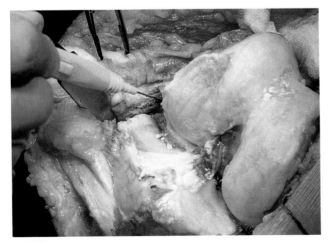

Figure 6. The lateral geniculate vessels can usually be identified and coagulated.

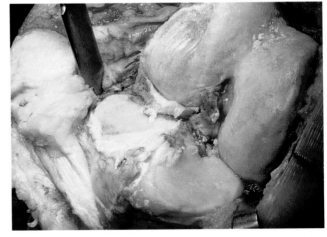

Figure 7. With external rotation and anterior displacement of the tibia, complete exposure to the tibial plateau and femoral condyles can be obtained.

TECHNIQUE

Bone Cuts

The total knee procedure comprises the same five bone cuts whether the prosthesis is cemented into place or fixed by porous ingrowth or press-fit techniques (Fig. 8). The procedure is also essentially the same whether the posterior cruciate ligament is sacrificed, saved, or substituted, the only difference being a sixth step of removing the intercondylar notch for the substituting prosthesis. The essential bone cuts are made regardless of the amount of bone loss, ligamentous imbalance, or osteophyte presence about the knee. For a routine total knee arthroplasty I will make these bone cuts, remove all osteophytes, and then evaluate and compensate for soft-tissue imbalance. In general, after the osteophytes are removed and normal anatomic planes have been reestablished, no specific releases or additional ligamentous balancing are necessary. However, for those knees with severe deformities and cases in which soft-tissue imbalance is a major problem, one should refer to the chapters on correction of these deformities.

The five essential cuts for any total knee replacement are:

Transverse osteotomy of the proximal tibia, tilted 5° posteriorly.
Resection of the distal femoral condyles, angulated at 5° to 7° of valgus alignment.
Anterior and posterior condylar resections to accept a prosthesis of the appropriate size.
Chamfers from the distal femur anteriorly and posteriorly, in order to conform to the internal prosthetic configuration.
Retropatellar osteotomy.
(Optional) resection of the intercondylar notch and posterior cruciate ligament for the posterior cruciate-substituting prosthesis.

The femoral and tibial osteotomies are independent of each other, and therefore either may be performed first. If the knee is relatively lax and has minimal deformity, and the tibia readily subluxes anteriorly, I usually osteotomize the tibia first, especially in cases of valgus knee deformity. On the other hand, if the knee is tight or there are large osteophytes in the back of the knee, and good exposure is difficult to obtain on the tibial plateau, I osteotomize the femoral condyles first. This releases some of the soft-tissue constraint within the knee and gives better access to the tibial plateau.

Osteotomy of the Proximal Tibia. I do this within an intramedullary guide. However, several extramedullary guides are also available and can give equally good results. I find the intramedullary (I.M.) system relatively easy to use, with a highly predictable end result. One of the keys of this technique is accurately choosing the entrance hole into the I.M. canal. This is best done by extending an imaginary line up the shaft of the tibia and exiting from the tibial plateau (Fig. 9). The exit site will usually be just lateral to the insertion of the anterior cruciate ligament. I place an osteotome at this location, check the alignment, and drill a hole there (Fig. 10). Next, I use a long intramedullary irrigator to irrigate the canal with antibiotic solution, removing some of the fat and marrow within the canal and hopefully reducing the potential for fat embolization. The drill hole is slightly larger than the size of the I.M. rod, in order to allow for venting of the intramedullary canal. A fluted I.M. rod with an appropriate transverse cutting jig is inserted into the tibial shaft (Fig. 11). This should be easy to accomplish; if it is not, the position of the entrance hole should be re-checked. The tibial rod should be inserted down to a snug position in the shaft of the tibia. The transverse cutting guide should slide down, and the cutting block may be fixed beneath the patellar tendon in a position that is transverse to the long axis of the tibia (Fig. 12). The outrigger device and intramedullary rod are then withdrawn and the tibial cutting guide is left on the anterior aspect of the proximal tibia. The depth of the tibial

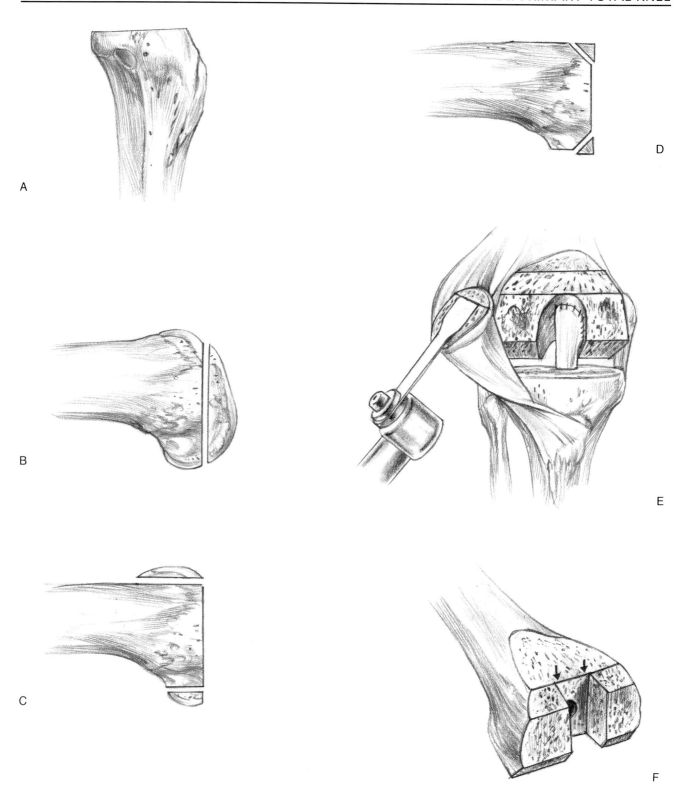

Figure 8. A total knee procedure comprises the same five cuts whether the prosthesis is fixed by methylmethacrylate, porous ingrowth, or press-fit techniques. A sixth step is added if the posterior cruciate ligament is to be substituted. The six steps are: **A:** Transverse osteotomy in the proximal tibia, tilted 5° posteriorly. **B:** Resection of the distal femoral condyles in 5° to 7° of valgus. **C:** Anterior and posterior condylar resections. **D:** Chamfers of the anterior and posterior condyles. **E:** Retropatellar osteotomy. **F:** (Optional) resection of the intercondylar notch of the posterior cruciate ligament for posterior-cruciate-sacrificing prostheses.

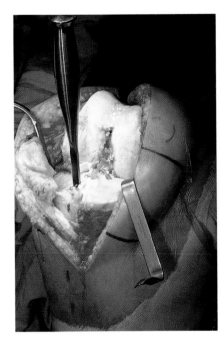

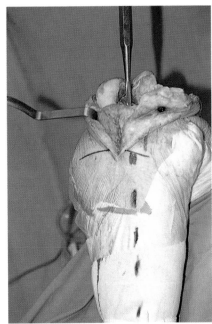

Figure 9. For an intramedullary guide, the entrance site into the tibial plateau is visualized by extending an imaginary line along the shaft of the tibia onto the tibial plateau.

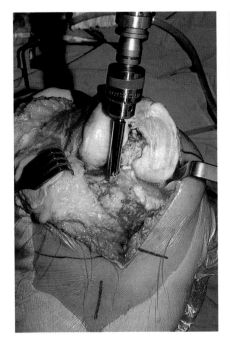

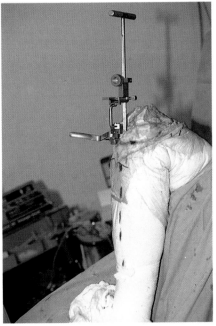

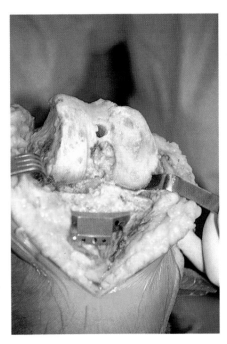

Figure 10. An osteotome localizes the entrance site in the tibial plateau. A large drill hole is made in this site.

Figure 11. A long intramedullary rod is inserted into the tibial shaft.

Figure 12. A tibial cutting guide is left on the anterior aspect of the proximal tibia and fixed in place.

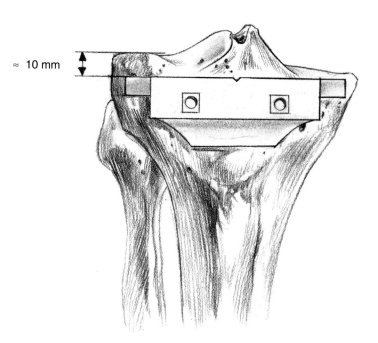

≈ 10 mm

Figure 13. The proximal tibial osteotomy should be taken 8 to 10 mm below the normal tibial plateau and transverse to the long axis of the tibia.

cut should correspond to the thickness of the tibial insert. In general, I try to place thicker polyethylene components than we had considered in the past. In most patients I try to insert a 10-mm-thick tibial plateau. Only in smaller women will I use an 8-mm-thick plateau. This cut will therefore usually be 10 mm below the level of a normal tibial plateau (Fig. 13), and the distance can be roughly measured with a ruler or rotating probe. Because of the deformities on the tibial plateau and their natural saddle shapes, a precise distance for making the cut cannot be measured, but a reliable estimate can be obtained. No effort should be made to remove enough bone to go to the bottom of all bone defects. However, if it appears that an additional 1 or 2 mm of tibial plateau thickness will completely eliminate a bone defect, then I would elect to make that additional cut. On the other hand, if the defect is deep, I will make the 10-mm osteotomy first and evaluate the defect later.

A power saw is used to cut the tibial condyles, with the blade resting on the top of the tibial cutting guide (Fig. 14). A Z-retractor should be placed beneath the medial collateral ligament and the bent Homan retractor placed laterally. The saw blade is advanced posteriorly until the last few millimeters of bone remain. The blade is then lifted off the surface, cracking the last millimeter of tibial plateau (Fig. 15). A clamp is placed on the tibial plateau and the osteotomized plateau is pulled forward. The remains of the posterior horn of the lateral meniscus, the medial meniscus, and a few anterior fibers of the posterior cruciate ligament are released from the tibial plateau. The posterior cruciate ligament is kept intact for those surgeons who prefer to retain this ligament. At this stage, osteophytes along the medial or lateral margins of the knee may be removed. The tibia is placed posteriorly under the femoral condyles, and attention is directed to the next series of cuts.

Osteotomy of the Distal Femur. An intramedullary guide is also used for the femur. A large drill hole is made in the midportion of the intercondylar notch just anterior to the insertion of the posterior cruciate ligament (Fig. 16). Fingers on the anterior shaft of the femur will provide an estimate of the direction of the drill. The canal is irrigated with antibiotic solution. The intramedullary guide, fixed at

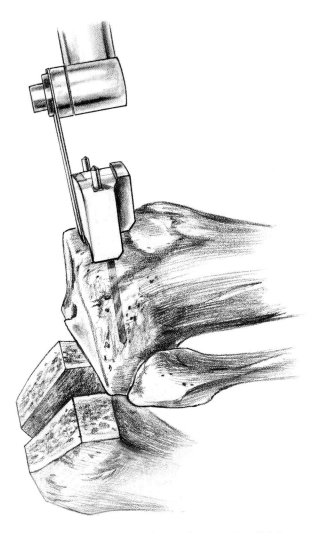

Figure 14. A power saw is used to cut the tibial condyle, with the blade resting on top of the tibial cutting guide.

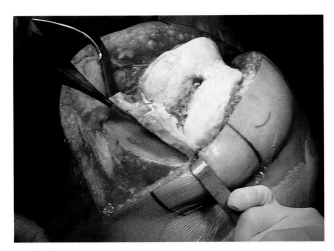

Figure 15. The proximal tibia is osteotomized, leaving the posterior rim intact. Raising the plateau cracks the last few millimeters of the tibial plateau, preserving the posterior cruciate ligament.

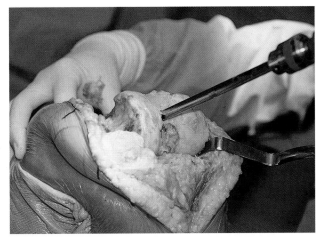

Figure 16. A drill hole is made in the midportion of the femoral condyle just above the intercondylar groove.

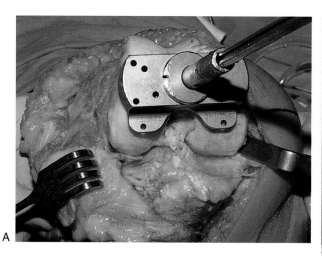

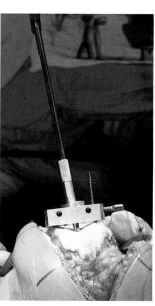

A

Figure 17. A, B: An intramedullary rod is inserted up into the shaft of the femur. A 5° or 7° varus alignment sleeve may be selected.

B

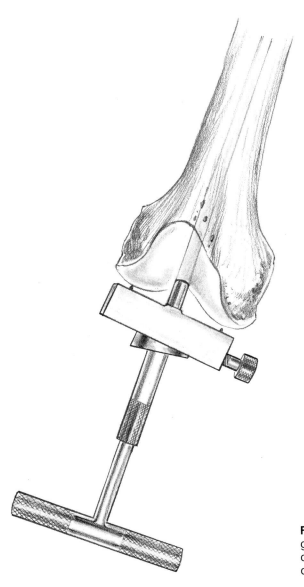

Figure 18. An intramedullary guide with a bushing at 5° or 7° of valgus is inserted into the distal femur.

5° to 7° of valgus, is placed up the shaft of the femur (Fig. 17 A,B). In general, I choose a 5° valgus alignment for preoperative varus or neutrally aligned knees, and 7° of valgus for valgus aligned knees (Fig. 18). The distal femoral cutting block is fixed to the anterior surface of the femur and the intramedullary system is removed (Figs. 19 and 20). The amount of bone to be resected should be equivalent to that which is to be replaced by the thickness of prosthesis measured from the lateral condyle, which is generally between 8 and 12 mm. I usually find that the appropriate resection depth corresponds to the entrance hole into the femur at the lowest portion of the trochlear groove (Fig. 21). The cutting block is used to

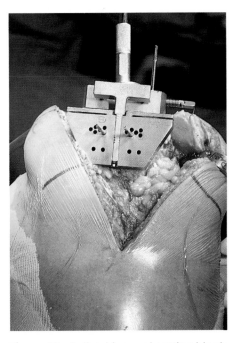

Figure 19. A distal femoral cutting block is fixed to the anterior surface of the femur at 5° or 7° of valgus. The amount of bone resected corresponds to the thickness of the prosthesis.

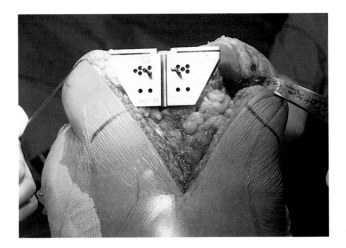

Figure 20. The distal femoral block is fixed to the distal femur.

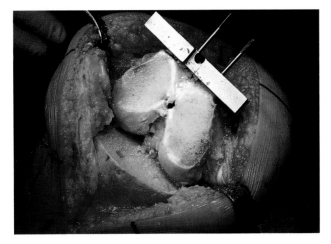

Figure 21. The distal femur is osteotomized. The depth of the osteotomy usually corresponds to the entrance hole into the femur at the lowest portion of the trochlear groove.

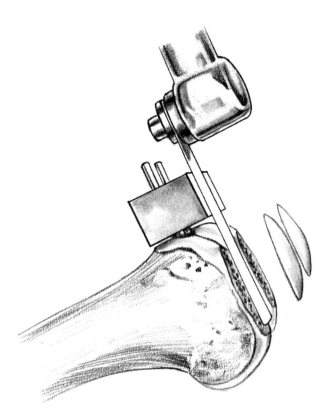

Figure 22. Osteotomies are completed in the distal femoral condyles.

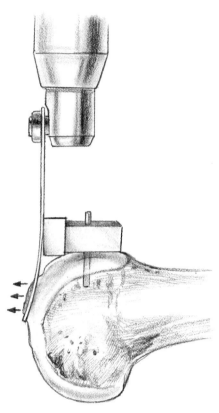

Figure 23. Care should be taken to avoid distortions that sclerotic bone will cause in a flexible saw blade.

guide the saw used to osteotomize the distal femoral condyles (Fig. 22). Care should be taken to avoid distortions that sclerotic bone causes in the saw blade (Fig. 23). The blade has a tendency to bend away from the sclerotic bone and thereby alter the alignment. Awareness of this pitfall is critical in achieving an accurate osteotomy.

Anterior and Posterior Femoral Condylar Osteotomies. These cuts are very important for a successfully functioning prosthesis. The height of the patellar flange should continue along the line of the anterior femoral cortex (Fig. 24). It should not be too high, tightening the retinaculum and preventing flexion or leading to subluxation. Nor should it be too low, notching the femur and creating a potential stress riser for a fracture (Fig. 25). The posterior femoral condyle cuts will be the guides used to set the rotation of the femoral component. It is important that the rotation be accurately judged, in order to prevent internal rotation of the prosthesis. One should appreciate that the posterior femoral condyle of the normal knee is longer medially than laterally. This means that more of the posterior femoral condyle should be removed from the medial side of the knee. There is a variation in the size difference of these two condyles, and therefore no precise difference can be described in the quantity of bone to be removed from each. In general, one can reliably estimate that 2 to 3 mm more bone should be removed from the posterior femoral condyle on the medial side than on the lateral side. Therefore, when the anteroposterior (AP) cutting guide is placed on the distal femur, it should be rotated so that additional bone is taken from the medial side of the knee, compensating when there are erosive changes under one of the condyles (Fig. 26). This is particularly important when the erosive changes are on the lateral femoral condyle, since the difference in the additional bone to be removed from the medial side is exaggerated.

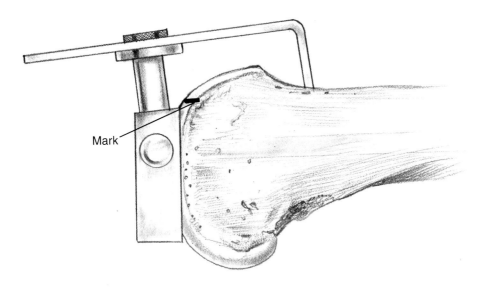

Figure 24. The level of the anterior femoral cortex can be determined with a guide crossing over the anterior femoral condyle.

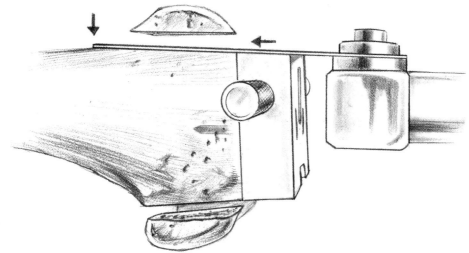

Figure 25. The anterior condylar osteotomy should continue along the line of the anterior femoral cortex.

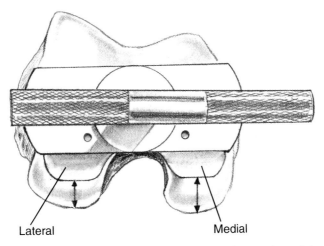

Figure 26. A normal knee has a posterior femoral condyle that is longer medially than laterally. Therefore, more of the posterior femoral condyle should be removed from the medial side of the knee.

The size of the prosthesis must then be determined. A guide can be placed to the distal femoral surface and measurements can be taken to choose the prosthesis of the appropriate size. The situation is best when the size corresponds exactly to the available stock; however, this is not always the case. Fortunately, there are only 2 or 3 mm separating the sizes in most designs of prostheses. I choose

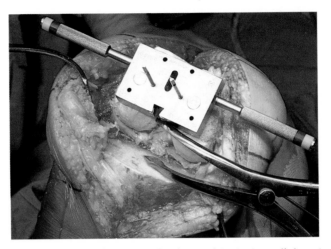

Figure 27. A lamina spreader is used to test medial and lateral ligament balance in flexion. The bottom of the cutting guide should be parallel to the osteotomy surface of the tibia. In a knee with minimal deformity, more of the posterior femoral condyle will be resected medially than laterally.

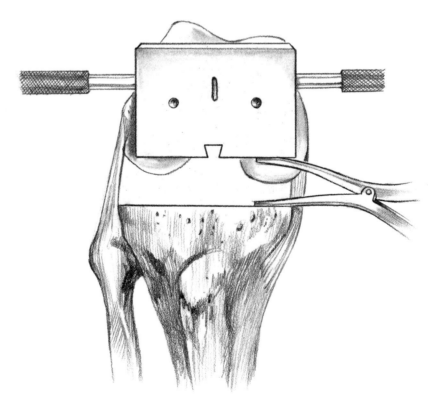

Figure 28. With tension from a lamina spreader, the posterior femoral condylar cutting block should produce a rectangular flexion gap.

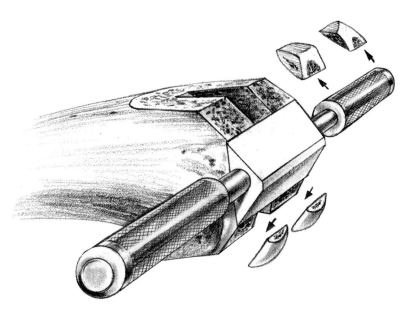

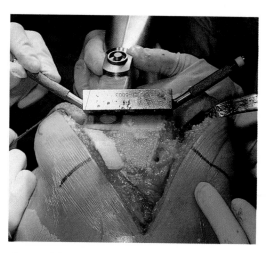

Figure 29. Chamfers are removed from the anterior and posterior condyles in order to create conformity with the internal surface of the prosthesis.

Figure 30. Anterior chamfers are taken to conform to the dimensions of the prosthesis.

the smaller size in order to prevent high riding of the patellar flange or excessive tightness in flexion.

If one saves the posterior cruciate ligament, increasing the thickness of the posterior osteotomy will slightly loosen this ligament. By substituting for the ligament, one avoids this problem. When in doubt, the size of the tibial tray can be checked to be sure that there will be no size mismatch between the femur and tibia.

After the size has been determined and the line marked that indicates the level of the anterior femoral cortex, I place the appropriate size distal femoral cutting block on the distal femur. One condyle is fixed with a pin and the guide is then rotated to the appropriate position (Figs. 27 and 28). The best position and rotation are those in which the cutting block will make the anterior osteotomy cut align directly with the anterior surface of the femur and the posterior condyles resected to produce a rectangular flexion gap. Approximately 8 mm of bone is then resected from the posterior medial condyle.

After the block is fixed to the distal femur, the anterior and posterior osteotomies are completed. Care is taken to protect the medial collateral ligament with a Z-retractor.

Anterior and Posterior Chamfers. These osteotomies are essential for the prosthesis to fit over the distal femur (Fig. 29). A chamfer guide is placed on the distal femur (Fig. 30). This is usually integrated into the same block as used for the anterior and posterior femoral cuts. The angle of this cut may vary with the style of prosthesis.

Retropatellar Osteotomy. The patella is everted. The synovium and fat are removed from the margins of the patella in order to determine its borders. Care should be taken to approximate the patient's own patellar thickness. Most patellae are approximately 25 mm thick and most patellar buttons are approximately 10 mm in height. Therefore, 15 mm of patella should remain. Obviously this varies with the size, shape, and dimensions of any given patella. A caliper can be used to check the dimensions of the patella before the osteotomy and after the button is in place (Fig. 31). A patella that is cut too thick tightens the retinaculum and contributes to lateral subluxation. A patella that is cut too thin is subject to in-

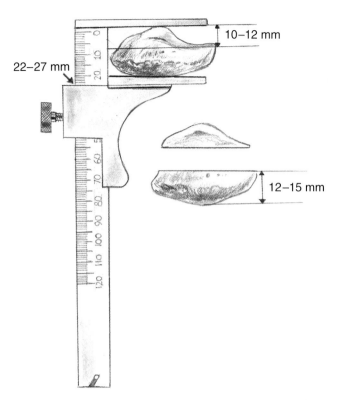

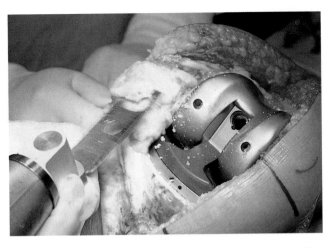

Figure 32. An osteotomy is taken across the retropatellar surface.

Figure 31. Normally, the thickness of the patella is between 20 and 30 mm. It is best to leave at least 15 mm of bone on the anterior surface of the patella for resurfacing.

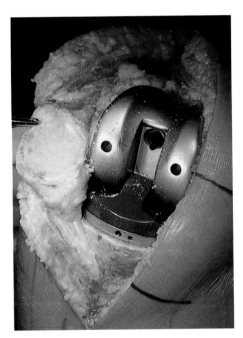

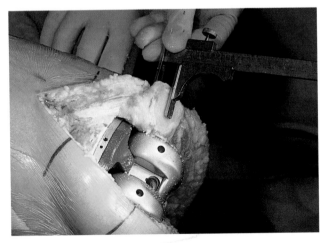

Figure 33. The remaining patellar thickness should be approximately 15 mm.

Figure 34. The retropatellar osteotomy should be approximately 1 mm above the level of the quadriceps tendon and parallel to its insertion.

creased risk of fracture. I take a free-hand osteotomy across the retropatellar surface (Fig. 32), although there are guides available. The free-hand cut is done in two or three stages. The first cut takes the median ridge from the patellar surface. The second pass removes the superior lateral corner. The osteotomy should be parallel to the anterior surface of the patella and to the insertion of the quadriceps tendon (Fig. 33). I check the appropriate alignment of the retropatellar osteotomy with my finger on the patellar edge of the quadriceps tendon. The osteotomy should be equally above (by approximately 1 mm) the level of the quadriceps tendon (Fig. 34). There should be no tilting and equal height should be noted above the tendon. Osteophytes should be trimmed from the patella and drill holes made with an appropriate guide. If size allows, I tend to set the patella slightly medially.

Posterior Cruciate Ligament: Save, Resect, or Substitute. The posterior cruciate ligament has been saved until this point. Those surgeons who would like to save the posterior cruciate ligament can proceed with fitting the prosthesis and seeking balance with the ligament attached. I have found that substituting for the posterior cruciate ligament has given me more consistent results with better range of motion than attempting to save the ligament. Therefore, I currently use an intercondylar cutting guide to resect the bone from the notch (Fig. 35 A,B).

Soft-Tissue Debridement and Balance

The most difficult part of a total knee replacement is achieving appropriate soft-tissue balance after the osteotomies have been completed. The first step in achieving such balance is to remove all osteophytes to an anatomic level. The osteophytes fold off the margins of the bone without difficulty after the osteotomies have been completed. The anatomic contours can be determined because there is a synovial layer against the cortical margin. It is easy to remove osteophytes from the patella, distal femur, and tibial surface. I do this with a curved rongeur. The most difficult location from which to remove osteophytes is the posterior femoral condyles. Exposure is achieved with the aid of a lamina spreader. This is placed into the medial side of the knee, over the posterior cortical edge, so that it will not crush the soft cancellous bone. With tension applied to the spreader, the posterior aspect of the knee on the opposite side can be well visualized. A rongeur can be used to trim off smaller osteophytes and an osteotome to trim larger osteophytes (Fig. 36). The remnants of the meniscus can be debrided and any proliferative synovium can be removed with a rongeur from the posterior compartment of the knee (Fig. 36). The same procedure is repeated on the medial side of the knee. The lamina spreader is set in the lateral compartment and the medial side is opened. A clamp is placed on the anterior border of the medial meniscus and pulled forward, exposing the medial compartment. The inner rim of the medial meniscus is trimmed, leaving the margin to protect the collateral

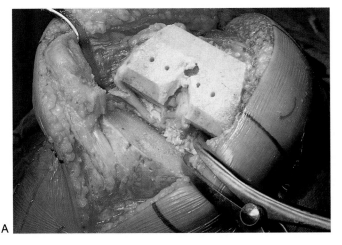
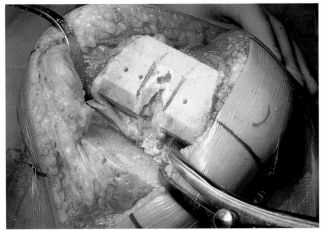

A

B

Figure 35. A: The posterior cruciate ligament may be preserved. A lamina spreader can be utilized to test its integrity. **B:** The posterior cruciate ligament may be resected. The vertical osteotomies are taken into the intercondylar grove to resect the notch and the cruciate ligament attachments.

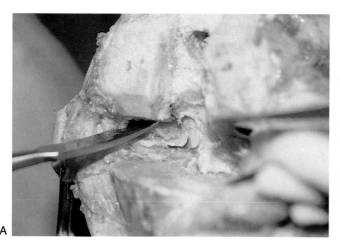
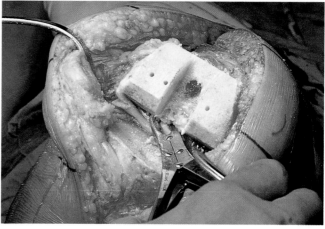

A   B

Figure 36. A: An osteotomy may be utilized to remove osteophytes in the posterior condylar area. **B:** A rongeur may be used to remove smaller osteophytes and synovial and meniscal remnants in the posterior compartment of the knee.

ligament (Fig. 37). Large osteophytes can then be removed from the posterior femoral condyle with an osteotome or rongeur. Synovial debris can also be removed. After the osteophytes are removed, attention can be directed toward inserting a trial prosthesis and determining ligament stability.

Trial Reduction

After the osteotomies have been completed, the soft-tissue debris and osteophytes are removed from around the knee, posterior aspect of the joint, and intercondylar areas. The knee is now ready for a trial reduction. In theory, the amount of bone taken from the distal femur is equivalent to the thickness of the distal femoral component of the prosthesis, and the amount of bone resected from the proximal tibia is equivalent to the thickness of the tibial plateau that is being replaced. As a result, additional balancing should not be required. The femoral

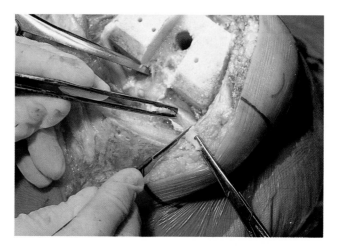

Figure 37. The inner rim of the medial meniscus may be removed while leaving a margin to protect the medial collateral ligament. Traction on the anterior aspect of the meniscal remnant gives good exposure to the posterior medial compartment.

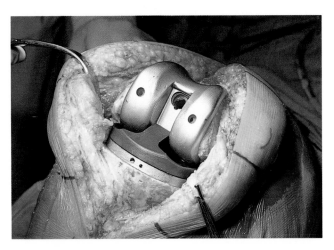

Figure 38. A trial reduction is completed by checking for appropriate tension in flexion and extension. The tibial component is rotated into correct alignment with the femur.

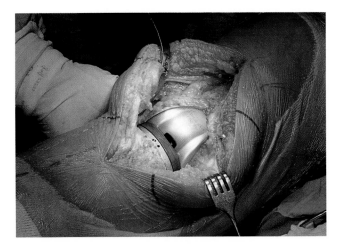

Figure 39. Varus and valgus stress on the tibia will test for ligament stability in full extension and in a few degrees of flexion.

component is placed onto the distal femur and fitted securely, without any toggle. Care should be taken to have the intercondylar box be of adequate size to prevent splitting of the condyles when inserting the femoral condyle of the prosthesis. If too much resistance is noted, the condylar dimension should be enlarged by a millimeter. The femoral component is then inserted onto the distal femur and the tibial plateau placed onto the tibial surface. With flexion and extension, the tibial plateau will tend to rotate itself into the correct alignment with the distal femur (Fig. 38). By applying varus and valgus stresses, the stability of the knee can be determined and the appropriate thickness of tibial insert can be determined (Fig. 39). With a severe preoperative varus deformity there may be some preoperative stretching on the lateral side of the knee, requiring a decision about whether this lateral laxity is excessive. In general I accept a few millimeters of lateral laxity as long as I have correct valgus alignment, a secure medial collateral ligament, and the knee is tracking well and feels secure in extension.

If there is a preoperative valgus deformity, and there has been some stretching of the medial collateral ligaments, I will not accept any medial laxity and will release the tight structures along the lateral capsule in order to achieve tension in the medial collateral ligament. The management of excessive varus or valgus deformity and ligament balancing is described in Chapter 19.

Rotation of the tibial component of the prosthesis on the tibial plateau is now checked. If the tibial component is internally rotated and the tibial tubercle is external to the midportion of this component, there will be a tendency for the patella to sublux or dislocate. Therefore, it is imperative to externally rotate the tibial component so that its midportion lies directly under the patellar tendon. A general guideline is to have the center of the tibial tray align over the medial one-third of the tibial tubercle (Fig. 40). The most common error in achieving adequate external rotation of the tibial component is poor exposure in the posterior lateral corner of the knee. In this corner the femoral condyle pushes against the tibial tray, driving it into internal rotation and creating this error. Therefore, good exposure and attention to the exposure in the posterior lateral corner of the tibia is important to maintaining adequate rotation. With the tibial tray placed on the tibial plateau in appropriate rotation, a central drill is inserted into the tibial plateau and a broach is used to make the opening for the tibial stem of the prosthesis (Figs. 41 and 42).

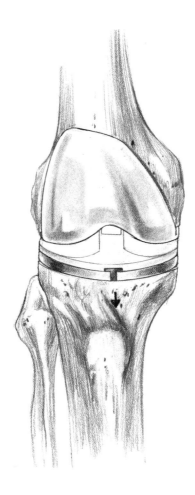

Figure 40. It is important to prevent external rotation of the tibial component. As a general rule, the center of the tibial tray should align over the medial one-third of the tibial tubercle.

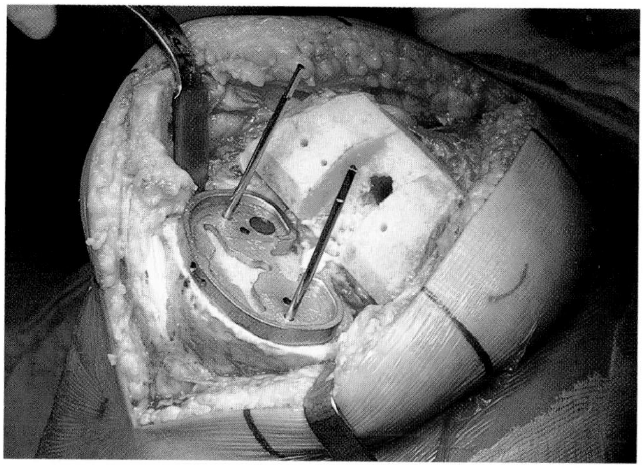

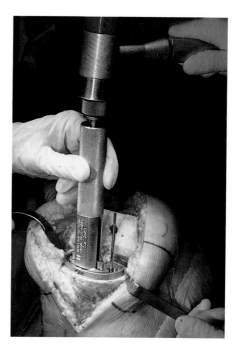

Figure 41. A guide plate is set onto the proximal tibia in order to receive the appropriate drill hole for the prosthetic stem.

Figure 42. A broach is used to control rotation and allow seating of the stem flanges into the tibial plateau.

Patellar stability is then checked. The knee is taken into flexion to be sure that the patella tracks centrally. If the rotation of the femoral component is appropriate, the patella will remain seated squarely in the intercondylar notch (Fig. 43). On the other hand, if the retinaculum is too tight laterally, the patella will begin to tilt or dislocate, requiring a lateral release. I accomplish this by placing the knee in full extension, pulling anteriorly on the patella, and feeling the tight structures in the lateral retinaculum. I release them in stages. First I remove the tight, thickened bands of synovium and then the distal portion of the lateral retinaculum. I advance more proximally in stages, as necessary.

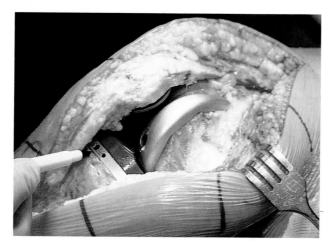

Figure 43. Trial reduction of the patella will demonstrate that it remains seated squarely in the intercondylar notch without a tendency to tilt or sublux.

Component Fixation

The components of the prosthesis can either be press fitted, have ingrowth surfaces, or be cemented in place with methylmethacrylate. I use cement. In order to cement the components, I thoroughly irrigate the bone with pressure and dry the bone completely (Fig. 44). I pour the methylmethacrylate in early, and when it has reached a doughy consistency I apply pressure to the tibial surface with my finger, pushing the cement into the clean cancellous bone (Fig. 45). I insert the tray of the tibial component into the tibia, trimming the excess cement as it exudes from under the plateau (Fig. 46). I then reduce the tibia under the cut femoral condyle and apply cement to the anterior femoral flange and back surface of the femoral component. Next, I place the femoral component over the distal femur and remove the excess cement extruding from under the prosthesis (Fig. 47). A trial tibial plateau is placed onto the tibial tray and the knee is extended in stages. As the excess cement begins to pour out from beneath the prosthesis, it is removed with a curette and a scalpel (Fig. 48). With the knee in full extension, the pressuri-

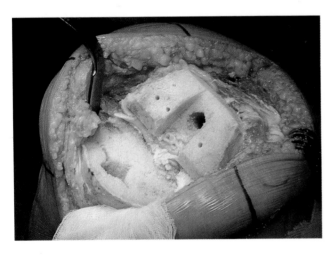

Figure 44. The bone should be pressure irrigated and dried prior to methylmethacrylate fixation of the components of the prosthesis.

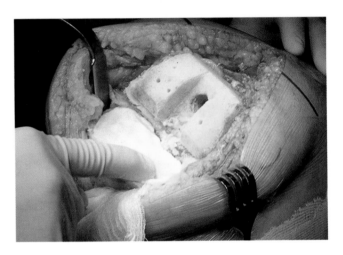

Figure 45. After it reaches a doughy consistency, methylmethacrylate is finger pressurized into the tibial plateau.

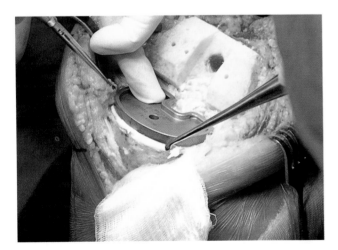

Figure 46. The tibial plateau is placed on the proximal tibia and the excess cement is carefully trimmed from around its margins.

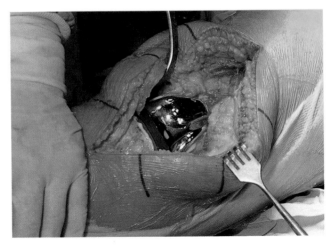

Figure 47. The femoral component is seated onto the distal femur, and as the knee is extended, the excess methylmethacrylate is expressed from beneath the prosthesis.

zation of the cement into the femur and tibia is quite dramatic (Fig. 49). While the knee is held in extension, the patellar component is cemented in place and held with a clamp. After the cement has hardened the patellar clamp is removed, the knee is flexed, the tibial trial insert is removed, and any excess cement is carefully trimmed. The real tibial component is then placed onto the tibial tray (Fig. 50). After the tibial tray is fixed into correct position, the knee is taken through a range of motion, stability and patellar tracking are carefully reassessed (Fig. 51), and the knee is prepared for closure.

Closure

The knee is copiously irrigated to be sure that no bone or cement fragments remain, and the wound is then closed. I use interrupted #1 Vicryl stitches to hold the quadriceps and medial retinaculum in place. I do a very careful subcutaneous closure, attempting to approximate the subcutaneous tissues. Sutures that are too

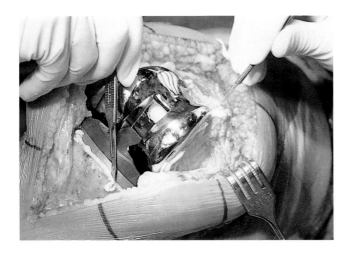

Figure 48. The excess cement is removed with a curette and scalpel.

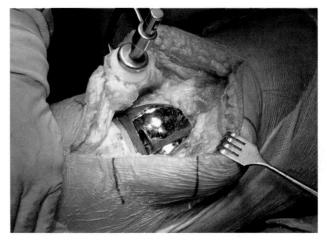

Figure 49. A pressure clamp is utilized to hold the patellar button in place while the methylmethacrylate polymerizes.

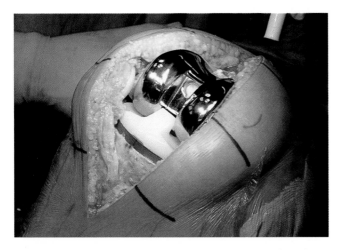

Figure 50. The trial tibial component is removed and the permanent polyethylene component is reinserted onto the tibial plateau. All extra cement is carefully removed from the posterior aspects of the knee.

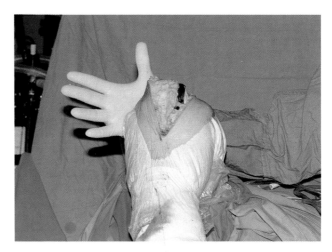

Figure 51. The patella should track centrally in the patellar groove and have no tendency to tilt or sublux. This is known as the "thumbs off" test.

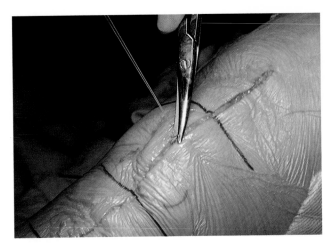

Figure 52. A very careful closure of the deep fascia and subcutaneous tissues is completed.

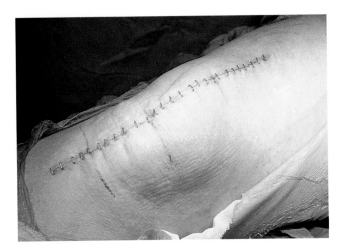

Figure 53. Staples are used for the skin closure.

tight may necrose the fat and lead to problems in wound healing. In the proximal portion of the wound I close the deep fascia as a separate layer with two or three sutures. The remaining subcutaneous tissues are closed as one layer unless the patient is very obese (Fig. 52). I prefer staples for the skin since they are quick to insert, but Steri-strips or nylon sutures are equally satisfactory (Fig. 53).

POSTOPERATIVE MANAGEMENT

Routinely, I place the patient in a splint for two days postoperatively and start motion on the third day. After the splint is removed, a dry sterile dressing and a pressure dressing are applied about the knee. Recently, if I have no special concerns about wound healing, I have been putting patients on a continuous passive motion (CPM) machine to 90° of flexion on the first night after surgery. This is particularly effective for patients who have a continuing epidural or long acting spinal anesthetic and those with patient-controlled analgesia. I am not yet ready to recommend this for all patients.

On the third day after surgery I remove the dressings and start active and passive range-of-motion exercises and increasing physical therapy. This continues with progressive activities as the patient improves. Patients may be discharged to a rehabilitation center after the fourth or fifth day, or may go home with supervised physical therapy after the sixth or seventh day. Some patients require longer hospitalization for a variety of reasons, but usually because they are failing to obtain adequate range of motion.

I advise patients to gradually increase their activities on crutches or a walker for at least 4 to 6 weeks. I do this to allow the bone around the prosthesis to adapt to the new stresses being applied through the prosthesis, or to allow ingrowth to occur. After 6 weeks, patients progress to walking with a cane and continue increasing their activities as tolerated. I generally advise them to plan on resuming normal activities by 10 to 12 weeks after surgery. However, I also caution them that their new knee will not reach its full healing and rehabilitation plateau until 9 to 12 months after surgery.

The functional results after total knee replacement do not replicate the function of a normal knee. The average range of motion will be 115°, which is less than normal flexion. Patients will notice a sense of tightness or aching after prolonged activity, and therefore some restriction in vigorous activity. However, the chief benefit of total knee replacement is relief of pain, and most patients will experience this goal. I tell my patients that they will be able to perform all normal activities compatible with someone aged 60 to 65 years. This includes dancing, swimming, golf, walking unlimited distances, and light tennis. I suggest that they avoid any impact sports or activities that require squatting or kneeling. With these guidelines I hope to obtain survival of 20 years or longer in more than 90% of my patients.

REHABILITATION

The specific rehabilitation program after total knee replacement is somewhat controversial. In general, I take a laissez-faire approach, encouraging patients to work on the range of motion of their prosthetic knee and gradually increase their activities as tolerated. I tend to avoid overzealous physical therapy or vigorous attempts to build muscles in the immediate postoperative period.

Physical therapists play an important role in supervising the postoperative course of patients who have undergone total knee replacement, encouraging them in range of motion exercises and extending our ability to observe their progress.

The goals of the population receiving total knee prostheses, generally the elderly, with an average age in the late sixties, are different than those of younger patients. They like to return asymptomatically to activities of daily living (ADL), and I therefore encourage them to resume these activities as soon as tolerated. I believe that this is the best form of rehabilitation.

COMPLICATIONS

Total knee replacement is a complex operation with innumerable potential complications. I will discuss the five most common problems directly related to surgical technique.

Malalignment

Malalignment is now less common than it once was, since there is a general awareness of its importance and the instrumentation systems for alignment have become more refined. It is clear that significant malalignment will lead to increased wear and loosening of a prosthesis. Therefore, care must be taken to become familiar with the instrument set that has been selected, and to be sure that the alignment is perfect. Malalignments can occur in many ways even with well-designed instruments. A few of these include inadequate exposure and inability to appreciate that the osteotomy cut is not following the guide's directions; failure of the final seating of the prosthesis to correspond to the trial reduction; and misjudgment of bone landmarks in obese or overdraped patients. Experience and attention to details will help prevent malalignment and its associated problems.

Malrotation with Patellar Subluxation

The patella has been associated with more than 50% of problems requiring additional surgery following total knee replacement. Patellar dislocation or subluxation can be a significant problem. One of the most important aspects in achieving consistent patellar tracking has been appreciation of the importance of correct rotation of the osteotomy in the posterior distal femur. The medial posterior femoral condyle is longer than the lateral, and more of this condyle must therefore be resected to place the femoral component of the prosthesis in external rotation and prevent patellar dislocation. In addition, keeping the anterior patellar flange at the level of the anterior femoral cortex avoids excessive tension on the patellar retinaculum, and also reduces the tendency to dislocate the patella. With attention to these two details, I believe that it is possible to reduce the need for a lateral retinacular release to less than 10%.

Loosening From Inadequate Fixation

Loosening of a prosthesis is a long-term complication that may be related to surgical technique. If a porous-ingrowth prosthesis is utilized, perfect osteotomy surfaces are required. Unless excellent approximation of the bone–prosthesis interface is obtained, cement should be considered for fixation. If cement fixation is chosen, adequate bone preparation with pulse-lavage irritation is required. Again, correct angular alignment protects against loosening.

Patellar Tendon Avulsion

Avulsion of the patellar tendon is a potential disaster in a total knee replacement. Therefore, attention to protecting the attachment of the patellar tendon to the tibial tubercle is essential throughout the entire treatment and rehabilitation period. There is a great tendency to hyperflex the knee before adequate exposure is obtained, and this will tend to avulse the patellar tendon. In addition, if adequate exposure has not been obtained, a Homan retractor pulling on the lateral border of the tibial plateau will also tend to avulse the patellar tendon. Adequate exposure will help prevent this complication. External rotation of the foot will externally rotate the tibial tubercle and also reduce the tension on the patellar tendon and the tendency for avulsion.

Wound Healing

Problems in wound healing may be a direct result of surgical technique. Many patients are obese, elderly, or immunosuppressed. Therefore, attention to details and careful closure techniques are especially necessary. In general, I advise residents and new fellows to avoid sutures that are too tight, to use suture material of appropriate size for the tissues to be repaired, to make sharp opening incisions with edges that lend themselves to ease of repair, and to approximate tissues into their anatomic planes in order to avoid shear across the incision surfaces. It appears that attention to good surgical technique and details does reduce problems with wound healing in the postoperative period.

ILLUSTRATIVE CASE FOR TECHNIQUE

A 69-year-old woman has long-standing osteoarthritis of the knee that has become progressively disabling during the past few years (Fig. 54). She has been on a variety of nonsteroidal and antiinflammatory medications, undergone attempts at physical therapy, and had occasional intra-articular injections without significant benefit during the past year. Initially, these conservative methods were quite effective, but as her deformity has increased, conservative measures have been less effective. She can now walk less than one or two blocks with discomfort, notes an increasing varus deformity, and presents with persistent pain and progressive disability.

Examination shows a varus deformity of approximately 185°. When the patient walks there is a 5° lateral thrust. The range of motion in the knee is 5° to 100°. There is moderate medial lateral instability, especially with a few degrees of flexion. There is mild synovitis and a small effusion.

Radiographs show severe medial femoral tibial osteoarthritis with complete loss of the medial joint space and early erosive changes down into the tibial plateau (Fig. 55). Moderate proliferative spurs are scattered throughout the joint, but principally in the medial compartment.

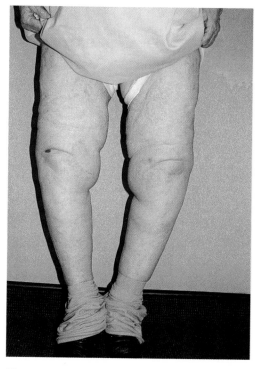

Figure 54. This 69-year-old woman has long-standing osteoarthritis and varus deformities of both knees.

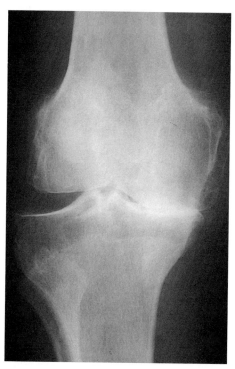

Figure 55. Radiographs show complete loss of the medial femoral tibial joint space with early subluxation, sclerosis, and moderate osteophyte production.

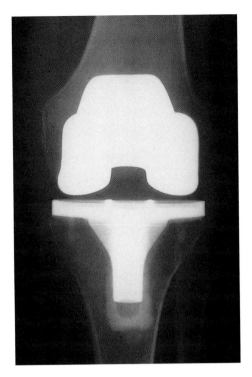

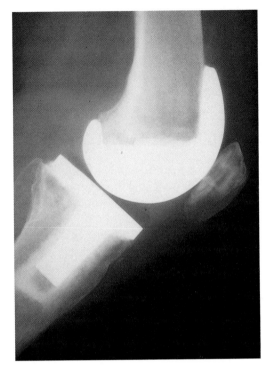

Figure 56. A total knee replacement in good position. The tibia sits squarely on top of the tibial plateau, the femur is in 5° of valgus alignment, and there is good cementation with a feathery pattern extending into the bony trabeculae.

Figure 57. A lateral view of a well-positioned total knee shows good conformity of the prosthesis to the ends of the bone. The tibia sits squarely on the tibial plateau, with a slight posterior tilt. There is no extra cement about the prosthesis. The patella sits centrally and the cementation under the patellar component of the prosthesis appears to be secure.

The patient has a total knee replacement, gradually resumes her activities, and at follow-up is pleased with her total knee. She has been encouraged to increase her activities as tolerated (Figs. 56 and 57).

RECOMMENDED READING

1. Stern, S. H., and Insall, J. N.: Posterior stabilized prosthesis: results after follow-up on none to twelve years. *J. Bone Joint Surg.*, 74A: 980–986, 1992.
2. Rand, J. A., and Ilstrup, D. M.: Survivorship analysis of total knee arthroplasty. *J. Bone Joint Surg.*, 73A: 397–409, 1991.
3. Wright, J., Ewald, F. C., Walker, P. S., Thomas, W. H., Poss, R., and Sledge, C. B.: Total knee arthroplasty with the kinematic prosthesis. *J. Bone Joint Surg.* 72A: 1003–1009, 1990.
4. Goldberg, V. M., Figgie, M. P., Figgie, H. E. 3d, Heiple, K. G., and Sobel, M. Use of a total condylar knee prosthesis for treatment of osteoarthritis and rheumatoid arthritis. Long term results. *J. Bone Joint Surg.* 70A: 802–811, 1988.

Master Techniques in Orthopaedic Surgery,
KNEE ARTHROPLASTY, edited by P. A. Lotke,
Raven Press, Ltd., New York © 1995.

7

Tips and Pearls of the Total Knee Replacement

Clifford W. Colwell, Jr.

In order to optimize the results of any surgical procedure, but with particular reference to a technologically demanding procedure such as a total knee replacement, a series of chronologic steps are necessary. These include a number of "tips and pearls" for helping the surgical procedure to go smoothly, with the best technical outcomes and fewest number of surgical complications. If these are added to the information previously outlined, they should yield a reproducible procedure with a high success rate.

PREOPERATIVE PLANNING

Standing coronal radiographs on a 51-inch cassette are extremely helpful in preoperative planning, making sure that the anatomic axis of the femur is approximately 6 degrees lateral to the mechanical axis and that the femoral neck, midshaft of the femur, or tibia contain no bony deformities that would change the overall alignment of the implant. Otherwise, one can effectively use intramedullary guiding systems in both the femur and the tibia. In the coronal plane, the distal-femoral cut is made 6 degrees from the anatomic axis, making it perpendicular to the mechanical axis. Using an intramedullary system in the coronal plane of the tibia allows the surgeon to make a cut perpendicular to the tibia with or without a posterior slope in the sagittal plane, depending upon the surgeon's desire to preserve the posterior cruciate ligament.

C. W. Colwell, Jr., M.D.: Division of Orthopaedic Surgery, Scripps Clinic and Research Foundation, La Jolla, CA 92037.

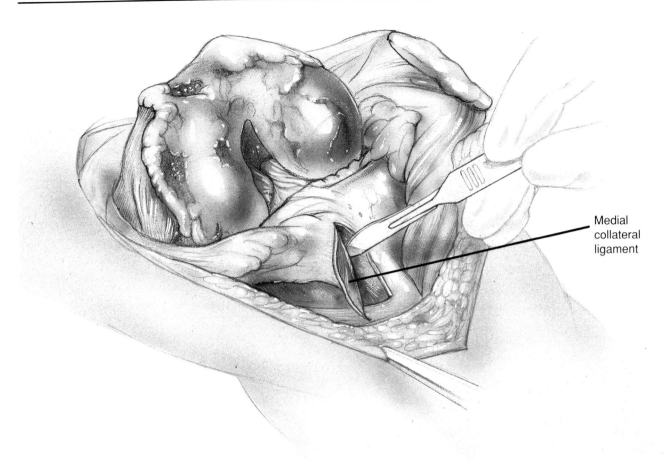

Medial
collateral
ligament

A

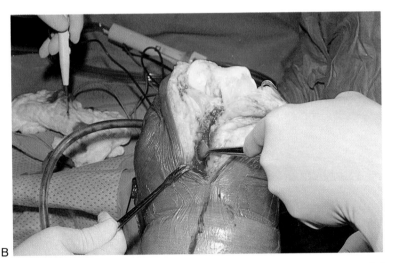

B

Figure 1. A,B: After elevation of the superficial fibers of the medial collateral ligament with a periosteal elevator, the deep fibers are shown elevated and removed by a sharp blade starting distally and moving proximally to avoid loss of medial collateral ligament fibers. Five millimeters of medial collateral ligament are left attached to the tibial tubercle for postoperative reattachment.

SURGERY

Exposure

The skin incision should be carried 1 cm below the tibial tubercle to prevent any skin necrosis by excess retraction, it should be centered in the middle third of the patella and then be carried at least 10 cm proximal to the patella into the area of the rectus femoris. This allows the patella to be everted without excess tension on the patellar tendon or quadriceps mechanism, and avoids the necessity of a temporizing screw to avoid a patellar tendon avulsion.

■ **Pearl**   In making the deep incision distally around the medial capsule and into the proximal tibia, 5 mm of periosteum is retained medial to the tibial tubercle (Fig. 1A). This allows a soft-tissue sleeve to be retained for adequate closure postoperatively, sealing the distal segment of the medial collateral ligament where any persistent synovial leak is usually located.

■ **Pearl**   The superficial fibers of the medial collateral ligament may be elevated without difficulty just superior to the pes anserinus attachment by using a periosteal elevator (Fig. 1B).

■ **Pearl**   The deep fibers are more adherent to the medial portion of the tibia and can be excised sharply by means of a scalpel moving from distal to proximal in order to maintain the medial collateral ligament as a single sleeve (Fig. 2). Any remaining fibers can be removed from overhanging osteophytes without difficulty

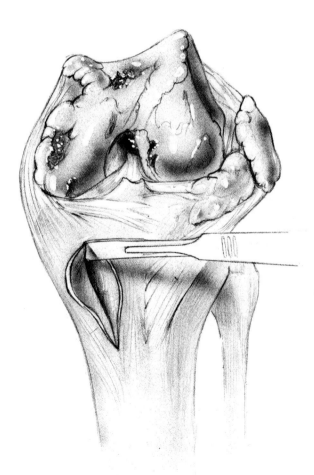

Figure 2. The coronal illustration of the elevation of the deep fibers of the medial collateral ligament from distal to proximal.

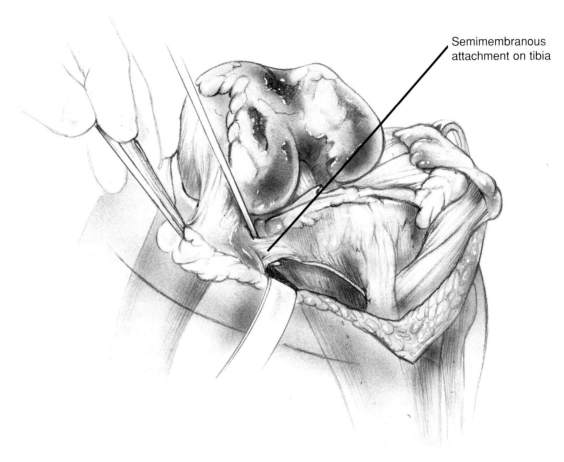

Semimembranous
attachment on tibia

A

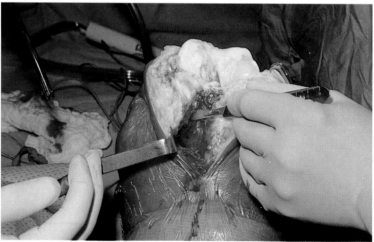

B

Figure 3. A,B: Elevation of the medial collateral ligaments in the sagittal plane as far posteriorly as the attachment of the semimembranous tendon on the superior aspect of the tibia.

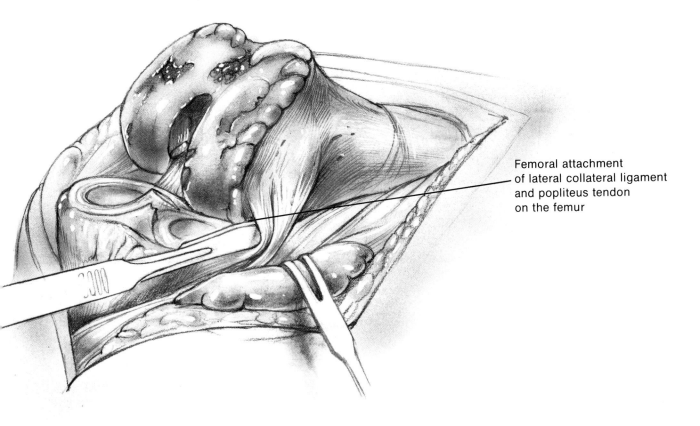

Femoral attachment
of lateral collateral ligament
and popliteus tendon
on the femur

Figure 4. Release of a popliteus tendon and lateral collateral ligament from the lateral femoral condyle in a valgus knee deformity.

or sacrifice of any of the medial collateral ligament. When the elevation of the medial collateral ligament is carried posterior to the midsagittal plane of the tibia, and upon excising the anterior cruciate ligament, the tibia should be able to be translated anteriorly without difficulty. If this can not be easily done, dissection should be carried posteriorly to include the attachment of the semimembranosus on the tibia (Fig. 3).

If a valgus deformity requires release of the lateral collateral ligament and the popliteus tendon, these can be elevated from the epicondyle of the femur in a fashion similar to that for the medial collateral ligament of the tibia (Fig. 4). If elevated in a subperiosteal fashion, it will resume its relative position in the midsagittal plane following completion of the total knee replacement.

For more accurate alignment, the intramedullary system, both of the femur and the tibia is advised.

■ **Pearl**   To avoid fat embolism one initially uses a Charnley Awl with multiple flutes (Fig. 5), enlarging the entrance hole to at least 3 mm greater than the size of the intramedullary rod and evacuating all blood and fat from the intramedullary canal by means of an irrigation system designed for water-picking the proximal femur in total hip replacement (Fig. 6). A water pick can also be used for opening and cleansing the intramedullary canal of the tibia prior to insertion of the intramedullary guiding system (Figs. 7 and 8).

When the surgeon removes the lateral meniscus by sharp dissection, the inferior lateral genicular vessels can be well visualized and cauterized to avoid excessive postoperative bleeding.

Text continues on page 102.

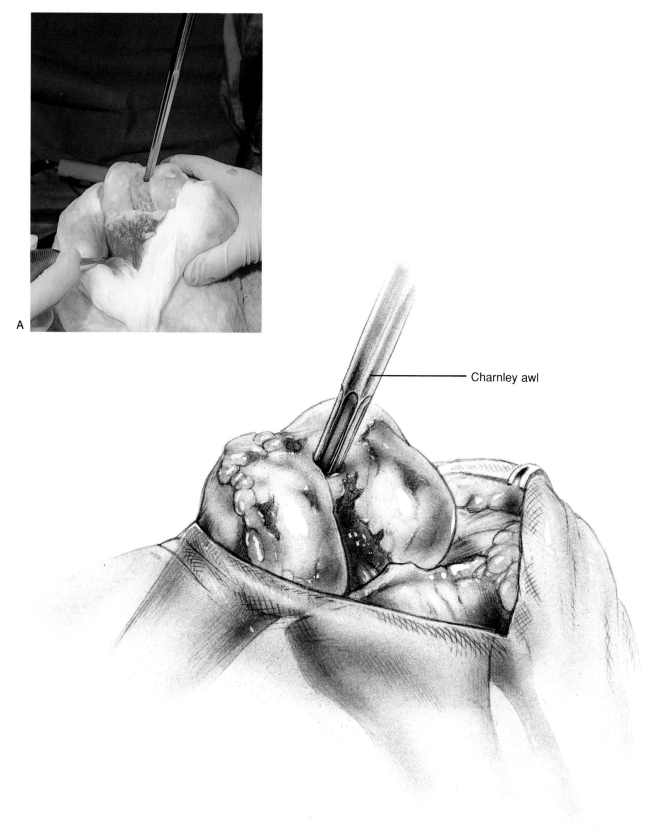

Charnley awl

Figure 5. A,B: Enlargement of the intramedullary canal with a Charnley awl to allow evacuation of intramedullary fat.

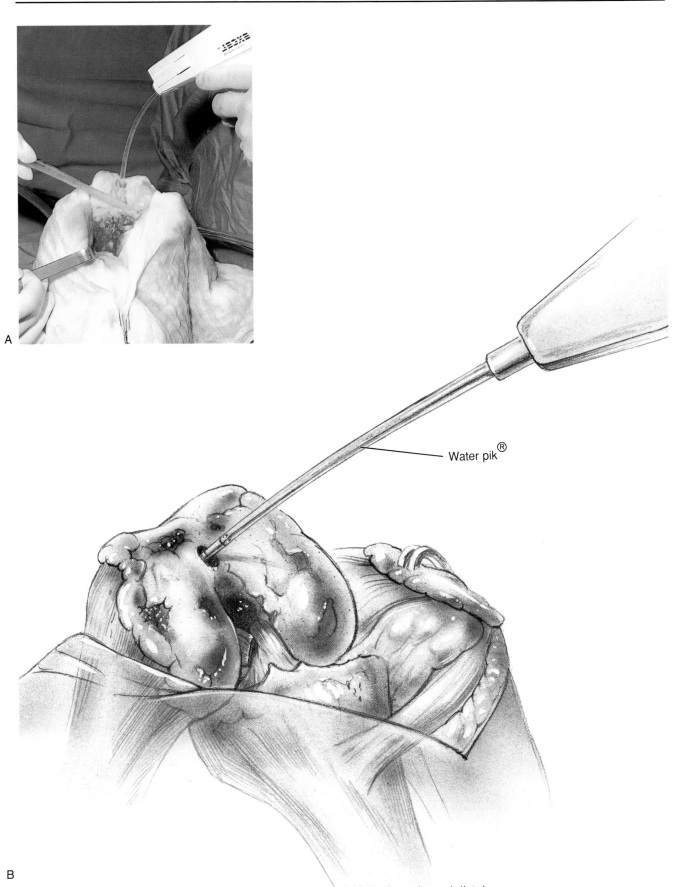

A

B

Figure 6. A,B: An elongated Water Pik system being inserted into the enlarged distal
femoral canal to evacuate any additional fat contents.

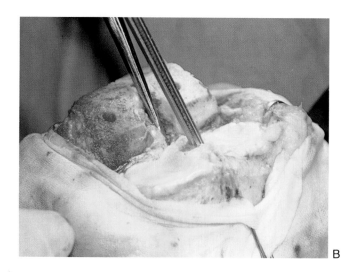

B

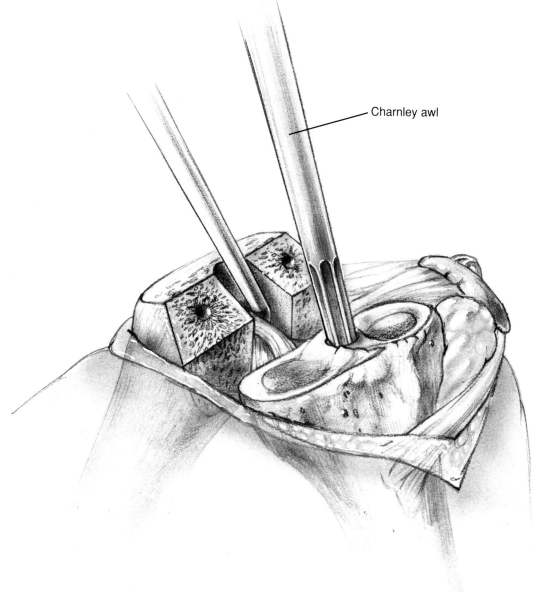

Charnley awl

A

Figure 7. A,B: A Charnley awl used to enlarge the opening in the proximal tibia for evacuation of fat contents.

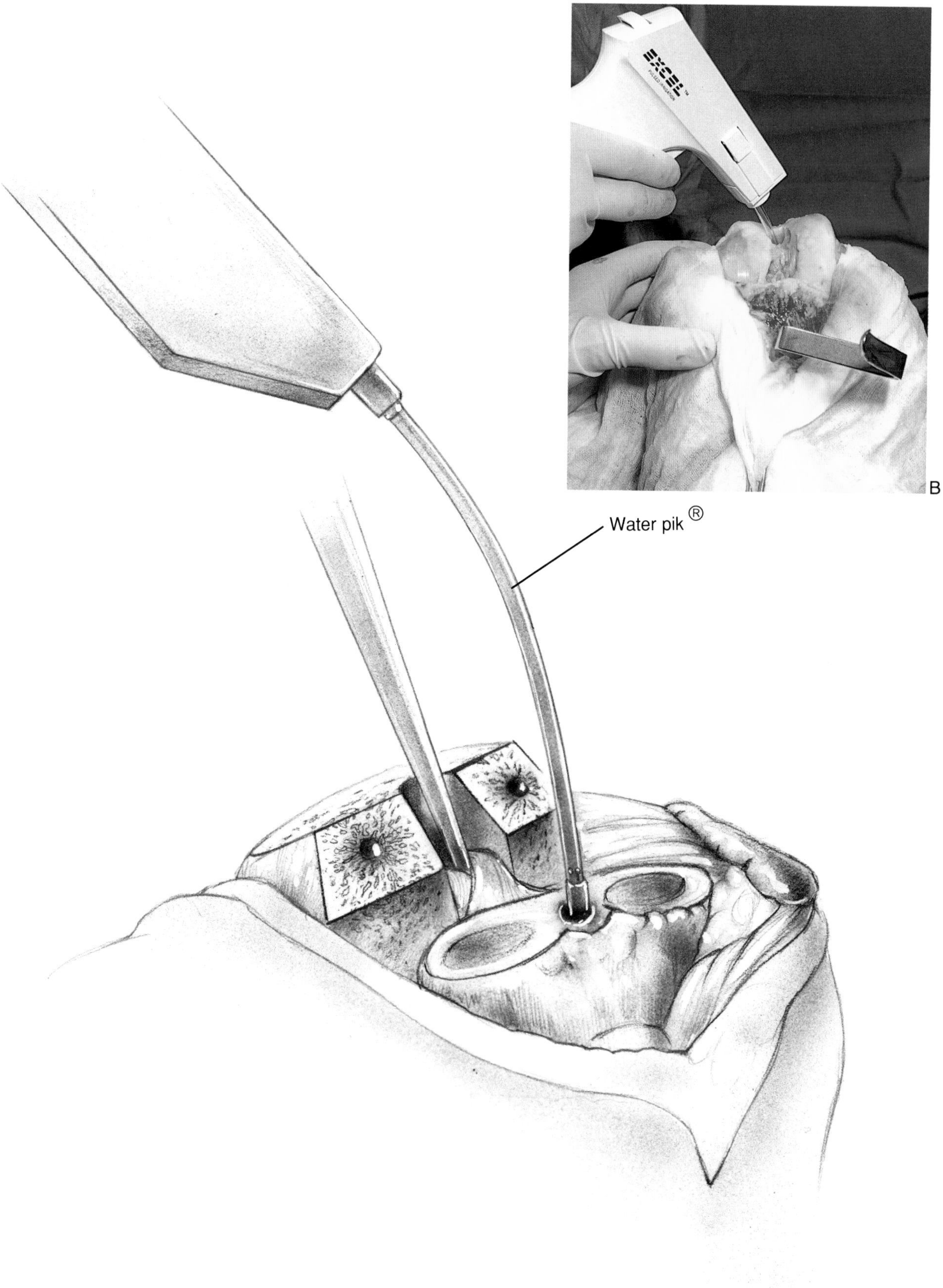

Water pik ®

Figure 8. A,B: The Water Pik system inserted into an enlarged proximal tibial opening for evacuation of remaining fat contents.

A

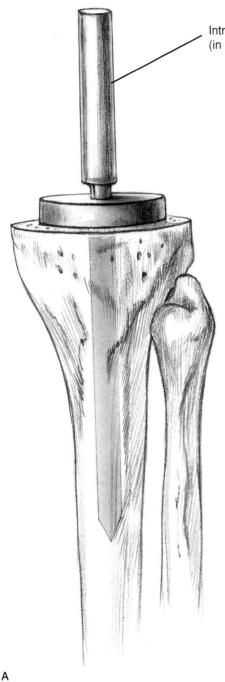

Intramedullary flatness accessor
(in coronal plane)

A

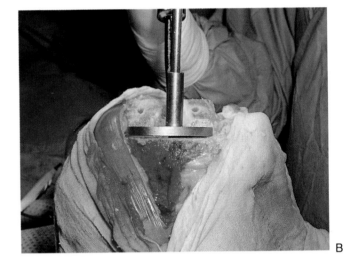

B

Figure 9. A,B: Tibial flatness accessor placed into the intramedullary canal of the tibia in order to document an absolute perpendicular cut in the coronal plane.

■ **Pearl**   To evaluate the accuracy of the tibial cut, because of the tendency for saw blades to "rise" in hard bone and "dive" in soft bone, a right-angle intramedullary device is utilized to confirm the perpendicular nature of the cut in the coronal plane (Fig. 9).

■ **Pearl**   If one has executed a posterior slope cut in the sagittal plane in the proximal tibia, a second device can be used over an intramedullary guide to document the sagittal slope of the tibia (Fig. 10). If the initial cuts were inaccurate, they may be corrected with either a saw or files prior to implantation.

■ **Pearl**   If any posterior osteophytes are present on the femur, they will inter-

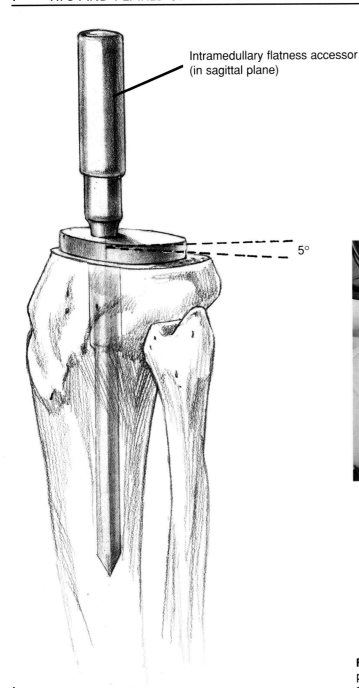

Intramedullary flatness accessor
(in sagittal plane)

5°

A

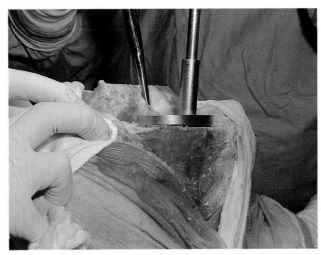

B

Figure 10. A,B: Tibial flatness accessor in the coronal plane, defining the accuracy of a perpendicular or sloped sagittal tibial cut.

fere with full extension postoperatively and should be removed along with posterior loose bodies. This is most easily done with a right-angle curette. The femur is elevated with the knee flexed at 90 degrees by an intramedullary rod in the femur (Fig. 11A). Additional osteophytes from either the medial or lateral femoral condyles the proximal tibia plateaus should also be removed to avoid excessive strain on the medial or lateral collateral ligaments (Fig. 11B).

If the surgeon is using cement, all hard subchondral bone should be drilled with a fine drill point to allow penetration of the cement (Fig. 11C). This is particularly important in the patella.

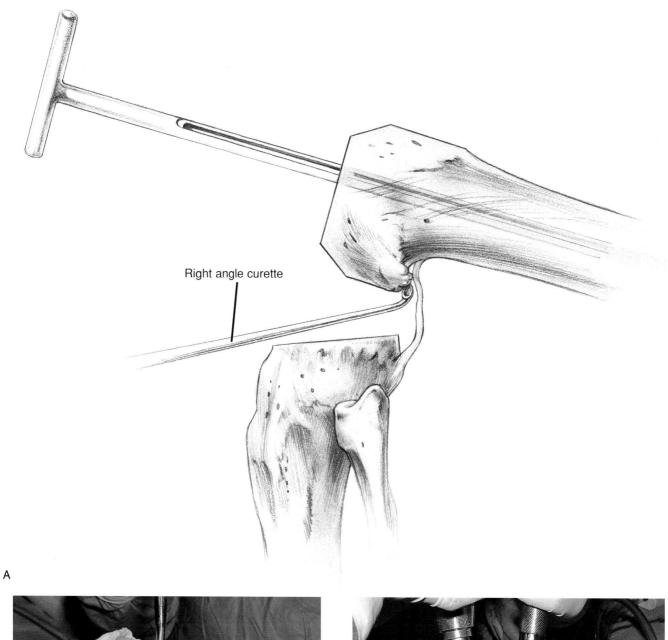

Right angle curette

A

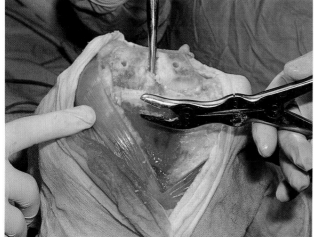

B

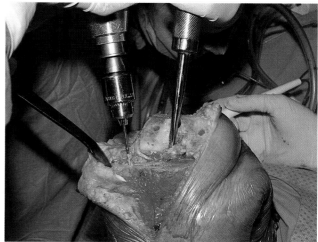

C

Figure 11. A: A posterior femoral osteophyte is removed with a right-angle curette, elevating the femur with an intramedullary rod. **B:** Additional osteophytes should also be removed to avoid excessive strain on the medial or lateral collateral ligaments. **C:** All hard subchondral bone is drilled with a fine-point drill to allow penetration of the cement.

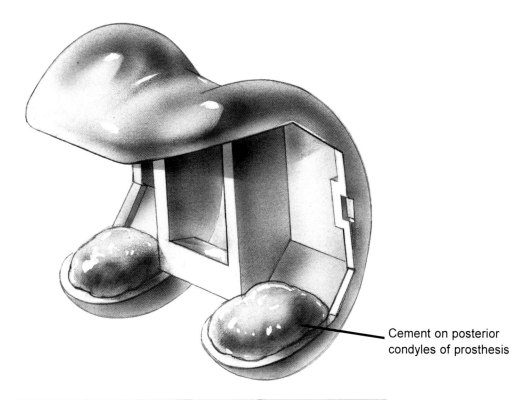

Cement on posterior
condyles of prosthesis

A

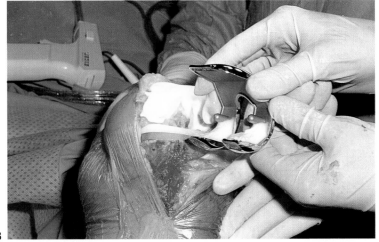

B

Figure 12. A,B: Cement applied to the posterior femoral condyles of the implant without being applied to the posterior condyles of the femur.

■ **Pearl**   To avoid any loss of cement into the posterior aspect of the knee, no cement should be directly applied to the posterior condyles of the femur; the cement should instead be added to the posterior condyles of the implant (Fig. 12). If one then starts the posterior condyles of the implant directly in contact with the posterior condyles of the femur, all excessive cement will be swept forward and can be removed without difficulty before hardening.

■ **Pearl**   A caliper must be used for measuring the thickness of the patella to ascertain adequate overall thickness following implantation of the patellar button (Fig. 13). If the patella is more than 25 mm thick, one can remove the articular surface to a 15-mm depth with a 10-mm patellar button to avoid excessive patello-femoral pressures caused by increased thickness (Fig. 14). If one is forced to leave

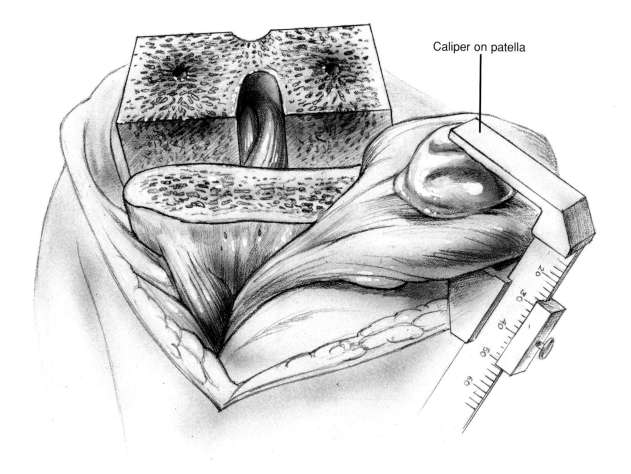

Caliper on patella

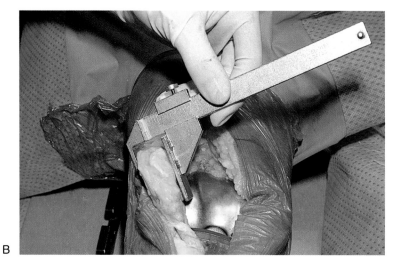

Figure 13. A,B: Caliper applied to the patella to assess the pre-cut patellar thickness.

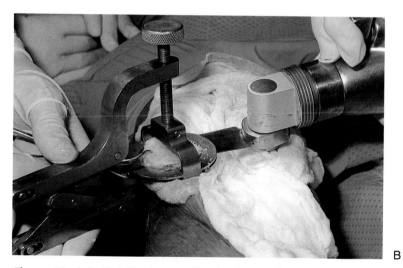

Patella clamp for
accurate cutting

15 mm

A

B

Figure 14. A,B: Patella clamp with slot for cutting exact thickness of remaining patella.

the patella at a thickness of less than 15 mm, this will increase bone strain anteriorly. A compromise may be necessary for the very thin patella seen in rheumatoid arthritis. The overall thickness should not exceed the initial thickness of the original patella (Fig. 15).

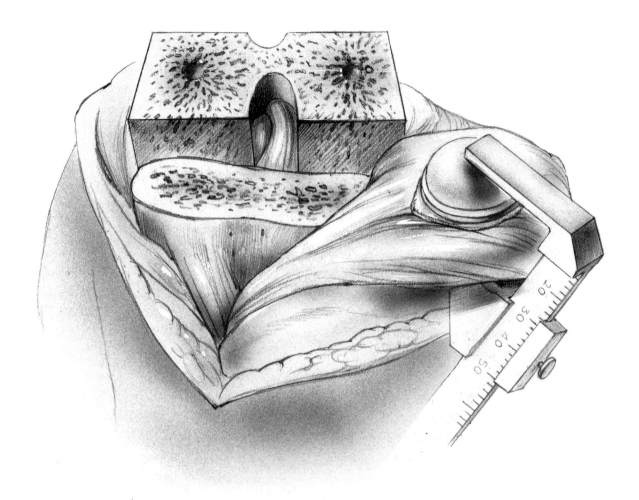

A

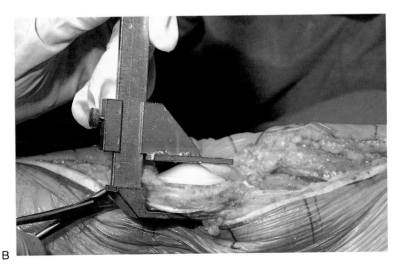

B

Figure 15. A,B: Reapplication of caliper on combined height of patellar bone and patellar implant, documenting matching pre-cut thickness.

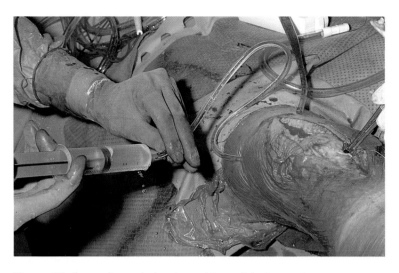

Figure 16. Intermittent irrigation with antibiotics maintains patency during closure.

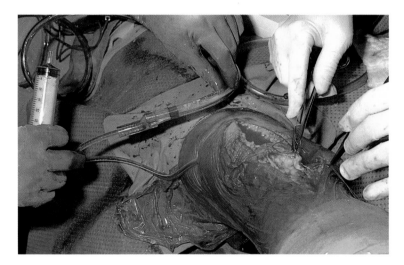

Figure 17. Evacuated blood can be stored in a cell saver.

■ **Pearl**   If the surgeon is using Constavac or Hemavac drainage, the irrigation tube should be carried through the vasus lateralis in an oblique manner, using intermittent irrigation with antibiotics to maintain patency during closure (Fig. 16). All blood evacuated after removal of the tourniquet can be stored in a cell-saver-reservoir at minimal expense (Fig. 17). In the case of excessive postoperative bleeding in which more than 500 cc of blood are retrieved, the reservoir may be connnected to a cell saver and blood returned to the patient. This may be done in the recovery room for up to 6 hours after completion of the surgery with either a filtered or washed-and-filtered retrievel system.

POSTOPERATIVE REHABILITATION

Range-of-motion exercises are started immediately postoperatively and should reach 90 degrees of flexion with an adequate straight leg raise by the third to fifth postoperative day. The flexion may be achieved more quickly with use of a CPM device, but this device has not shown an advantage over active range-of-motion exercises in terms of overall functional outcome at 3 months, 6 months, or 1 year of follow-up.

Additional modalities, such at TENS units, continuous cooling pads, or PCA have not proven effective in improving functional outcome or decreasing the use of pain medication during hospitalization.

RECOMMENDED READING

1. Bourne, M. H., Rand, J. A., and Ilstrup, D. M.: Posterior cruciate condylar total knee arthroplasty: five-year results. *Clin. Orthop.*, 234: 129–136, 1988.
2. Insall, J. N., Lachiewicz, P. F., and Burstein, A. H.: The posterior stabilized condylar prosthesis: a modification of the total condylar design. Two- to four-year clinical experience. *J. Bone Joint Surg.*, 64A: 1317–1323, 1982.
3. Krackow, K. A.: *The Technique of Total Knee Arthroplasty*. St. Louis, Mosby-Year Book, Inc., 1990.
4. Ranawat, C. S., and Boachie-Adjei, O.: Survivorship analysis and results of total condylar knee arthroplasty: eight- to eleven-year follow-up period. *Clin. Orthop.*, 226: 6–13, 1988.
5. Rand, J. A.: *Total Knee Arthroplasty*. Raven Press, New York, 1993.
6. Scott, W. N., Rubinstein, M., and Scuderi, G.: Results after knee replacement with a posterior cruciate-substituting prosthesis. *J. Bone Joint Surg.*, 70A: 1163–1173, 1988.

Master Techniques in Orthopaedic Surgery,
KNEE ARTHROPLASTY, edited by P. A. Lotke,
Raven Press, Ltd., New York © 1995.

8

Fixed Varus and Valgus Deformities

Giles R. Scuderi and John N. Insall

INDICATIONS/CONTRAINDICATIONS

Fixed angular deformity about the knee necessitates special consideration in order to restore normal alignment during a total knee arthroplasty. With fixed angular deformity, one ligament is shortened or contracted while the opposite ligament is usually elongated. There is usually an associated flexion contracture with involvement of the posterior structures. The cruciate ligaments, being in the center of the knee, usually retain their normal length, but it is usually difficult to elongate the contracted side without releasing the cruciate ligaments. The ideal postoperative alignment is independent of the original anatomy, and should not be compared to that of the opposite, normal knee, since it most likely has a similar angular deformity. This ideal alignment, which is achieved by balancing the soft tissues and placing the components of the prosthesis in proper position, is 5° to 10° of valgus. The tibial component should be placed at 90 ± 2° to the long axis of the tibial shaft in both the coronal and sagittal planes, while the ideal placement of the femoral component is 7 ± 2° of valgus angulation in the coronal plane and 0° to 10° of flexion in the sagittal plane (7). When the alignment is not sufficiently corrected, the components of the prosthesis will be unequally loaded and subjected to excessive stress, resulting in eventual loosening of the prosthesis (14). Intraoperatively, it is imperative to reassess each step of the soft-tissue release as it is performed so as not to overcorrect the deformity and create an unwanted instability. When using an unconstrained or semiconstrained knee prosthesis, it is the intact collateral ligaments and not the prosthesis alone that gives stability to the knee (1).

G. R. Scuderi, M.D., and J. N. Insall, M.D.: Office of the Director, Insall Scott Kelly Institute for Orthopaedic & Sports Medicine, New York, NY 10128.

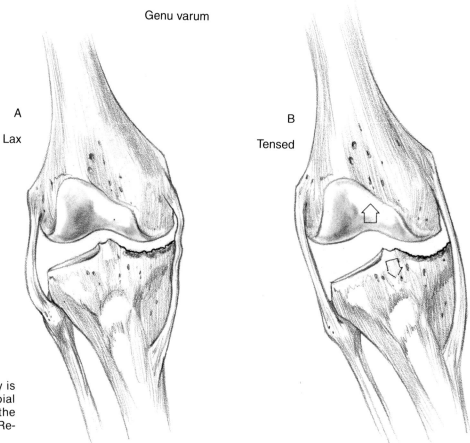

Figure 1. A, B: Varus deformity is usually caused by medial tibial bone loss and contracture of the medial supporting structures. (Redrawn from ref. 1.)

Varus deformity is usually caused by medial tibial bone loss with contracture of the medial collateral ligament, posterior medial capsule, pes anserinus, and semimembranosus muscle (Fig. 1A, B). Medial femoral bone loss is usually minimal because this bone is stronger than the tibia. Elongation of the lateral collateral ligament is a late event, and rupture of the ligament is rare.

Because of the articulation of the lateral femoral condyle with the posterior aspect of the tibia, valgus deformity usually involves a posterior tibial defect with sparing of the anterior tibial margin. The lateral femoral condyle is also eroded in a valgus deformity because of its articulation with the tibia and wear from a laterally tracking patella. Additionally, a fixed valgus deformity is due to contracture of the iliotibial band and biceps femoris, lateral collateral ligament, popliteus, and lateral posterior capsule (Fig. 2A, B). Elongation of the medial collateral ligament is a late secondary event. Those knees with rheumatoid arthritis and valgus deformity usually have an external deformity of the tibia caused by contracture of the iliotibial band.

PREOPERATIVE PLANNING

A careful physical examination should determine the degree of deformity, range of motion, and muscle strength of the knee. Ligamentous instability is rarely a problem in the degenerative knee with a fixed angular deformity. The anterior cruciate ligament is usually deficient, but this is not a problem in total knee arthroplasty. However, the integrity of the posterior cruciate ligament (PCL) will determine the choice of prosthesis. If the PCL is deficient or needs to be resected

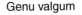

Genu valgum

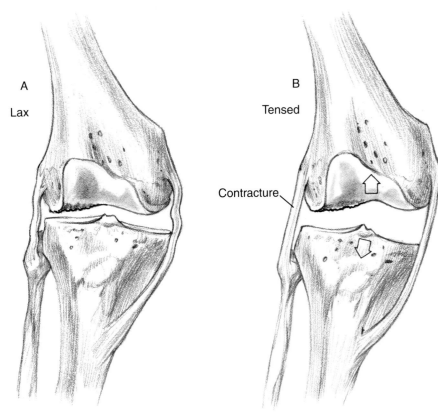

Figure 2. A, B: Valgus deformity is usually caused by lateral femoral bone loss and contracture of the lateral supporting structures. (Redrawn from ref. 1.)

in order to correct the fixed deformity, then a PCL-substituting prosthesis should be implanted. For those cases with severe contracture requiring extensive ligamentous release and difficulty in balancing the soft tissues, a constrained condylar prosthesis should be utilized.

For accurate preoperative planning, a full-length standing anteroposterior (AP) radiograph should be made of the entire limb. The objective in correcting fixed angular deformities is to restore the mechanical axis of the leg to 0°. This mechanical axis consists of a straight line from the center of the femoral head through the center of the knee and to the center of the ankle. Preoperative radiographs should also demonstrate any bony defects that may need augmentation, while the tangential view should be used to assess patellar tracking.

SURGERY

Surgical Procedure

The anterior midline approach allows full exposure of the distal femur and proximal tibia. Since it is our objective to produce a knee that has approximately equal soft-tissue tension medially and laterally, as well as in flexion and extension, appropriate soft-tissue and ligamentous releases are performed prior to bone cuts. The straight anterior incision is extensile and can be extended proximally and distally to expose the distal femur and proximal tibia. This anterior incision also allows exposure of the medial and lateral supporting structures.

Following the skin incision, a medial parapatellar arthrotomy is performed through a straight incision extending over the medial one-third of the patella and

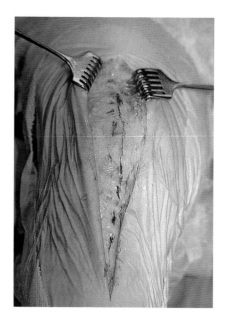

Figure 3. The medial parapatellar arthrotomy extends from the quadriceps tendon over the medial one-third of the patella, and continues along the medial border of the tibial tubercle.

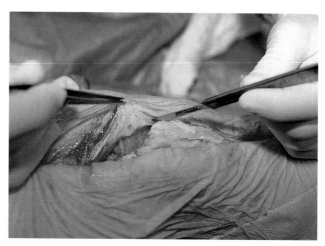

Figure 4. The quadriceps expansion is sharply dissected from the medial border of the patella.

continuing along the medial border of the tibial tubercle (Fig. 3). The quadriceps expansion is peeled from the anterior surface of the patella by sharp dissection until the medial border of the patella is visualized (Fig. 4). The synovium is divided and the fat pad is split along the midline. The patella is then everted and dislocated laterally. To avoid avulsion of the patellar tendon, it can be subperiosteally dissected to the crest of the tibial tubercle, releasing tension while the knee is flexed. This approach is the most versatile and allows the broadest exposure to the knee joint.

Varus Deformity

To correct a fixed varus deformity, progressive release of the tight medial structures is performed until they reach the length of the lateral supporting structures (1). The release is begun by excising osteophytes from the medial femur and tibia. These osteophytes tent the medial capsule and ligamentous structures, and their removal can produce a minimal amount of correction before the soft-tissue release is begun. Posteromedial osteophytes may need to be removed after the proximal tibia is resected. With the knee in extension, a subperiosteal sleeve is elevated from the proximal medial tibia, including the deep medial collateral ligament, superficial medial collateral ligament, and insertion of the pes anserinus tendons. A medial subperiosteal sleeve is sharply elevated from the proximal tibia (Fig. 5A, B) and the elevation then continued with a periosteal elevator (Fig. 6) to free the posterior fibers. Retraction of this subperiosteal sleeve for better exposure during the release is performed with a Homan retractor (Fig. 7). Placement of this retractor also allows traction on the medial soft tissues, facilitating the subperiosteal release. The extent of the release can be monitored by inserting lamina spreaders within the femorotibial joint and judging alignment with a plumb line. The cruciate ligaments may inhibit the correction, and should be resected if they do. Attempts to retain the PCL in cases of severe varus deformity usually result in

Patella displaced laterally

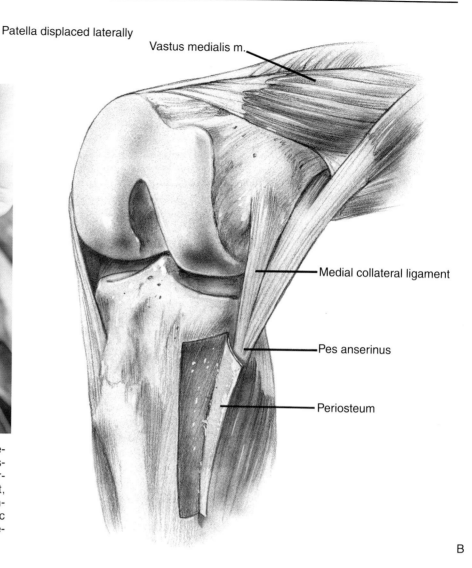

Vastus medialis m.

Medial collateral ligament

Pes anserinus

Periosteum

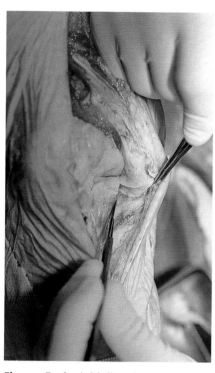

A

Figure 5. A: Initially, the varus release is begun with sharp subperiosteal dissection of the deep and superficial medial collateral ligament, along with the insertion of the pes anserinus tendons. **B:** Diagrammatic representation of the initial varus release. (Redrawn from ref. 1.)

B

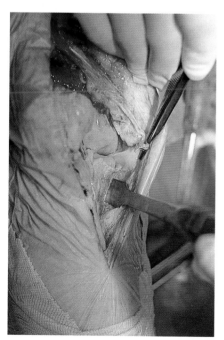

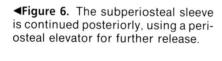

◄**Figure 6.** The subperiosteal sleeve is continued posteriorly, using a periosteal elevator for further release.

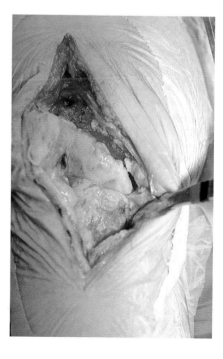

►**Figure 7.** A Homan retractor is placed beneath the subperiosteal sleeve for better exposure.

an inability to correct the deformity. Though conceptually it would be appealing to progressively release the PCL or perform a PCL recession from the tibial tubercle, we prefer to resect the PCL and insert a posterior-cruciate-substituting prosthesis. Besides preventing the correction of a fixed varus deformity, a tight PCL will limit motion and cause the knee to open like a book, preventing the more normal gliding and rolling that occurs with knee flexion. With the cruciate ligaments resected, the knee can be flexed and the tibia externally rotated. The insertion of the semimembranosus muscle is released from the posterior medial corner (Fig. 8A, B), with posterior osteophytes being removed at the same time. Distally the release includes the deep fascia of the soleus and popliteus muscles. With severe varus deformity, the medial subperiosteal dissection is continued posteriorly and distally, maintaining continuity of the medial structures (Fig. 9A, B). Correction should be periodically checked with lamina spreaders. The medial side is surgically released and lengthened to the same degree as the lateral side has been stretched preoperatively. When a flexion contracture is present, it may be necessary to further release the posterior capsule, which can be stripped subperiosteally from the femur and tibia after the bone cuts are made. In severe cases with extensive subperiosteal dissection, the proximal medial tibia appears skeletonized (Fig. 10).

When the medial release is complete and normal alignment has been achieved, the standard bone cuts are made (8). The level of the tibial cut is constant, conservative, and perpendicular to the long axis of the tibia. It should be 5 mm or less

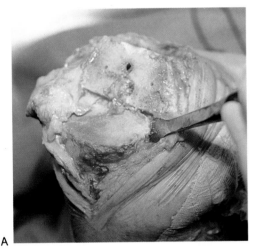

A

Figure 8. A: The insertion of the semimembranosus muscle is released from the posterior medial corner. **B:** Diagrammatic representation of the release of the posteromedial corner. (Redrawn from ref. 1.)

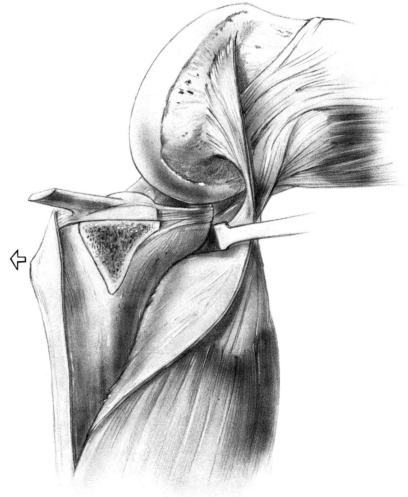

B

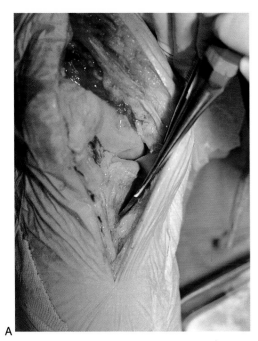

A

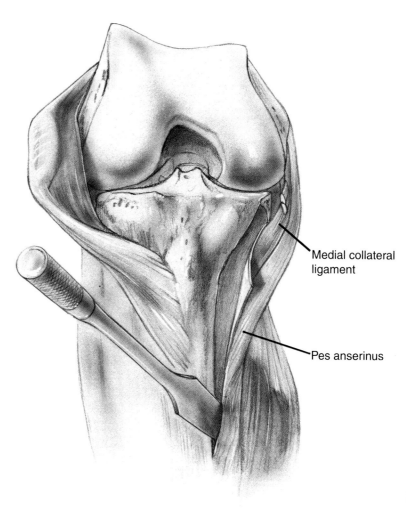

Medial collateral
ligament

Pes anserinus

B

Figure 9. A: In severe varus deformity, the medial subperiosteal dissection is continued posteriorly and distally, maintaining continuity of the medial structures. **B:** Diagrammatic representation of more distal medial release. (Redrawn from ref. 1.)

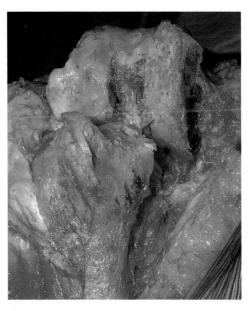

Figure 10. In severe cases of varus deformity, with extensive subperiosteal dissection, the proximal medial tibia appears skeletonized.

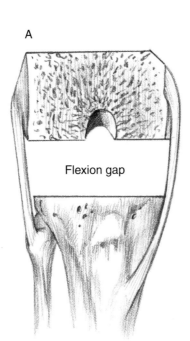
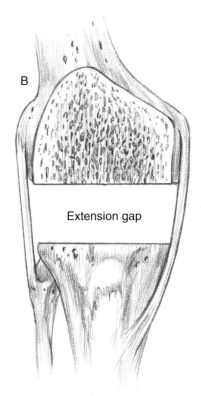

Figure 11. **A, B:** The flexion and extension gaps should be equal and rectangular in shape. (Redrawn from ref. 1.)

below the tibial plateau because tibial cancellous bone weakens rapidly as the distance from the articular surface increases. In a knee with a varus deformity more bone is resected from the lateral than from the medial tibial plateau. Once the tibia is cut, resection of the femur is undertaken. The flexion gap produced should be rectangular rather than trapezoidal in shape (Fig. 11A, B). In order to achieve this, the femoral template is externally rotated on the distal femur until it becomes parallel to the cut tibial surface. This results in more bone resection from the posterior medial femoral condyle than from the posterolateral femoral condyle. Up to 10° of rotation is permissible; if more rotation is needed, the medial soft-tissue release is probably inadequate.

When in cases of varus deformity a large tibial defect is present after the bone cut, several options are available. The defect can be filled with polymethylmethacrylate (PMMA) or PMMA reinforced with screws or mesh. The disadvantage of PMMA alone is that it cannot be pressurized to insure good trabecular penetration, while the use of mesh may produce lamination, resulting in subsequent cement fragmentation and failure. Autogenous bone grafting of the proximal tibial defect in primary total knee arthroplasty is a biocompatible and bioadaptive means of restoring the proximal tibial surface (5). Occasionally, a custom prosthesis or a metal tibial wedge component may be successfully implanted and is biomechanically superior to PMMA alone.

Valgus Deformity

By comparison with that of a varus release, the principle of a valgus release is to stretch the contracted lateral structures to the length of the medial structures. The difference is that the valgus release detaches the lateral ligamentous and capsular structures from the femoral rather than the tibial side of the knee. Though lateral osteophytes may be present and should be removed, they do not bowstring the lateral collateral ligament in the same way as osteophytes on the medial side, because the distal insertion of the lateral collateral ligament into the fibular head brings the ligament away from the tibial rim. The knee is approached in a fashion similar to that described for a varus deformity, but with the knee flexed the fat pad is removed to allow a Bennett retractor to be placed beneath the lateral femoral condyle, stretching the lateral supporting structures. (Fig. 12). The lateral collateral ligament, lateral capsule, arcuate complex, and popliteus muscle are cut transversely at the joint line (Fig. 13A, B). This release extends around the posterolateral corner; occasionally also, the lateral head of the gastrocnemius requires division (Fig. 14A, B). The extent of the release can be evaluated with lamina spreaders (Fig. 15). We prefer to release the lateral collateral ligament and popliteus muscle first. If further correction is needed or if there is an associated external rotational deformity, the iliotibial band should be released. Previously, we found transverse division of the iliotibial band to be suitable for this release, but we have recently begun to strip the iliotibial band from the proximal lateral tibia and Gerdy's tubercle, as in the subperiosteal medial release (Fig. 16). This allows the iliotibial band to stretch proximally, lengthening the lateral side. Another alternative is to pie crust the iliotibial band from within using a 15-blade and then stretch the lateral side with a laminar spreader. Rarely is division of the biceps femoris required.

After a valgus release, the resultant space between the femur and tibia is usually larger than it normally is when the medial collateral ligament is tensed, and for this reason a thicker tibial component is usually needed. Release of the lateral structures does not cause any functional instability, but since the cruciate ligaments are resected to correct the alignment of the knee, a posterior-cruciate-substituting prosthesis is recommended. In addition, erosion and deficiency of the lateral femoral condyle should raise the consideration of bone grafting or metal augmentation of the femoral component of the prosthesis. Special consideration should also be given to the alignment of the patella, since subluxation usually exists preoperatively in cases of valgus deformity. A lateral retinacular release is often necessary to restore normal patellar alignment and tracking. This is accomplished by incising the lateral retinaculum in line with its fibers, at 1 cm from the patella. This should be done in stages, extending the incision as necessary. If possible, the lateral superior geniculate vessels should be preserved in order to avoid avascular necrosis of the patella. If the patella still appears to be tracking laterally after lateral release, a proximal patellar realignment may be performed during closure of the arthrotomy. Recurrent patellar subluxation or dislocation following total knee arthroplasty is due to errors in surgical technique (4).

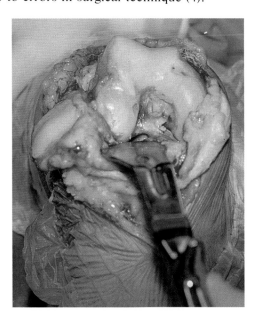

Figure 12. To initiate the valgus release, a Bennett retractor is placed beneath the lateral femoral condyle, stretching the lateral supporting structures.

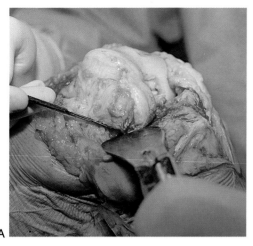

Figure 13. A: The lateral collateral ligament, lateral capsule, arcuate complex, and popliteus muscle are cut transversely at the joint line. **B:** Diagrammatic representation of the valgus release. (Redrawn from ref. 1.)

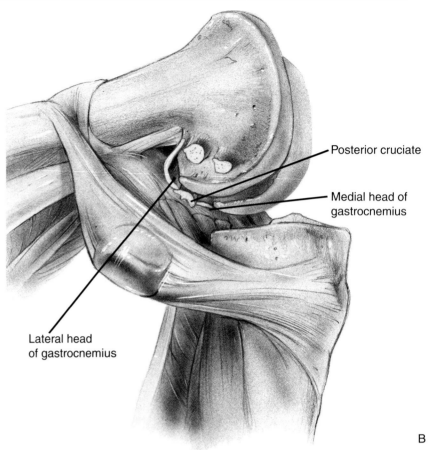

Posterior cruciate

Medial head of gastrocnemius

Lateral head of gastrocnemius

B

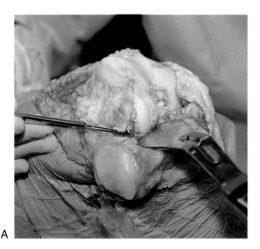

Figure 14. A: The release extends around the posterolateral corner. **B:** Diagrammatic representation of the release with extension to the posterolateral corner. Occasionally, the lateral head of the gastrocnemius requires division.

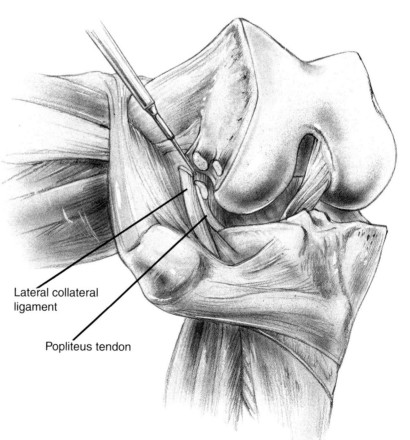

Lateral collateral ligament

Popliteus tendon

B

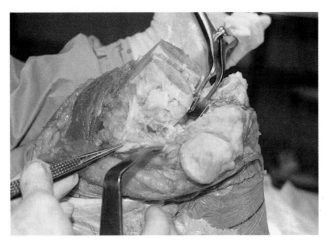

Figure 15. While the release is being performed, its extent can be evaluated with lamina spreaders.

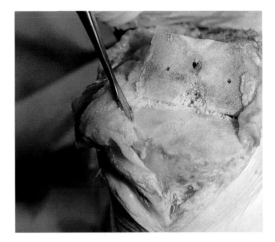

Figure 16. The iliotibial band can be released by subperiosteal dissection from the proximal lateral tibia and Gerdy's tubercle.

After appropriate ligament balancing is achieved and the flexion and extension gaps are equal, the components of the prosthesis are fixed into place. The trial components are removed, the tourniquet released, and major vascular sources of bleeding are cauterized. The tourniquet is then reinflated, the wound copiously irrigated, and the components of the prosthesis fixed in place. The wound is closed in a routine manner and compressive dressings are applied.

POSTOPERATIVE MANAGEMENT

Postoperatively, patients who have undergone ligament releases for fixed deformities of the knee are managed in a manner similar to those who have had routine total knee arthroplasties. A soft dressing is applied and the patient is immediately placed in a continuous passive motion (CPM) machine in the recovery room. We have found CPM to be a useful adjunct to rehabilitation, that has reduced the time required to achieve 90° of flexion. Some patients are unwilling to participate aggressively in their postoperative therapy and have difficulty obtaining 90° of flexion by the second to third week postoperatively. For these patients, manipulation under general or epidural anesthesia is usually required. Avoiding a flexion contracture is also critical in the early postoperative period, for which reason it is recommended that the patient sleep in a knee immobilizer with the knee in extension. Patients are instructed to stand with the assistance of the physical therapist on the second postoperative day, and to resume walking with full weight-bearing, using crutches or a walker, on the third postoperative day. The use of modular augmentation wedges has reduced our use of bone grafts, and does not alter the weight-bearing status of the patient during ambulation. Contained tibial bone grafts are also treated in the same way as a standard total knee arthroplasty. In cases with large uncontained bone grafts, partial weight-bearing with crutches is recommended for a period of 4 to 8 weeks, or until the bone graft has been incorporated into the tibial shaft.

Patients usually remain in the hospital until they walk independently with crutches or a cane, can climb stairs, and have achieved 90° of flexion.

Prophylaxis for deep-vein thrombosis is individualized to the patient. Patients undergoing bilateral surgery or who have a history of prior thrombophlebitis or factors predisposing to thrombosis are started on aspirin the night before surgery and have pneumatic sequential stockings applied in the operating room on the uninvolved limb and then continued bilaterally beginning in the recovery room. The stockings are disconnected while the patient is walking, but are otherwise connected until the results of the venogram are available on the fifth to seventh postoperative day. If the venogram is negative the pneumatic stockings are removed and the patient is continued on aspirin alone. If the venogram is positive the pneumatic stockings and aspirin are discontinued and warfarin therapy is begun, maintaining the serum prothrombin time at 15 to 16 seconds. The warfarin therapy is continued for 2 months. Those patients undergoing bilateral surgery or who have a history of prior thrombophlebitis or factors predisposing to thrombosis are begun on warfarin therapy the night before surgery. This therapy is monitored by the serum prothrombin time, as described above, and continued for 2 months.

Clinical Results

Our surgical technique for releasing the medial structures of the knee, balancing the collateral ligaments, and restoring normal alignment has been successful since we began performing total knee arthroplasties. The results of our survivorship analysis (6) and clinical studies (2,9,10,13) have supported our technique for correcting fixed varus deformities, and have proven enduring and predictable. In our series of total condylar replacements, 63 knees had a varus deformity, including 23 with more than 10° of fixed deformity (13). Stability was maintained at 10 to 12 years of follow-up, with 88% of the knees continuing to have good or excellent results. In one case proper balancing of the soft tissues was not achieved and varus instability recurred. Although initially rated as showing a good result, this knee deteriorated to yield a poor result owing to progressive instability, and required revision at 8½ years after the original total knee arthroplasty.

Although we feel that complete excision of the cruciate ligaments and use of a posterior-cruciate-substituting prosthesis is helpful in correcting a fixed varus deformity, Tenney has found that routine excision of the PCL is unnecessary (12). Instead, a posterior-cruciate-sparing prosthesis would be used, which has been shown to be stable even when a PCL recession is performed.

A review of the results of total knee arthroplasty in valgus knees with lateral ligamentous release from the femur has shown that they are comparable to the results of arthroplasty in knees with lesser deformity (11). A review of 168 arthroplasties for valgus deformity demonstrated 91% good and excellent results, 6% fair results, and 3% poor results, with an average follow up of 4.5 years. There were no revisions for recurrent instability, and the postoperative tibial femoral alignment was maintained at an overall average of 7° of valgus. Although valgus deformities represented a greater challenge in terms of intraoperative balancing, the results showed total knee arthroplasty to be a reliable and durable procedure.

COMPLICATIONS

Several complications may arise from the correction of fixed angular deformities. These are discussed in the following sections.

Instability

Instability in extension can be either symmetric or asymmetric. Symmetric instability occurs when the extension gap is incompletely filled by the components of the prosthesis and there is residual laxity of the collateral ligaments in extension. This problem can result from the resection of too much bone from the distal femur because of miscalculation, or from improper soft-tissue balance. The problem can sometimes be solved by inserting a thicker tibial component, but when the flexion gap is too tight to accommodate such a thicker component, it may be necessary to build up the distal femur prior to implantation of the femoral component of the prosthesis. This can be achieved with screws and cement or, with the current modular designs of prosthesis, through the attachment of distal augmentation blocks on the femoral component.

It is inappropriate to perform a ligament release after making the bone cuts for an arthroplasty, because this will effectively increase the extension gap and results in instability in extension. In a medial release for varus deformity, it is possible to solve this problem by implanting a thicker tibial component, since both the flexion and extension gaps tend to be larger. However, this is not so easily done after a lateral release for a valgus deformity, because in this case only the extension gap tends to enlarge. The best way to avoid this problem is to perform ligament releases prior to the bone cuts and, especially in the case of valgus deformity, to initially underestimate the degree of the release.

Asymmetric instability commonly occurs when a tight ligament is inadequately released. If the bone cuts are made without regard to the fixed angular deformity, the total knee arthroplasty will be unstable on one side. Consequently, it is imperative to balance the soft tissues prior to bone resection.

Apart from the special case of inadvertent division of the medial collateral ligament, the absence of collateral ligaments is unusual, even in rheumatoid arthritis or following trauma. Although the collateral ligaments may be incompetent prior to arthroplasty, they tend to be present and elongated. Sometimes, stretching of the collateral ligaments to obtain a tight fit is impractical because of the degree of leg lengthening needed to equalize the ligaments. In such cases it is more practical to implant a constrained condylar prosthesis.

Excessive tibial bone resection can result in instability in flexion. To avoid this problem it is preferable to resect the tibia at a level of 5 mm from the normal joint surface and not at the level of the tibial defect. Tibial bone defects can be augmented with cement, cement and screws, bone grafts, or metal wedges. Instability in flexion can also occur when too little bone is resected from the distal femur. It is tempting to insert a thinner tibial articular surface to fit in extension, but this will result in instability when the knee is flexed. In this situation, the flexion and extension gaps can be equalized by cutting additional bone from the distal femur. Correction of a fixed angular deformity also complicates this problem, because ligamentous release does not affect the flexion and extension gaps equally. The ligamentous release is intended to equalize the length of the leg bilaterally and provide symmetry in extension, but asymmetry may be present in flexion. A medial release to correct a varus deformity balances the knee in extension, but the lateral supporting structures often remain lax in flexion. To avoid this asymmetry, the femoral cutting guide should be externally rotated so that the posterior femoral condyles are cut parallel to the cut tibial surface. By externally rotating the femoral component and removing an asymmetric amount of bone from the posterior femoral condyles, the soft-tissue length on either side of the knee is equalized and the resulting space is rectangular. A lateral release for valgus deformity results in lateral instability in flexion. A solution to asymmetric instability in flexion after the correction of varus and valgus deformities is to implant a posterior-cruciate-substituting prosthesis.

Rotatory instability can occur because of instability in flexion, or more commonly from malposition of the tibial components causing a mismatch at the femoral–tibial articulation. Apparent malrotation of the tibial component is seen when the popliteus is too tight and flexing of the knee causes internal rotation of the tibia. The simple solution to this problem is to cut the popliteus tendon, allowing the lateral tibial plateau to drop back in flexion and restoring congruent tracking.

Patellar Instability

Recurrent subluxation or dislocation of the patella following ligamentous release to correct a fixed deformity, especially with a fixed valgus deformity, is due to errors in surgical technique. Internal rotation of the tibial component of a prosthesis with respect to the tibia will cause external rotation of the tibia when the knee is reduced, resulting in lateral displacement of the tibial tubercle. This displacement increases the valgus vector and the tendency of the patella to sublux laterally. Correct rotational positioning of the tibial component is best achieved by aligning the intercondylar eminence of the tibial component with the tibial crest. External rotation of the femoral component, as discussed above, will also improve patellar tracking. Other sources of patellar instability are a tight lateral retinaculum or malalignment of the extensor mechanism of the prosthesis. In these cases a lateral retinacular release is necessary to restore normal patellar tracking. If possible, preservation of the lateral superior geniculate vessels should be attempted in an effort to maintain the patellar circulation. However, this may sometimes be possible because the vessels and soft-tissue bridge may continue to tether the patella and keep it tracking laterally. In these extreme cases the vessels should be sacrificed. If the patella still appears to be tracking laterally after a lateral retinacular release, a proximal patellar realignment should be performed during closure following the arthrotomy.

Avulsion of the Tibial Tubercle

Avulsion of the tibial tubercle can easily occur during exposure of the stiff knee with a fixed angular deformity. When the patella is everted and dislocated laterally, considerable traction is exerted on the patellar tendon at the tibial tubercle. Repairing a transverse tear of the patellar tendon and periosteum is a difficult process, and the best way to avoid this intraoperative complication is with meticulous technique during exposure of the knee. The joint is exposed through a medial parapatellar arthrotomy that is continued onto the tibia to a point 1 cm medial to the tibial tubercle. This allows a cuff of periosteum to be dissected subperiosteally from the tibial tubercle, along with the insertion of the patellar tendon. As the knee is flexed and the patella dislocated laterally, this periosteal sleeve may pull further away from the tibial tubercle, along with the patellar tendon. This technique permits distal continuity of the soft tissue and prevents a horizontal tear.

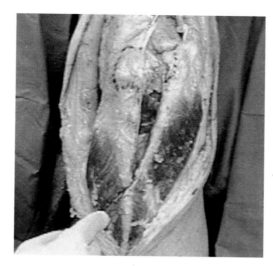

Figure 17. The quadriceps snip.

If there is a chance of avulsion of the patellar tendon, a V-Y quadricepsplasty should be performed. Over the past few years we have begun to use the quadriceps snip, in which the quadriceps tendon is cut proximally, obviating lateral dissection (Fig. 17). This technique provides excellent exposure and allows eversion of the patella.

Peroneal Nerve Injury

The risk of inadvertent and unavoidable stretching of the peroneal nerve as it courses around the fibula head is an issue of concern in valgus release and lengthening of the lateral side of the knee, since the leg is being lengthened. Peroneal nerve palsy remains a significant worry with a valgus knee, and has been seen postoperatively in 3% of patients (11). The peroneal nerve can be injured with either undercorrection or overcorrection of the valgus deformity. Inadequate soft-tissue release necessitates forceful manual correction, which will stretch the nerve, while overcorrection creates a ''bowstring'' effect with probable nerve injury. Although direct injury to the nerve has always been suggested, we believe that ischemic injury to the peroneal nerve can also occur, and may especially be the source of injury in patients with arteriosclerotic disease. To avoid the deleterious affects of peroneal nerve injury, it had been previously suggested that the nerve be dissected and visualized, freeing it from the fascial sheath behind the head of the fibula. However, we no longer advocate exploration of the peroneal nerve. Recently, patients have been placed in CPM machines in the recovery room, which tends to keep the knee in a flexed position, avoiding stretching of the peroneal nerve and reducing the incidence of this complication. In order to avoid excessive stretching of the lateral side, we also suggest consideration of implanting a constrained prosthesis with a tibial articular surface slightly smaller than the one that will fully elongate the medial structures. The constrained prosthesis provides inherent stability and can be used for primary implantation.

ILLUSTRATIVE CASE FOR TECHNIQUE

Varus Deformity

A 71-year-old man had severe osteoarthritis of the right knee and a fixed varus deformity of 10° (Fig. 18). At the time of total knee arthroplasty, a medial soft-

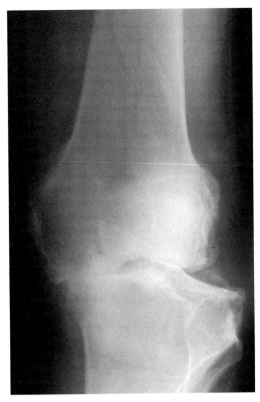

Figure 18. Preoperative radiograph of a knee with severe osteoarthritis and fixed varus deformity.

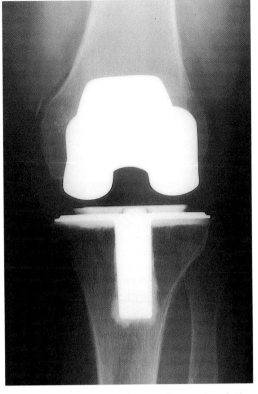

Figure 19. Postoperative radiograph of the total knee arthroplasty.

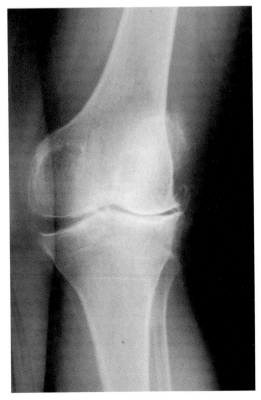

Figure 20. Preoperative radiograph of a knee with severe osteoarthritis and a fixed valgus deformity.

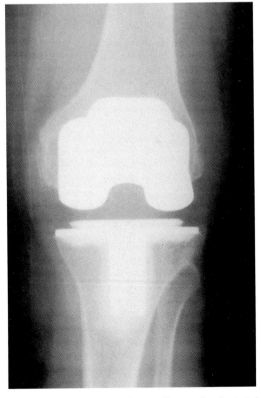

Figure 21. Postoperative radiograph of a total knee arthroplasty.

tissue release was performed, as described above, and a posterior stabilized prosthesis was implanted (Fig. 19).

Valgus Deformity

A 77-year-old woman had severe osteoarthritis of her left knee and a fixed valgus deformity of 15° (Fig. 20). At the time of total knee arthroplasty, a release of the lateral structures was performed, as discussed above, and a posterior stabilized prosthesis was implanted (Fig. 21).

RECOMMENDED READING

1. Insall, J. N.: Total knee replacement. In: *Surgery of the Knee,* edited by J. N. Insall, pp. 587–696. Churchill Livingstone, New York, 1984.
2. Insall, J. N., and Hood, R. W., Flawn, L. B., and Sullivan, D. J.: The total condylar knee prosthesis in gonarthrosis. *J. Bone Joint Surg.,* 65A: 619–628, 1983.
3. Laskin, R. S.: Soft tissue techniques in total knee replacement. In: *Total Knee Replacement,* edited by R. S. Laskin, pp. 41–54. Springer-Verlag, New York, 1991.
4. Merkow, R. L., Soudry, M., and Insall, J. N.: Patella dislocation following total knee replacement. *J. Bone Joint Surg.,* 67A: 1321–1327, 1985.
5. Scuderi, G., Haas, S. B., Windsor, R. E., et al.: Inlay autogenous bone graft for tibial defects in primary total knee arthroplasty. *Clin. Orthop.,* 248: 93–97, 1989.
6. Scuderi, G. R., Insall, J. N., Windsor, R. E., and Moran, M. C.: Survivorship of Cemented Knee Replacements. *J. Bone Joint Surg.,* 71B: 798–803, 1989.
7. Scuderi, G. R., and Insall, J. N.: The posterior stabilized knee prosthesis. *Orthop. Clin. North Am.,* 20(1): 71–78, 1989.
8. Scuderi, G. R., and Insall, J. N.: Cement technique in primary total knee arthroplasty. *Techniques Orthop.,* 6(4): 39–43, 1991.
9. Scuderi, G. R., and Insall, J. N.: Total knee arthroplasty. Current clinical perspectives. *Clin. Orthop.,* 276: 26–32, 1992.
10. Stern, S. H., and Insall, J. N.: Posterior stabilized prosthesis. Results after follow-up of nine to twelve years. *J. Bone Joint Surg.,* 74A: 980–986, 1992.
11. Stern, S. H., Moeckel, B. H., and Insall, J. N.: Total knee arthroplasty in valgus knees. *Clin. Orthop.,* 273: 5–8, 1991.
12. Tenney, S. M., Krackow, K. A., Hungerford, D. S., and Jones, M.: Primary total knee arthroplasty in patients with severe varus deformity. *Clin. Orthop.,* 273: 19–31, 1991.
13. Vince, K. G., Insall, J. N., and Kelly, M. A.: The total condylar prosthesis 10 to 12 year results of a cemented knee replacement. *J. Bone Joint Surg.,* 71B: 793–797, 1989.
14. Windsor, R. E., Scuderi, G. R., Insall, J. N., and Moran, M. C.: Mechanism of failure of the femoral and tibial components in total knee arthroplasty. *Clin. Orthop.,* 248: 15–20, 1989.

■ COMPLEX TOTAL KNEE

Master Techniques in Orthopaedic Surgery,
KNEE ARTHROPLASTY, edited by P. A. Lotke,
Raven Press, Ltd., New York © 1995.

9

Bone Grafting

Thomas P. Sculco

INDICATIONS/CONTRAINDICATIONS

Bone loss occurs most commonly on the tibial side of the knee joint in angular deformity. It is generally localized posteriorly on the tibial plateau, owing to the frequently associated flexion contracture present in patients with severe knee deformity. There may be concomitant fragmentation of the tibial plateau, but as a rule the tibial surface is concave, extremely sclerotic, and devoid of cartilage (Fig. 1). Because there is often also subluxation of the femur on the tibia, a peripheral rim of tibial bone is not present. Consequently there is a steep descent from the middle of the tibial surface to the periphery. Femoral deficiency is infrequently present except in severe valgus deformities, where it is seen in combination with lateral tibial bone loss.

The management of bone deficiency in total knee arthroplasty will vary according to the degree of bone loss. Various management methods have been employed with success, including the use of methylmethacrylate alone (4), methylmethacrylate reinforced with mesh or screws (5), and bone grafting (1,2,5). Wedges and other metallic augmentations are also gaining some support for this problem.

Except in the mildest of bone defects (less than 8 mm), the tendency to resect additional bone from the tibia must be resisted. When excess tibial bone is resected the flexion gap is increased, requiring a thicker tibial component for stability. This will alter the patellofemoral kinematics, since the patella, tethered by the patellar tendon, will descend and may come into frank contact with the tibial implant itself. Furthermore, the tibial component becomes seated on poor-quality cancellous bone when the upper tibial resection is made far into the tibial shaft. Sizing problems will likewise occur because of the diminished cross-sectional area as one progresses down the tibia distally. Lowering the resection line on the tibia to deal

T. P. Sculco, M.D.: Department of Orthopaedic Surgery, Hospital for Special Surgery, New York, NY 10021.

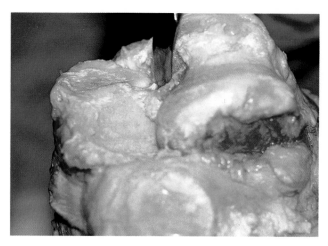

Figure 1. Bone deficit on the tibial surface is usually posterior, with a concave and sclerotic surface.

with bone loss is an unsatisfactory method and should be utilized only for the smallest defects.

Tibial Defects of 6 to 12 Millimeters

When tibial bone loss is less than 12 mm in depth and encompasses less than one-half of the tibial surface, several techniques are available for restoration of the upper tibial surface. Resection of tibial bone to a depth of up to 8 mm can be done without difficulty, and removal of this segment of the upper tibia may leave only a small defect. The remaining sclerotic bed is fenestrated with a ⅛-inch drill to allow penetration of bone cement into the subchondral bone. The tibial component can also be shifted to the noninvolved tibial plateau to better support the component on a more stable surface. Up to 3 mm of remaining void can be filled with methylmethacrylate cement. Small amounts of unsupported methylmethacrylate will provide ample stabilization of the implant and will not fail. Larger columns of methylmethacrylate, however, may fracture and initial support may be lost. This is especially true in the patient in whom proper knee-joint alignment has not been achieved.

If, after resecting the tibial plateau, a defect of 3 to 5 mm remains, screws can be used to reinforce the methylmethacrylate column. Two cortical screws are usually used in the area of bone deficiency. The heads of the screws are placed just below the metallic tray of the tibial component. The screws are surrounded with acrylic cement to fill the bone deficit. Synergistic metals must be used for the screws and the metal tibial tray, should contact of their surfaces occur (Fig. 2).

Tibial Defects Greater than 12 Millimeters in Depth

For defects greater than 12 mm in depth, and those encompassing up to one-half the upper surface of the tibia, bone grafting is recommended. Although wedge augmentation of the tibial tray may be used in these cases, I prefer biologic support in the form of grafting. Metallic wedges have several significant disadvantages in the primary knee replacement. First, they add considerable expense to the prosthesis. Moreover, the method of fixation of these wedges to the undersurface of the tibial component may be problematic; methylmethacrylate may fatigue with time; screw fixation of the wedges can produce corrosive metallic byproducts and

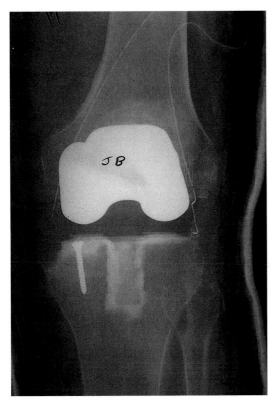

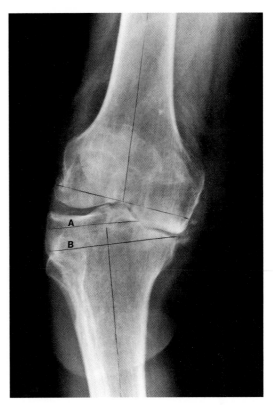

Figure 2. Screw augmentation may be used with methylmethacrylate to reinforce the cement.

Figure 3. Lines drawn on radiograph to determine the degree of bone loss after upper tibial osteotomy. *Line A* represents the correct level and *line B* shows the incorrect level.

debris, and with time may promote osteolysis. Creep of polyethylene into the screw holes can also occur, and increased polyethylene wear is seen as a result of this plastic migration.

Contraindications to autogenous bone grafting of the tibia include defects in which there is inadequate autogenous bone for reconstitution of the upper tibial surface. Although it has been suggested that this technique should not be used in the elderly, it has been my experience that consolidation of the graft occurs without problem in these patients.

In femoral condylar bone loss the concepts are similar. At the time of resection of the distal femur to restore valgus alignment to the knee, there may be no distal femoral condyle (usually lateral) to resect. If the amount of bone is less than 5 mm, methylmethacrylate alone can be used to fill the void. Generally, this has not been augmented with screws or mesh. In defects exceeding 5 mm, bone grafting is recommended.

PREOPERATIVE PLANNING

Weight-bearing anteroposterior radiographs of the knee must be taken preoperatively to determine the extent of the angular deformity and the degree of bone deficit. Lines may be drawn on these radiographs to determine the degree of bone loss after upper tibial osteotomy has been performed (Fig. 3). Also, the level of femoral resection should be planned to allow ample femoral condylar bone for autogeneous grafting of the tibia. Cancellous or cortical screws, made of a metal synergistic to the tibial component, must be available in the operating room. Because the deformities that require bone grafting of the tibia and femur are complex and associated with major soft-tissue contractures and insufficiencies, it is imperative that a constrained condylar-type knee system be available, with augmentations should they be needed.

SURGERY

The patient is placed in the supine position and draped in the usual fashion for total knee arthroplasty. A pneumatic tourniquet is routinely used on the thigh and inflated prior to the skin incision.

Technique

A mildly curved medial incision is used just next to the patella. The interval between the vastus medialis and the quadriceps tendon is identified and the knee joint entered, leaving several millimeters of tendon on the vastus medialis. This allows a tendon-to-tendon closure at the conclusion of the procedure. The knee joint is then exposed in the usual manner by elevating a medial flap and dislocating the tibia anteriorly on the femur. The patellofemoral ligament must be released laterally to allow the patella to evert without tension.

The defect will usually occupy the posterior two-thirds of the tibial surface, and the bed of the defect will be sclerotic. The peripheral rim is almost always absent in these patients. The initial tibial proximal cut is made with a standard tibial cutting guide. The upper tibial osteotomy should be at a right angle to the tibial shaft (unless there is bowing of the tibia). A guide perpendicular to the upper tibial cut should bificurate the ankle joint and point to the interval between the first and second metatarsal. No more than 8 mm should be resected from the upper surface of the tibia. An oscillating saw is then used to create an oblique osteotomy on the side of the tibial defect. The sclerotic, concave surface of the defect must be removed with this osteotomy to expose a cancellous bed (Fig. 4A). There may be cystic areas in this bed once the sclerotic surface has been removed, and these may be curetted and filled with cancellous bone from the femur or tibial peg hole. It is important not to be timid in the removal of this sclerotic bed, since consolidation of the graft will be greatly impeded if there is no cancellous bed onto which to place the donor femoral bone (Fig. 4B). The cut should be planar and smooth, so that a flattened graft will fit intimately onto this bed (Fig. 5).

If the tibial implant to be used has a central peg hole, this hole should now be made. This will insure that the screws that fix the graft into place will not violate the peg hole when the implant is inserted. For implants with peripheral fixation peg holes, this step is of less importance.

The next step is to remove the distal femoral bone. Generally, the resected distal medial femoral bone is larger than the lateral condyle and therefore tends to be better graft material. Having resected the distal femoral condyle, this segment of bone is rotated so that its cancellous surface faces against the cancellous surface of the recipient bed. The defect should be filled completely by the donor bone. There will be an overhanging segment of bone which protrudes above the cut surface of the tibia. If there is any gaping between the bone and the recipient bed, the bed must be planed with the oscillating saw. There should be perfect coaptation between the graft and the underlying bed. Once this seating is precise, two K-wires may be used to stabilize the graft to the proximal tibia (Fig. 6). The wires should be inserted from the periphery and below the level of femoral condylar bone that is above the surface of the tibia. If these pins are too superior they will impede resection of the overhanging bone and lose their fixation. After the graft is fixed in position, the overhanging bone should be removed, using the tibial

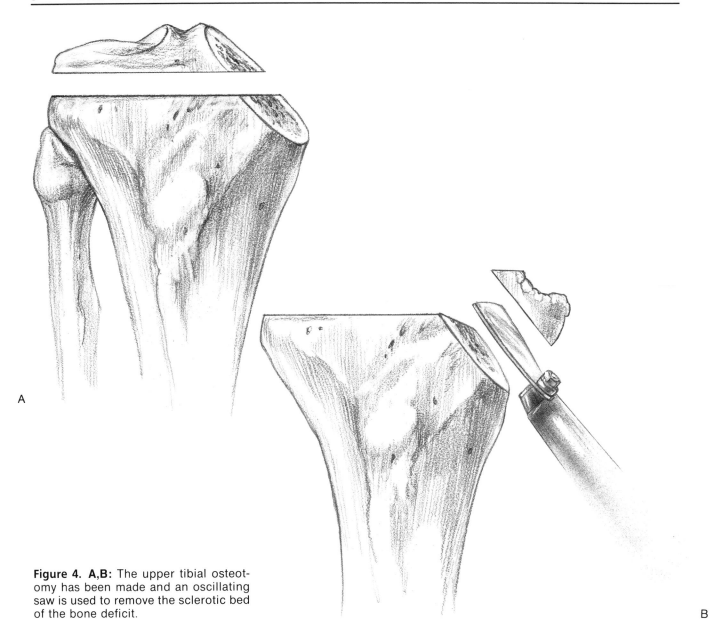

A

B

Figure 4. A,B: The upper tibial osteotomy has been made and an oscillating saw is used to remove the sclerotic bed of the bone deficit.

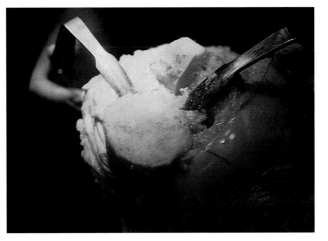

Figure 5. The excision of the sclerotic bone from the deficit must be extensive enough to expose a flat cancellous bed.

cut surface on the more normal side of the tibia as the cutting guide. Having resected this excess femoral bone from the tibia, the upper surface of the tibia should be reconstituted. On observing the tibia from the top, the subchondral bone of the femoral condylar bone graft will act as the peripheral tibial bone of

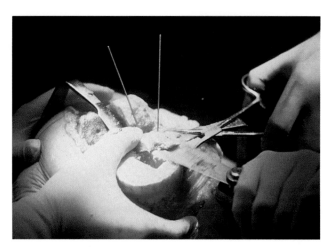

Figure 6. Graft is stabilized with two K-wires and excess bone is excised utilizing the tibial surface as a guide.

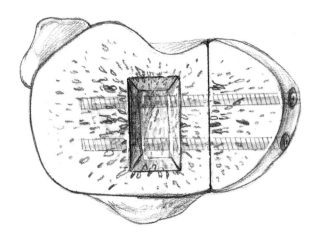

Figure 7. Superior view of the graft demonstrates a reconstitution of the peripheral rim of the tibia by the subchondral femoral graft bone.

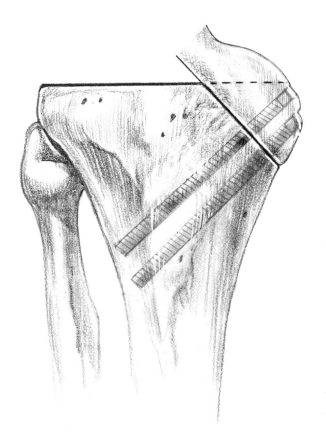

Figure 8. Level of bone cut through femoral condyle is illustrated. Femoral condyle (single) is placed over the defect with cancellous surfaces coapted. Fixation is rigid with two screws.

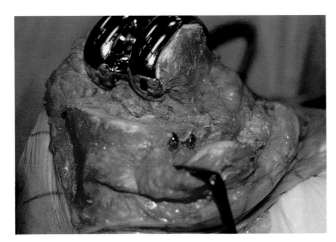

Figure 9. Caulking of the graft–tibia interface has been done with femoral cement.

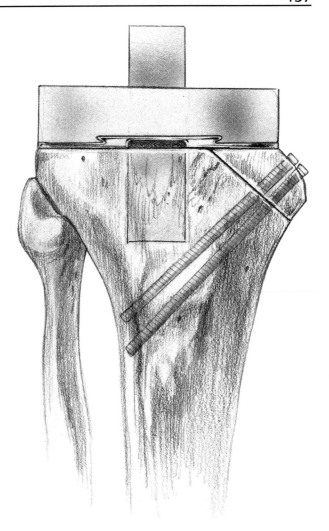

Figure 10. Graft in place, fixed with two screws to upper surface of tibia.

the upper tibia (Fig. 7). There should be no gap between the graft and the bed. Autogenous cancellous bone may be used to fill any small voids.

The K-wires are then individually removed and replaced with screws. Cancellous malleolar screws may be used for fixation, or alternatively one can use cortical screws and overdrill peripherally to allow a lag effect. The peg hole should be examined when the holes are drilled and their depth measured. The screws should not violate or contact the post of the tibial prosthesis.

Once the screws have been tightened, the graft should be securely fixed to the tibia (Fig. 8). It is now of utmost importance that cement not be allowed to enter the space between the graft and the recipient bed. An excellent method of preventing this is to cement the femoral component first and to use a small piece of cement from this batch to caulk the upper surface of the tibia along the line of the graft and the tibial host bone (Fig. 9). This will harden and prevent penetration of cement into the graft–tibia interface when the tibial cement and component are inserted (Fig. 10).

For femoral grafting, the sclerotic surface of the distal femoral condyle is removed to a cancellous bed. Condylar bone removed from the unaffected side is moved to the defect and screwed into position. The implant is then inserted over this composite. The knee is reduced and checked for stability and alignment. A routine closure is completed.

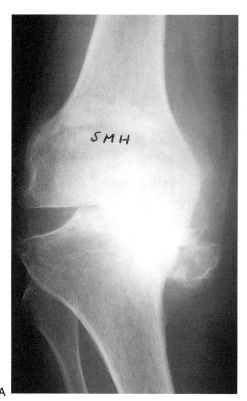
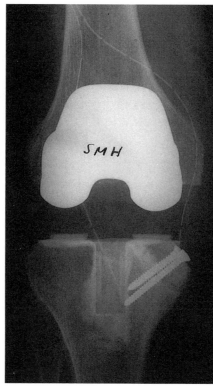
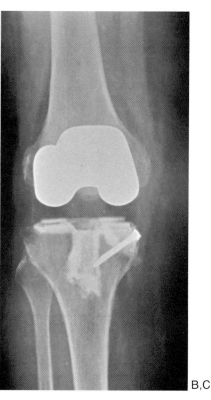

A   B,C

Figure 11. A: Preoperative radiograph of severe varus deformity with large medial tibial defect. **B:** Radiograph at 3 months postoperatively, demonstrating partial cement penetration into graft–tibial interface. **C:** Radiograph at 13 years postoperatively. Note sclerosis of the graft without resorption or loss of implant position.

POSTOPERATIVE MANAGEMENT

Postoperative management for these patients is the same as for patients without bone grafting. A constant passive-motion machine is used on the first postoperative day and the patient is allowed protected weight bearing on postoperative day two. This is permitted because the tibial and femoral implant support is maintained on the more normal side of the femur and tibia, and because the graft is securely fixed to the underlying bone. The patient is advanced from a walker to a single cane at the time of discharge. All patients are expected to be able to transfer in and out of bed, walk with a cane, climb and descend stairs, and flex to 80 to 90 degrees prior to discharge.

I have used this technique of postoperative management in over 35 knee replacements over the past 13 years. The results have been excellent, with no patient experiencing collapse of the graft. Because of the complex nature of these deformities, a more constrained prosthesis has been used in seven patients. Revision surgery has been necessary in two patients. One patient fell two years after total knee replacement with grafting, and incurred a complete disruption of her medial collateral ligament with severe valgus deformity. She underwent revision with a constrained implant; at that time the bone graft was noted to be intact and consolidated. A second patient with rheumatoid arthritis developed a late deep infection five years after her knee replacement. At the time of removal of the implant and subsequent reimplantation, the bone graft was noted to be stable and consolidated.

COMPLICATIONS

The most common complication of autogenous bone grafting would be resorption of the graft with loss of implant position. To date this has not occurred. However, if the graft is too small, the bed not cancellous, or fixation is poor, this complication could occur. This would require revision of the tibial component and utilization of a wedge augment on the tibial component to fill the bone deficit.

It is necessary to expose the upper tibial surface thoroughly to allow proper preparation of the graft bed and coaptation of the graft. Injury to neurovascular structures, especially the popliteal artery, might result if injudicious dissection is performed posterior to the tibia. Should this happen, vascular consultation should be obtained for arterial repair.

In that these deficits are most common in severe angular deformities, ligamentous instability is frequently present. The use of a constrained implant may be necessary to accommodate persistent soft-tissue imbalance after appropriate releases have been made. If this is not done, the knee may be unstable postoperatively, resulting in pain or implant failure. Revision of a total knee replacement should be done if this complication develops.

ILLUSTRATIVE CASE FOR TECHNIQUE

N.J. is a 69-year-old woman with advanced rheumatoid arthritis. She had been increasingly disabled because of pain in her right knee. Associated with her pain was a progressive severe valgus deformity of the knee. She used a walker to ambulate, could not climb stairs, and had become homebound.

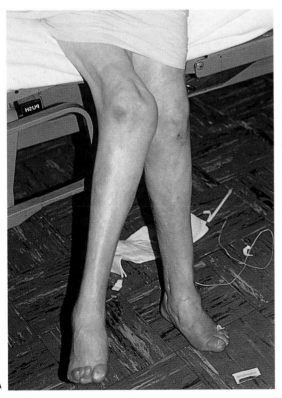
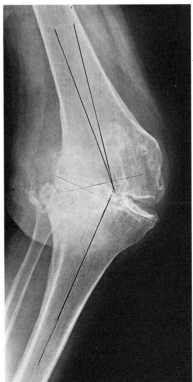

Figure 12. A: Severe valgus deformity on weight-bearing. **B:** Radiographs show severe loss of lateral tibial bone.

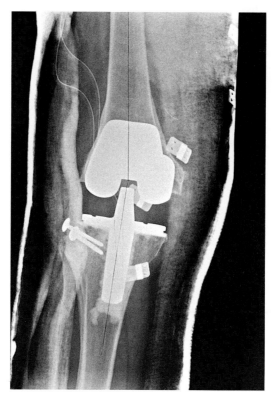

Figure 13. Postoperative radiograph showing graft in place and correction of deformity.

On physical examination she stood with a 30-degree valgus alignment to the knee. She supported the medial joint line on the contralateral knee as she stood. Her range of motion was preserved, at 10 to 100 degrees. The knee was unstable medially on valgus stress, although the medial collateral ligament was competent. Her neurovascular status was intact.

Radiographs demonstrated severe valgus deformity of the knee joint, with marked lateral compartment destruction (Fig. 12). A large tibial deficit was noted in the lateral tibial surface. Osteopenia was also present.

The patient underwent total knee replacement with autogenous tibial bone grafting from the medial distal femoral condyle. At the time of surgery, a constrained implant was used because of persistent medial instability despite complete lateral soft-tissue release. Postoperatively the patient ambulated without difficulty, and was discharged home on the tenth postoperative day. Alignment of the limb was restored and the patient has continued to function without problem (Fig. 13).

RECOMMENDED READING

1. Altchek, D., Sculco, T. P., and Rawling, B.: Autogenous bone grafting for severe angular deformity in total knee arthroplasty. *J. Arthroplasty*, 4: 151–156, 1989.
2. Dorr, L. D., Ranawat, C. S., Sculco, T. P., and McCaskill, B.: Bone graft for tibial defects in total knee arthroplasty. *Clin. Orthop.*, 205: 153–165, 1986.
3. Laskin, R. S.: Total knee replacement in the presence of large bony defects of the tibia and marked knee instability. *Clin. Orthop.*, 248: 66–70, 1989.
4. Lotke, P. A., Wong, R., and Ecker, M. L.: Use of methylmethacrylate in primary total knee replacements with large tibial defects. *Clin. Orthop.*, 270: 288–294, 1991.
5. Ritter, M.: Screw and cement fixation of large defects in total knee arthroplasty. *J. Arthroplasty*, 1: 125–130, 1986.
6. Windsor, R. E., Insall, J. N., and Sculco, T. P.: Bone grafting of tibial defects in primary and revision total knee arthroplasty. *Clin. Orthop.*, 205: 132–137, 1986.

Master Techniques in Orthopaedic Surgery,
Knee Arthroplasty, edited by P. A. Lotke,
Raven Press, Ltd., New York © 1995.

10

The Stiff Knee
Ankylosis and Flexion

Chitranjan S. Ranawat and William F. Flynn, Jr.

INDICATIONS/CONTRAINDICATIONS

Knees with less than a 50° arc of motion are considered "stiff," but there is a wide variation in presentation. One may be faced with a knee ankylosed in extension or one with flexion of 0° to 50°. The surgeon who is to successfully correct such problems with an arthroplasty must have a clear plan in mind.

The approach to total knee arthroplasty in the patient with a stiff knee is similar to planning the revision of a total knee arthroplasty. One must first identify the reason for the lack of motion. Some of the most common causes are previous surgery on the knee; previous injury to the knee; ankylosis, particularly in rheumatoid or psoriatic arthritis; reflex sympathetic dystrophy; severe pain; neuromuscular disorder; and previous infection.

The underlying cause of stiffness of the knee can have a profound effect on the success of the proposed surgery. Mechanical problems (bony deformity, ligamentous and capsular contracture) can usually be addressed successfully. Severe pain may limit motion with an alert patient; the same patient anesthetized may have a much better range of motion. Patients with severe reflex sympathetic dystrophy may have very limited motion, and surgery in these patients should be approached very cautiously since it can exacerbate this disorder. Patients with neuromuscular disorders, including those who have had a stroke, should also be approached with caution, since one cannot correct their underlying disorder. Patients with a history of knee sepsis may also have a stiff knee. Before considering arthroplasty, one must absolutely rule out low-grade sepsis.

C. S. Ranawat, M.D.: Department of Orthopedic Surgery, Cornell University Medical College; Combined Arthritis Service, The Hospital For Special Surgery, New York, NY 10021.

W. F. Flynn, Jr., M.D.: Adult Reconstructive Service, The Hospital For Special Surgery, New York, NY 10021.

PREOPERATIVE PLANNING

The pathologic anatomic conditions encountered in cases of stiffness of the knee may include shortening and tightness of the ligaments and muscles, fibrosis of the quadriceps muscle, intra- or extra-articular fibrosis, and intra- or extra-articular bony blocks from malalignment or new bone formation. The surgeon must be able to address any or all of these conditions.

Preoperative planning for arthroplasty of the stiff knee must include a thorough clinical and radiographic evaluation of the knee. The preoperative range of motion of the knee must be documented, along with any contractures, scars, or angular deformity. The circulation and sensation in the limb, and its motor function, particularly with regard to the quadriceps muscle, must be assessed. In addition, as in the case of any surgery, the patient's overall condition must be evaluated preoperatively, including the patient's desire and ability to comply with postoperative therapy.

Radiographic evaluation must include anteroposterior (AP), lateral, and patellar views, with additional studies such as computed tomography (CT), bone scans, or scanograms added as needed. As in a revision situation, alignment, bone loss, and bone quality must also be assessed. Additionally, any hardware present about the knee and which will have to be removed must be identified so that appropriate instrumentation for accomplishing this will be available at the time of surgery.

Finally, the surgeon must decide which prosthesis to use. A wide variety of modular systems are available and can accommodate almost any situation, but

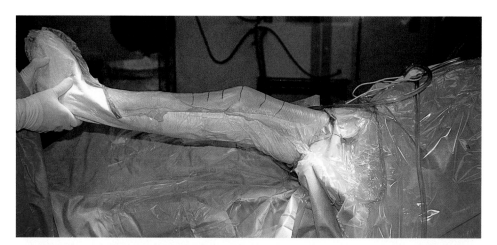

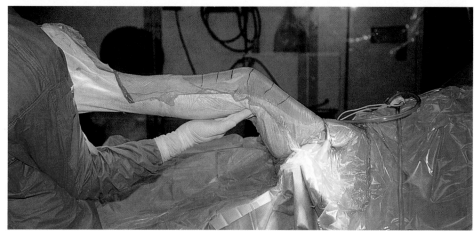

Figures 1 and 2. Preoperative extension ($-20°$) and flexion ($50°$). Note that the leg is draped free.

occasionally a custom prosthesis must be fabricated for a very small or large knee or a knee with severe bone loss or malalignment. Careful consideration must be given to expected soft-tissue deficiencies. With severe deformity, the posterior cruciate ligament is usually abnormal and the prosthesis must substitute for it. Additionally, the collateral ligaments may be deficient or may become functionally deficient if extensive soft-tissue releases are required, and a constrained option must be available.

SURGERY

Once preoperative planning is complete and an appropriate prosthesis has been selected, the surgeon can proceed. In a laminar flow operating room, the patient is put in the supine position with a tourniquet on the thigh of the leg that will undergo surgery. The leg is draped free, and Vi-drape is used to isolate the operative field. We utilize epidural anesthesia in all knee replacements. This technique is very safe and effective, and provides the additional benefit of permitting the patient to be maintained postoperatively on continuous infusion. This dramatically decreases the patient's postoperative pain and narcotic usage.

The patient's range of motion and ligamentous stability should be assessed under anesthesia prior to incision (Figs. 1 and 2). If there is no previous incision, a

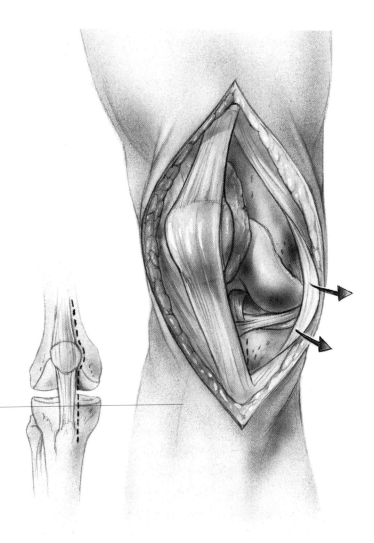

Figure 3. Initial incision and approach.

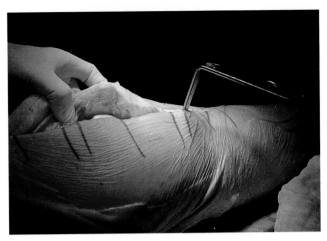

Figure 4. Lateral flap, with femur at left. Flap is full thickness, and a Kocher clamp is used to hold the edge.

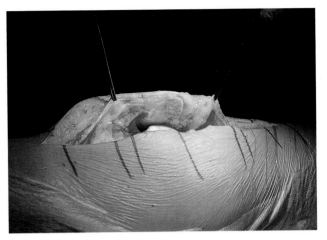

Figure 5. Early dissection of the lateral flap.

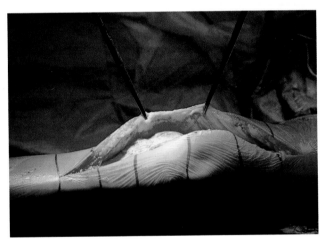

Figure 6. Medial flap. Note subperiosteal dissection of the tibia (left).

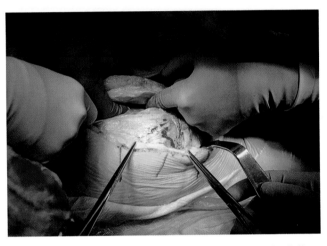

Figure 7. Lateral flap mobilization, femur at left. Adhesions in the gutter are released completely.

straight midline or slightly paramedian incision should be used. Old incisions should be incorporated as much as possible into new ones, making sure to leave no avascular islands or narrow strips of skin.

A medial parapatellar arthrotomy is then performed along the junction of the quadriceps tendon and vastus medialis muscle (Fig. 3). If the patella is ankylosed, it may be osteotomized at this time. Any adhesions between the quadriceps and femur on either side of the patella and gutter are released, and the quadriceps is mobilized from the femur (Figs. 4–9). Flexion of the knee is now assessed. If the knee cannot be flexed more than 30° to 40°, we perform a quadriceps release rather than a V-Y turndown or tibial tubercle osteotomy. A V-Y turndown devascularizes the extensor mechanism, and adjusting the final length of the quadriceps mechanism is difficult. Small tubercle osteotomies may create problems with nonunion or loss of fixation, and large osteotomies require substantial fixation. In addition, any tubercle osteotomy can change the position of the patella, and the final adjustment of quadriceps tension is again somewhat problematic.

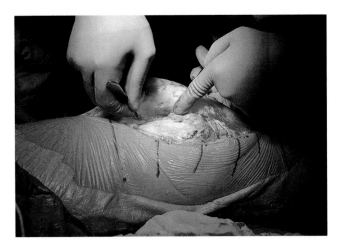

Figure 8. Lateral flap mobilization.

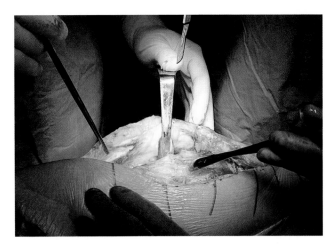

Figure 9. A small, angled Homan retractor is used for continued lateral mobilization.

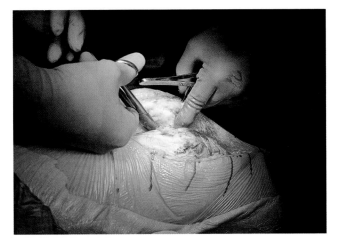

Figure 10. Beginning of lateral release, performed from the inside out. Complete retinacular release.

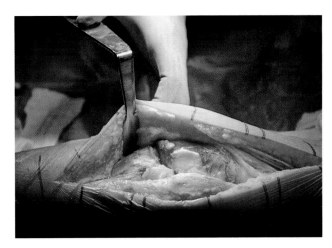

Figure 11. Beginning of deeper medial dissection, femur at right. An angled retractor is used.

Quadriceps Release

With the knee in extension, the patella is everted and the patellofemoral ligaments are released with electrocautery. Next, we routinely perform a lateral retinacular release from the inside out (Fig. 10). If preservation of the superior genicular artery prevents an adequate release, we sacrifice the artery.

Following this, a careful dissection is done, releasing the vastus medialis, medial capsule, and superficial medial collateral ligament from the medial and anterior femur, and leaving the superior attachment of the deep medial collateral ligament, thus forming a long sleeve subperiosteally (Fig. 11). The dissection of the medial collateral ligament is done subperiosteally to about the midplane of the tibia. If the tibia and femur are ankylosed, an osteotomy is performed at the joint line; in other cases, scar tissue in the joint is excised with a scalpel and the cruciate ligaments and menisci are released (Fig. 12). If the knee cannot be flexed at least 30° to 40° because of a tight quadriceps mechanism, a controlled Z-lengthening is

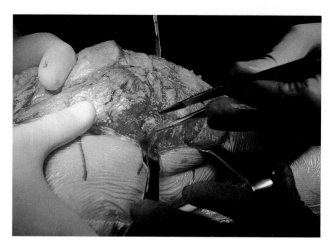

Figure 12. Excising scar tissue at medial joint line, femur to left.

done of the rectus femoris and vastus intermedius muscles, using six to eight small incisions made with a #11 blade. The rectus is first separated from the vastus, and the knee is then flexed to keep tension on the tendon. With each Z, the flexion of the knee increases in a controlled fashion, until 70° to 80° of flexion is reached (Figs. 13–15).

Once this is accomplished, the knee is flexed with the patella everted, occasionally without dislocation, and the tibia is externally rotated to avoid avulsing the tendon from the tubercle (Fig. 16). The subperiosteal medial release is then continued as the knee is further flexed and the tibia externally rotated. The release is carried around medially and posteriorly to at least the midplane of the tibia (Figs. 17–19). The attachment of the medial collateral ligament to the femur is not detached subperiosteally unless it interferes with the balance of the soft-tissue sleeve once the trial implant is in place. Any remnant of the medial meniscus is carefully released.

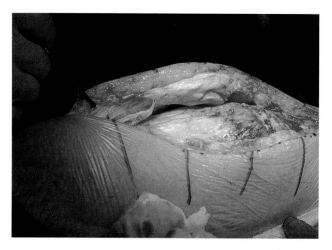

Figure 13. Beginning separation of rectus in preparation for Z-plasty. The easiest way to create this type of incision is with a scalpel.

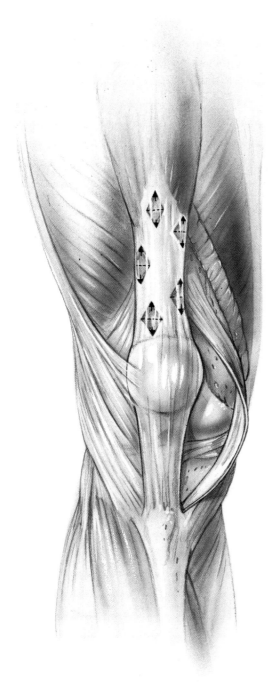

Figure 14. Anterior view of Z-lengthening.

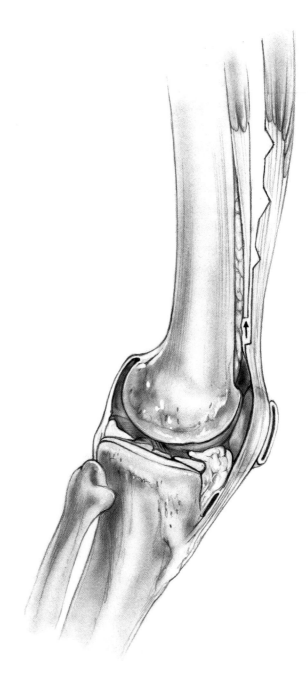

Figure 15. Lateral view of Z-lengthening. Note that the rectus is separated from the underlying vastus.

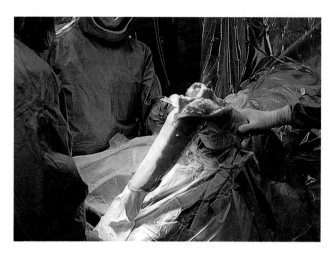

Figure 16. Tibia flexed up. Assistant externally rotates the foot to exert tension on the patellar tendon.

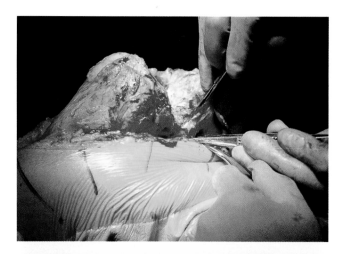

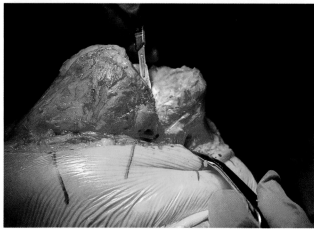

Figures 17 and 18. Continuation of medial release. This subperiosteal dissection continues all the way to the posterior capsule.

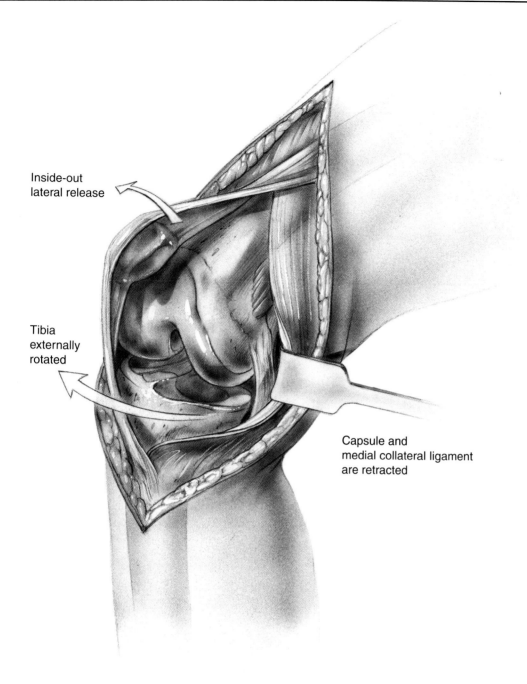

Inside-out
lateral release

Tibia
externally
rotated

Capsule and
medial collateral ligament
are retracted

Figure 19. Deep exposure of the medial side. The tibia is externally rotated as flexion
proceeds.

Dissection is now done laterally with the knee flexed. The remaining patellofemoral ligaments are released (Figs. 20 and 21). The insertion of the iliotibial band is identified and preserved. The lateral capsular structures, including the popliteus and lateral collateral ligament, are released from the femur subperiosteally, using either a knife or an osteotome (Figs. 22–24). Lastly, if necessary, the iliotibial band is lengthened in a Z fashion. We then cut the proximal tibia, taking between 6 and 10 mm of bone and slightly more if a flexion contracture is present. The alignment of the cut is checked to be sure that it is neutral (0° varus/valgus, 2° to 3° posterior slope) to the axis of the ankle (Figs. 25 and 26).

Intramedullary instrumentation is then placed in the femur and the distal femoral cut is made, removing 9 to 10 mm of bone from the lateral condyle in order to properly align the mechanical axis of the knee (Figs. 27 and 28). We generally make the femoral cut in 5° of valgus, unless the patient had a severe valgus deformity. In this situation we choose 3° or even 0° of valgus.

Thus, we create a rectangular gap approximately 20 mm in height, with medial and lateral soft-tissue sleeves.

The extension gap is checked using lamina spreaders or spacer blocks (Figs. 29 and 30). If the medial side is tight, the medial release is extended. In cases of

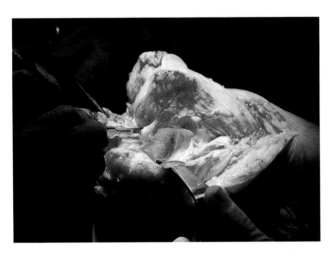

Figure 20. Lateral view of excision of lateral meniscus remnants.

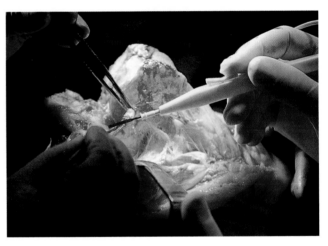

Figure 21. Final release of patellofemoral ligaments with cautery. This is an important and often overlooked step.

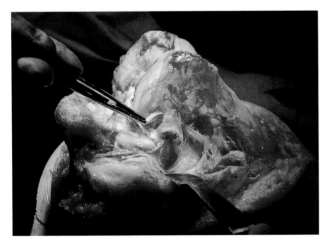

Figure 22. Lateral mobilization. Note external tibial rotation. If necessary, the subperiosteal dissection continues to or beyond the lower collateral ligament.

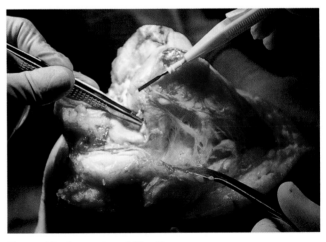

Figure 23. Lateral mobilization.

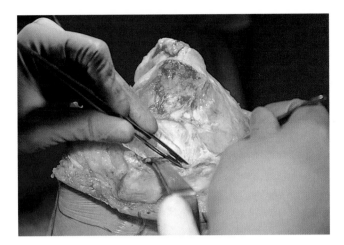

Figure 24. Extent of lateral mobilization.

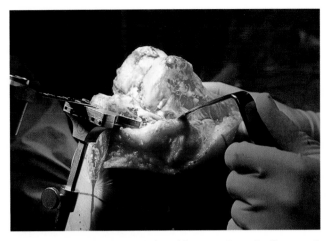

Figure 25. Cutting the tibia with an external alignment guide. Intramedullary guides may be used, but with attention to the possibility of bowed tibiae.

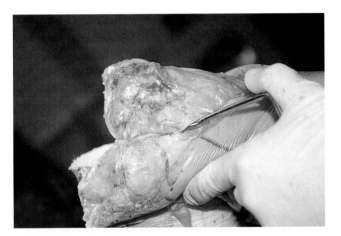

Figure 26. Lateral view after tibial resection. We typically resect the tibia first.

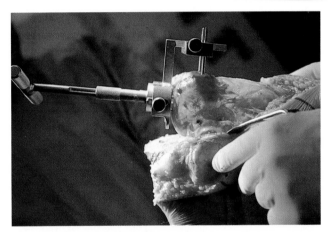

Figure 27. Femoral intramedullary instrumentation for distal resection. We enlarge the entry hole and irrigate and suction the femur to minimize the risk of fat embolization. The use of extramedullary guides for the tibia minimizes the chance of fat embolization from this bone.

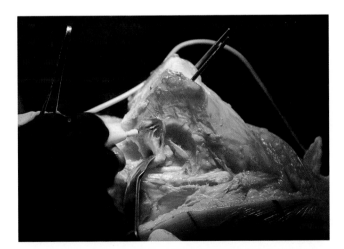

Figure 28. After resection. The pins are left in, should recutting prove necessary. Typically, patients with a flexion contracture will require more than a "standard" distal femoral resection. Leaving the pins in while checking the gap allows for easier replacement of the cutting guide.

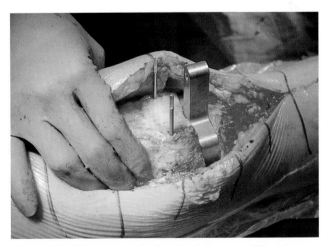

Figure 29. Spacer to check extension gap. We also use lamina spreaders, one applied medially and one applied laterally, to assess soft-tissue tension.

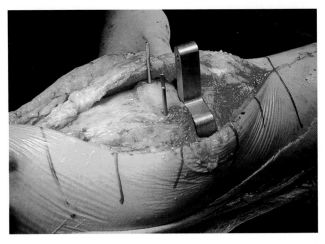

Figure 30. Valgus pressure to assess medial release and stability.

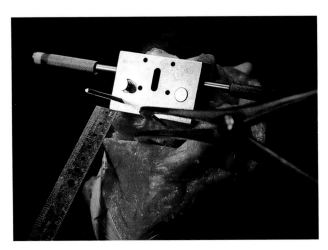

Figure 31. Anteroposterior cutting guide. The rectangular flexion gap is also checked with lamina spreaders.

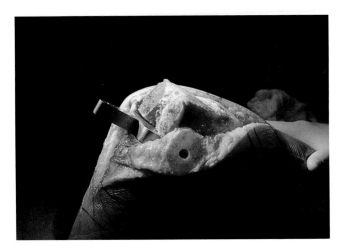

Figure 32. Spacer to check flexion gap.

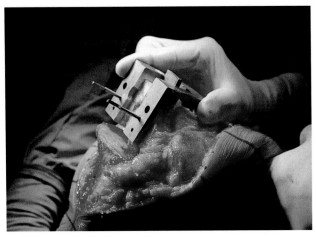

Figure 33. Notch guide placement. Proper placement of the guide is important in order to leave sufficient bone medially and laterally as not to weaken the condyles.

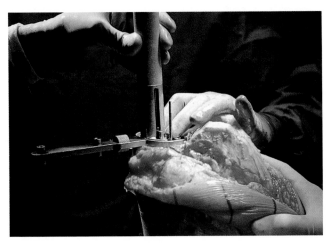

Figure 34. Tibial instrumentation. Care should be taken not to internally rotate the tibia relative to the tubercle.

severe valgus/flexion deformity, release of the lateral head of the gastrocnemius may occasionally be needed. If the knee lacks extension, the posterior capsule is released from the femur as needed. Occasionally, capsulotomy may be required.

Following this, the anterior and posterior femoral cuts are made. The cutting blocks are placed so as to equalize the flexion gap medially and laterally, and are then slightly externally rotated (Fig. 31). This helps to keep the flexion gap equal as flexion increases, and also aids patellofemoral tracking.

If desired, spacer blocks can now be placed to assess the flexion and extension gaps. The intercondylar notch cut and chamfer cuts are made, and a femoral trial component is put in place (Figs. 32 and 33).

The tibial trial component is emplaced with the appropriate instrumentation. Care should be taken to ensure that the component is neutral or slightly externally rotated and aligned with the tubercle (Fig. 34). As determined either by measurement or spacer block, a tibial trial insert of the proper thickness is then placed, and the knee joint is reduced. A careful assessment of flexion and extension gaps, varus/valgus stability, and range of motion must be made at this time. If the quadriceps mechanism is still tight and does not allow 30° to 40° of flexion with the implant in place, even with the tourniquet released, further controlled Z lengthening is done (Fig. 35). It should be noted that in the stiff knee with a flexion contracture, there may be a disparity in the flexion and extension gaps, with the flexion gap

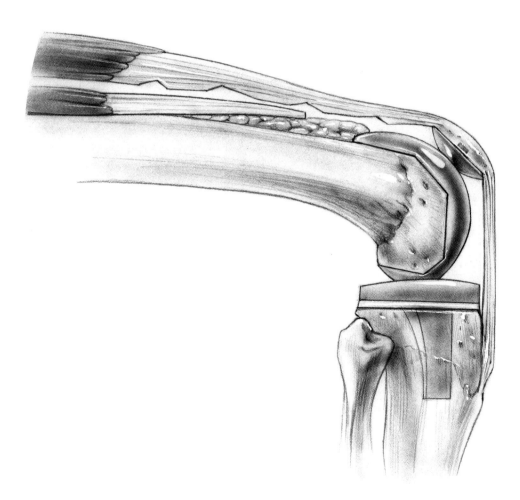

Figure 35. Lateral view with components in place. Note that if flexion is insufficient, further Z-lengthening of the rectus may be done.

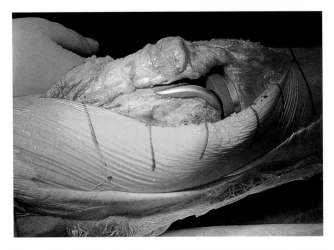

Figure 36. Trial reduction of femur and tibia. Flexion and extension should be checked.

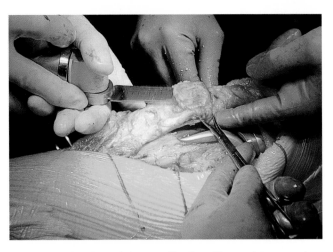

Figure 37. Cutting of the patella. A cutting guide may also be used. The patellar height should be measured before resection and after patellar trial placement to ensure that the height of the patella is not increased.

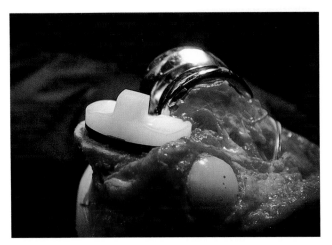

Figure 38. Placement of final components of prosthesis prior to reduction. The extensor mechanism should be protected by externally rotating the tibia. Care must be taken not to place the patella too far medially, and also to assess patellar tracking.

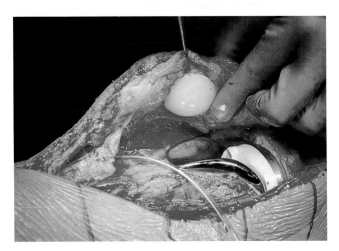

Figure 39. Extent of lateral release. The retinaculum is completely released, as is the insertion of the vastus lateralis.

the greater of the two. When this occurs, one must consider a constrained insert that provides stability in flexion as well as augmenting the function of the collateral ligament. In many cases the posterior stabilized insert will allow appropriate stability.

If the trial components are satisfactory, they can be left in place while the permanent prosthesis is opened and the patella is cut. We always resurface the patella with an all-polyethylene tibial component, taking care not to increase the overall height of the patella (Figs. 36 and 37). Trial reduction of all three components is done, and the knee is taken through a range of motion. The patella should track easily, without tilting, using the "no thumb" technique.

Jet lavage is used to clean the bony beds of the patella, femur, and tibia, which are then carefully dried with a lap sponge. Once the cement is at a consistency of dough or toothpaste, it is finger pressured into the patella and femur. The patellar component of the prosthesis is held with a special clamp, and the femoral component is impacted using the appropriate tool. Any excess cement is removed

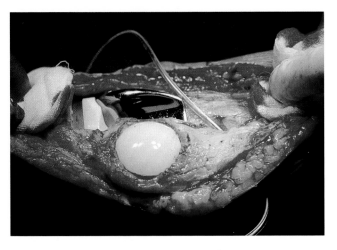

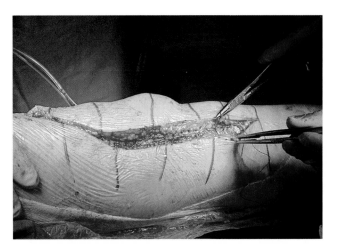

Figure 40. Drain placement. We pass a drain once, from the inside out, and leave the drain in the lateral gutter.

Figure 41. Arthrotomy closure with Tevdek and Vicryl sutures, spaced approximately 1 cm apart.

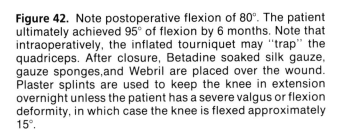

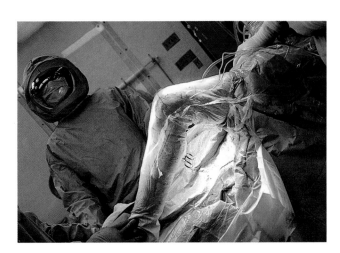

Figure 42. Note postoperative flexion of 80°. The patient ultimately achieved 95° of flexion by 6 months. Note that intraoperatively, the inflated tourniquet may "trap" the quadriceps. After closure, Betadine soaked silk gauze, gauze sponges,and Webril are placed over the wound. Plaster splints are used to keep the knee in extension overnight unless the patient has a severe valgus or flexion deformity, in which case the knee is flexed approximately 15°.

with curettes. While this is occurring, an assistant mixes the second batch of cement for the tibia. Once this cement reaches the correct consistency, the tibial baseplate is cemented in position after finger pressurization of cement into the plateau. A trial polyethylene tibial component is placed, and the knee joint is reduced into extension. This "lever" action further pressurizes the cement, extruding some of it, which is removed with curettes. Once the cement has completely polymerized, the knee is flexed. Any excess cement is removed with osteotomes. The trial polyethylene tibial component is replaced with the real polyethylene insert, and the knee is reduced (Fig. 38). The knee is copiously irrigated with jet lavage.

At this point we release the tourniquet and coagulate any bleeding vessels, paying particular attention to the area of the lateral release (Fig. 39). The limb is then re-exsanguinated with an Esmarch bandage and the tourniquet reinflated. More irrigation is performed. Two Constavac drains are placed. The arthrotomy is closed with #0 Tevdek and Vicryl sutures (Figs. 40 and 41). Subcutaneous tissues are closed in one layer with #0 Vicryl and the skin is closed with a running 3-0 nylon suture. Several interrupted vertical mattress sutures are added. Subcutaneous closure with #0 and 3-0 Vicryl followed by staples is preferred by some surgeons. Flexion and extension are again assessed (Fig. 42).

The wound is dressed with Betadine silk gauze, plain gauze, and soft padding. Two plaster splints are placed medially and laterally keeping the knee in extension, and an Ace bandages is placed. A radiograph is made in the recovery room. In cases of correction of valgus with flexion contracture, the knee is immobilized in 15° of flexion in order to reduce the risk of peroneal nerve palsy.

POSTOPERATIVE MANAGEMENT

Drains and splints are removed on the first postoperative day and the patient is placed in a continuous passive motion (CPM) machine. Initially this is set for a range of from 0° to 30°, which is increased as tolerated, usually by about 10° per day. If the patient had a preoperative flexion contracture or if the knee was tight in extension in the operating room, the patient is taken out of the CPM at night, and must sleep with a knee immobilizer. On the afternoon of the first postoperative day or the morning of the second, the patient, accompanied by a physical therapist, begins to ambulate with a walker. Ambulation is increased daily, and the patient is progressed to crutches or a cane as tolerated. The therapist also assists the patient with knee flexion exercises and straight leg raises.

The expectations of both the surgeon and the patient must be realistic. Even the most educated patient often hopes for a "normal" knee following arthroplasty, and the surgeon cannot paint too gloomy a picture. However, the surgeon must explain that the goal will be to improve the range of motion and function of the knee, and not to make it normal or near normal. In patients with 50° or less of knee motion preoperatively, 70° to 80° of motion without pain should be considered a successful outcome.

COMPLICATIONS

The following sections are devoted to major problems that may be encountered intraoperatively in arthroplasty of the stiff knee.

Avulsion of the Tibial Tubercle

This can be avoided with careful subperiosteal mobilization, with the tibia externally rotated, as the knee is flexed. This complication can usually be avoided. The emphasis is again on external rotation of the tibia along with flexion.

Unequal Flexion/Extension Gap

As mentioned, an unequal flexion/extension gap requires a constrained polyethylene insert, and is associated with the correction of a flexion contracture or loss of condylar bone from previous surgery. We do not hesitate to release the medial collateral ligament from the femur if this facilitates exposure and soft-tissue balance.

Bone or Ligament Loss

Compensation for loss of bone or ligament can usually be made with a modular knee system. Both kinds of loss must be considered preoperatively, and the surgeon should be prepared to deal with any possible loss. Remember, however, that the patient with limited motion has "aggressive fibroblasts" and will rarely end up with instability.

Other major problems encountered after arthroplasty of the stiff knee are as follows (excluding the usual concerns with deep-vein thrombosis, infection, etc.).

Loss of Range of Motion

Despite what the surgeon achieves in the operating room (i.e., 80° to 90° of flexion), the patient may have difficulty achieving motion postoperatively, usually because of pain. Continuous epidural anesthesia can diminish the pain, and appropriate physical therapy may help, but sometimes manipulation may be required. If the patient has not achieved 60° of flexion by 6 weeks, we manipulate the knee under anesthesia.

Abnormalities in Wound Healing

Aside from the usual concerns, any knee that has had prior surgery, especially with multiple incisions, may be subject to drainage, or worse, to skin sloughing. Skin sloughing may often require a flap for reconstruction, and this possibility should always be considered preoperatively. Consultation with a plastic surgeon may prove helpful. We put patients who have persistent drainage on bedrest, with a clean, sterilely applied compressive dressing. We allow no CPM or therapy until the drainage ceases.

Patient Expectations

Once having achieved an improved range of motion, the patient may begin to expect that improvement will continue, resulting in a near-normal range of motion. The patient must be reminded of preoperative goals and that the maximum benefit of the total knee replacement is only achieved by 8 to 10 months postoperatively.

ILLUSTRATIVE CASE FOR TECHNIQUE

The patient whose surgery is shown in Figures 43 and 44 was 81-year-old man who had had a total medial and lateral meniscectomy of the left knee in 1963. Over the 5 years before his initial visit, he had been experiencing increasing pain, more in the left than in the right knee. If the year prior to his presentation the pain had become moderate to severe. He also noted increasing stiffness. He could walk one or two blocks using a cane, with a limp, and could not reciprocate on stairs. Because of the increasing severity of his symptoms, he presented for an evaluation.

His physical examination revealed a range of motion of 20° to 40°, with fixed flexion contracture. His quadriceps strength was 4+/5, and his sensory examination was normal. No instability was noted, but he had a moderate varus deformity (Fig. 43). Total knee replacement was recommended, and the patient was informed that he could expect perhaps 70° of flexion. He was asked to donate 2 units of autologous blood.

His surgery was performed in April 1992. The procedure required 90 minutes, and a cemented Johnson & Johnson PFC prosthesis was implanted, with a constrained tibial insert. The range of postoperative flexion of the knee, as seen in Figures 43 and 44, was 80°. The patient remained in the hospital for 8 days, and a routine venogram revealed no deep-vein thrombosis.

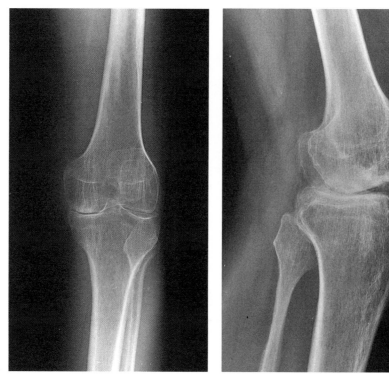

A

B

Figure 43. Preoperative AP **(A)** and lateral **(B)** radiographs of an 81-year-old male patient who presented with moderate to severe pain.

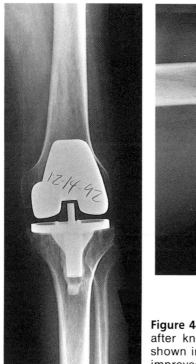

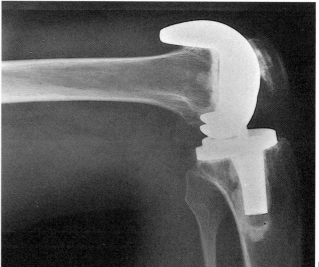

A

B

Figure 44. AP **(A)** and lateral **(B)** radiographs 6 months after knee replacement in the patient whose knee is shown in Figure 43. The patient's range of motion was improved and he walked without a limp.

At 6 weeks postoperatively the patient's wound was benign, and his range of motion was 10° to 70°. At 3 months he was walking without a cane or limp, and had a range of motion of 7° to 90°. His range of motion at 6 months was 5° to 100°, and has not changed since that time. The patient describes himself as "very satisfied."

RECOMMENDED READING

1. Aglietti, P., Windsor, R. E., Buzzi, R., and Insall, J. N.: Arthroplasty for the stiff or ankylosed knee. *J. Arthroplasty,* 41(1): 1–5, 1989.
2. Rand, J. A.: Revision total knee arthroplasty: surgical technique. In: *Total Knee Arthroplasty,* edited by J. A. Rand. Raven Press, 1993, 155–176.
3. Scott, R. D.: Revision total knee arthroplasty. *Clin. Orthop.,* 226: 65–78, 1988.
4. Scott, R. D., and Siliski, J. M.: The use of a modified V-Y quadricepsplasty during total knee replacement to gain exposure and improve flexion in the ankylosed knee. *Orthopedics,* 8(1): 45–48, 1985.
5. Sculco, T. P., and Faris, P. M.: Total knee replacement in the stiff knee. *Tech. Orthop.,* 3(2): 5–8, 1988.
6. Vince, K., and Dorr, L. D.: Total knee arthroplasty: Principles and controversy. *Tech. Orthop.,* 1(4): 69–82, 1987.
7. Whiteside, L. A., and Ohl, M. D.: Tibial tubercle osteotomy for exposure of the difficult total knee arthroplasty. *Clin. Orthop.,* 260: 6–9, 1990.
8. Windsor, R. E., and Insall, J. N.: Exposure in revision total knee arthroplasty: the femoral peel. *Tech. Orthop.,* 3(2): 1–4, 1988.

Master Techniques in Orthopaedic Surgery,
Knee Arthroplasty, edited by P. A. Lotke,
Raven Press, Ltd., New York © 1995.

11

Patellar Malposition, Erosion, and Absence

David S. Hungerford

INDICATIONS/CONTRAINDICATIONS

Patellar complications in total knee replacement comprise up to 50% of all complications in some reported series (3). This is in spite of the fact that most patients presenting for total knee replacement have either minimal or no patellofemoral joint involvement. It is well known that several technical problems in total knee replacement may conjoin to produce patellar subluxation or dislocation, patellar fracture, avulsion of the patellar tendon, or rupture of the quadriceps tendon (2). Three technical errors increase the ''Q'' angle, leading to lateral patellar subluxation: a) internal rotation of the tibial component, which lateralizes the tibial tubercle; b) internal rotation of the femoral component of the prosthesis, which medializes the trochlear groove; and c) lateralization of the patellar resurfacing component, which lateralizes the central ridge, requiring the patella to ride more medially in order for the articular surface to track congruently in the trochlea. Skiving the patellar resection so that the lateral facet is under-resected increases the lateral thickness of the replaced patella, increasing tension on the lateral retinaculum and leading to patellar subluxation. Under-resection of the patella or oversizing of the femoral component of the prosthesis has the same effect. Over-resection of the patella weakens the bone and predisposes it to fracture. Exposure problems in patients with a stiff knee or in obese patients may put excessive tension on the patellar tendon, leading to its avulsion. Over-resection of a proximal margin of the patella may compromise the quadriceps insertion into the patella, leading to rupture of the tendon.

From this brief overview, it can be seen that there is a great potential for patellar complications despite what is often a relatively normal patellofemoral joint preop-

D. S. Hungerford, m.d.: Department of Orthopaedic Surgery, Johns Hopkins University School of Medicine, Baltimore, MD 21239.

eratively. Many surgeons have advocated not resurfacing the patella if its articular cartilage is reasonably intact. However, even in such cases, malalignment of the femoral or tibial components of the prosthesis could lead to subluxation or dislocation of the unresurfaced patella.

SURGERY

Those patients who present with significant malposition or erosion of the patella or its absence require special surgical handling. Although these problems are similar and the special techniques for handling them somewhat overlap, each problem must nonetheless be addressed separately because of the features unique to these conditions.

Patellar Malposition

There are four categories of patellar malposition: patella alta; patella baja; mild, moderate and severe subluxation; and long-standing permanent dislocation. Patella alta is not often a problem and patella baja is rare. Most cases of patellar malposition consist of moderate patellar malposition with severe subluxation and long-standing permanent dislocation.

Patella Alta and Baja. Since the trochlear groove for all modern femoral components of knee prostheses extends significantly more proximally than the anatomic patellar groove, patella alta does not really constitute a clinical or technical problem. Patella baja is not, generally speaking, a condition that occurs spontaneously or as an anatomic variant. It occurs in the knee that has undergone multiple operations, and is due to scarring and contracture in the fat pad and the patellar tendon itself, secondary to both the trauma of prior surgery and prolonged quadriceps inactivity. In some cases of patella baja there may also be an associated extension contracture of the knee, making exposure at the time of total knee replacement extremely difficult. In such cases, adjunctive exposure of the knee is indicated. My preferred technique for this is a tibial tubercle osteotomy.

Tibial Tubercle Osteotomy For Enhanced Exposure

The tibial tubercle osteotomy (TTO) for enhancing exposure of the knee at the time of total knee replacement applies not only in patella baja but also in any situation in which the knee has limited flexion and exposure is difficult. A TTO gives better exposure of the knee than does a quadriceps turndown because the entire quadriceps mechanism, rather than its proximal portion only, is turned laterally (Fig. 1A, B). Moreover, the repair of the TTO is such that no special postoperative handling is required. A TTO is vastly preferred to avulsing the patellar tendon, and should be considered when the surgeon is struggling for exposure. The TTO recommended here is different from the TTO used with medialization of the tibial tubercle for patellofemoral instability.

The patellar tendon insertion into the tibial tubercle is carefully identified, and a transverse cut is made to a depth of 1 cm in the bone just proximal to the tibial tubercle, using an osteotome. Next, a thin oscillating saw is used to create a coronal osteotomy paralleling the crest of the tibia for a distance of 5 to 7 cm. The osteotomy will be approximately 1 cm posterior to the tibial tubercle because of the prominence of the tubercle, but at its distal extent will be approximately 4 to 5 mm posterior to the tibial crest (Fig. 1C). The oscillating saw is carried laterally to, but not through, the lateral cortex. At the distal margin, another transverse osteotomy, parallel to the proximal transverse osteotomy, is carried posteriorly

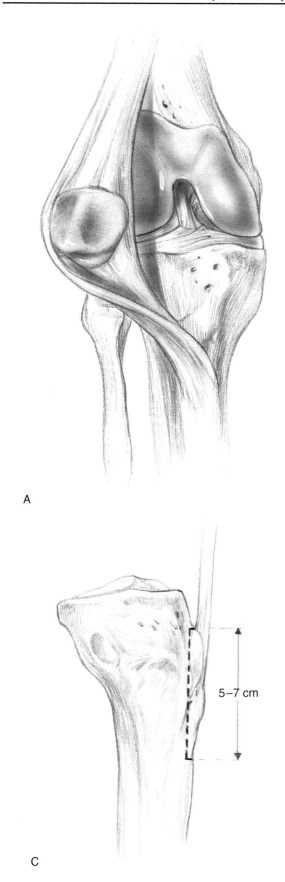

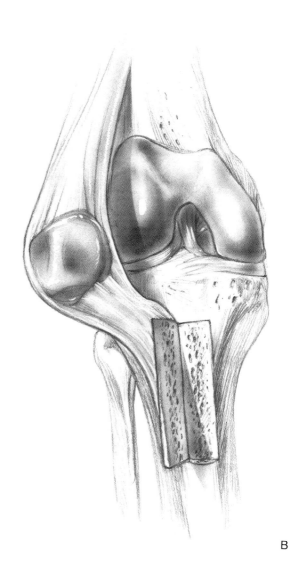

Figure 1. A: Typical exposure in a patient with patella baja, obesity, or extension contracture. The patellar tendon and fat pad obscure the lateral femoral condyle and lateral tibial plateau. **B:** With the tibial tubercle, patellar tendon, and fat pad rotated laterally, the distal femur and proximal tibia are completely exposed. **C:** View of the proximal tibia from the medial side shows the outline of the osteotomy.

5–7 cm

to the level of the coronal osteotomy. At this point, osteotomes are inserted into the coronal osteotomy to the level of the lateral cortex. The entire osteotomized fragment must be supported by osteotomes. Failure to support the entire fragment may result in fracture of the fragment, significantly reducing the stability of the knee. At this point, the osteotomes are rotated anteriorly, turning the osteotomized fragment laterally and cracking the lateral cortex, but leaving the attachment of the anterior compartment muscles intact on the lateral side of the osteotomy fragment. This turns the entire quadriceps mechanism laterally and vastly improves exposure. In this way the osteotomy fragment is opened like a book and turned laterally. When the book is closed by repositioning the osteotomized fragment into its prepared bed, the proximal transverse osteotomy acts as a stop to prevent the osteotomy from being pulled proximally. The fragment is held in the closed position by two cerclage wires. Postoperatively the patient is managed with routine physical therapy, including passive and active range-of-motion exercises. However, I protect patients by having them ambulate in a knee immobilizer splint for 6 weeks. The knee immobilizer is removed several times a day for physical therapy.

Patellar Subluxation—Preoperative Planning. Forewarned is forearmed. Therefore, the patient with patellar subluxation must be carefully examined preoperatively for the position and tracking of the patella, for range of motion of the knee, and particularly for any limitations of flexion. Good quality anteroposterior (AP) and lateral radiographs, but most specifically those that provide a "skyline" view of the patellofemoral joint, are required (4) (Fig. 2A, B).

When problems related to malposition of the patella have been identified, I change from a slightly median parapatellar incision to a midline incision. Although most balancing of the extensor mechanism can be done from inside the joint, in extreme instances it may be desirable to approach the lateral side of the knee from outside the joint. If this is the case, the midline incision provides easier access to the outside of the lateral retinaculum and the vastus lateralis without creating an excessive anterior and lateral skin flap. Although it may be tempting to use a lateral parapatellar incision, particularly in dealing with severe valgus deformity with patellar malposition, most surgeons will find this unfamiliar territory and more difficult. Moreover, since medial plication may be necessary to balance the extensor mechanism, the argument that the lateral approach preserves

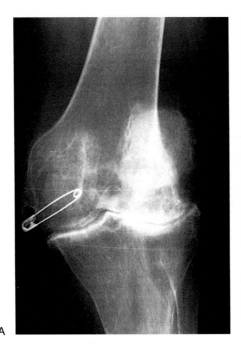

A

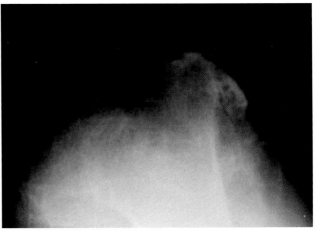

B

Figure 2. A: This AP radiograph of the knee suggests that the patellofemoral joint is severely arthritic and subluxed. **B:** However, the "skyline" view shows the degree to which the patella is eroded and laterally subluxed to the point of near dislocation.

the blood supply to the patella on the medial side is often invalid. Finally, if one is doing an extensive lateral release and the skin approach is lateral and parapatellar, the intra-articular hematoma resulting from the release is directly contiguous with the subcutaneous tissue and the skin incision. With an anterior incision there is some distance between the skin incision and the lateral release.

The medial retinaculum and the quadriceps tendon are opened in a routine fashion and the patella dislocated laterally. The femoral and tibial cuts are made in a routine way and trial tibial and femoral components are inserted. It is an advantage not to fix rotation of the tibial component until the rotational relationship of the tibial component to the tibial tubercle and collateral ligament balance are shown at trial reduction. It is often possible to laterally rotate the tibial component in order to medialize the tibial tubercle, without affecting the medial/lateral or flexion/extension balance between the femoral and tibial components. I do not do a routine lateral release until the trial reduction demonstrates that a lateral release is necessary. By debriding the lateral gutter of fibrosis, hypertrophic synovial tissue, and the lateral plica; removing patellar, femoral, and tibial osteophytes; and choosing a femoral component of appropriate size in cases of mild and even moderate patellar subluxation, the need for a lateral release may be eliminated.

With the trial femoral and tibial components in place, the rotational alignment of the tibial component temporarily fixed, and the knee flexed to 90°, the patella is exposed and held for resection at the appropriate level and orientation (Fig. 3). Prior to resection, the synovial fringe around the patella is resected and osteophytes are removed. The patella is palpated for thickness and measured with a caliper, and the articulating facets are resected. Appropriate resection of the patella leaves an anterior wafer of the patella that is equally thick proximally, distally, medially, and laterally. This is accomplished first by orienting the saw blade parallel to the central ridge (Fig. 4). The first pass of the saw then moves from medial to lateral, with care taken not to over-resect the lateral facet. The proximal and distal patellar thicknesses are then evaluated between the thumb and the index finger, and any discrepancies are adjusted with the second pass of the saw blade (Fig. 5). Because the lateral facet will usually be intentionally under-resected with the first pass, the second pass is concentrated on "truing" the medial/lateral resection level. The final result is a flat saw cut that leaves the patellar remnant equally thick throughout.

The drill guide for the patellar resurfacing prosthesis is aligned parallel to the line of resection of the saw, which is perpendicular to the now resected central

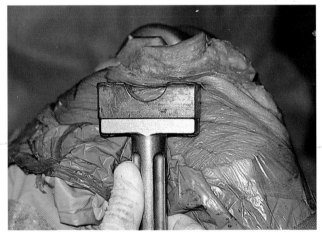

Figure 3. With the trial components in place, the knee flexed 90°, and the patella everted, the patella is held steady by an assistant pushing up on the subcutaneous patellar surface with the femoral impactor.

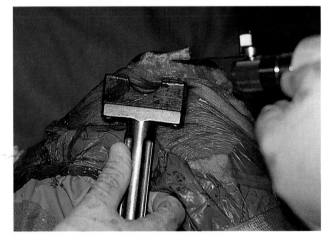

Figure 4. Proper orientation of the saw blade for the first pass.

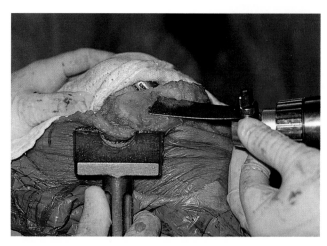

Figure 5. After digital assessment of the patellar thickness, the oscillating saw is passed a second time, usually to additionally resect the lateral facet and "true-up" any variation in overall thickness.

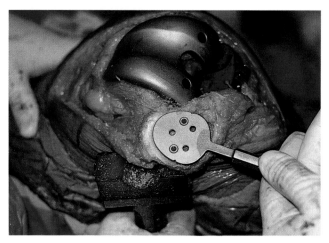

Figure 6. The patellar prosthesis must not be lateralized. Therefore, the drill guide is coapted with the medial margin of the cut surface, even if this means a little uncovering of the lateral patellar surface.

ridge. The medial margin of the drill guide is coapted with the medial margin of the saw cut (Fig. 6). The drill bit of the appropriate size is chosen, but since the patella is always wider in the medial/lateral plane than in the proximal/distal plane, there may be some overhang of the lateral bone. This does not represent a problem. Drill holes for the trial of the patellar component are made, the trial component inserted, and the extensor mechanism reduced. A single suture or towel clip is placed in the tendon of the vastus medialis at the proximal medial corner of the patella, and the knee put through a range of motion. Careful observation of the position of the patella as it enters the trochlear groove and throughout the range of motion is mandatory. If there is any tendency for the patella to sublux laterally, or if the medial margin of the patella does not contact the lateral margin of the femoral condyle in full flexion (Fig. 7), lateral patellar retinacular release will be needed. The lateral release should be titrated to the degree of the problem. Minimal subluxation requires incision only of the patellofemoral ligament at the midlateral portion of the patella. This can easily be done from inside the joint and does not violate the superior lateral retinacular vessel to the patella.

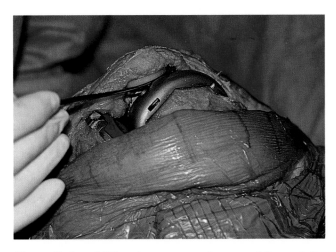

Figure 7. In addition to proper entrance of the patella into the trochlear groove, the medial facet of the patellar component must contact the lateral margin of the medial femoral condyle, with the knee in 90° flexion.

For severe lateral subluxation an extensive lateral release may be necessary. Such a lateral release would extend laterally along the anterior margin of the iliotibial tract, down as far as Gerdy's tubercle, and proximally along the posterior margin of the vastus lateralis. I do not believe that it is ever necessary to incise the tendon of the vastus lateralis that inserts into the superior lateral corner of the patella. I have seen one case on referral in which this was done and resulted in quadriceps rupture. Isolation of the superior lateral retinacular vessel, which provides a significant blood supply to the patella has been recommended (3). However, in most cases in which such an extensive lateral patellar release is necessary, it requires a significant repositioning of the patella from its original preoperative position, making it unlikely that the patella will function even if the vessel is left intact. Moreover, there is no convincing evidence that sectioning this vessel leads to patellar necrosis. However, if an extensive lateral release is done, the tourniquet should be deflated prior to wound closure to make sure that there is no pulsatile bleeding from lateral retinacular vessels. Such vessels can then be identified and coagulated. It must be recognized that with an extensive lateral release the knee is open to the subcutaneous space. While it may be arguable that the standard total knee arthroplasty does not require drainage, or even that it should not be drained, I believe that it is safer to use a drain and a good compression dressing when performing an extensive lateral release.

Patients with severe lateral subluxation of the patella may also have a laterally oriented tibial tubercle. In most instances it should be possible to "cheat" a little on tibial rotation and externally rotate the tibial component of the prosthesis so that the tibial tubercle is aligned more medially. However, there will be rare instances in which medialization of the tibial tubercle will be necessary. This is much more likely to be the case in permanent lateral dislocation of the patella, and will be addressed in the appropriate section below. It will be rare that subluxation of the patella requires medial capsular imbrication, but if this is needed to make the patella track centrally, it should be done. If the components of the prosthesis are correctly placed and the extensor mechanism is appropriately balanced, with the deeper trochlear grooves and more appropriate patellar component shapes in current total knee systems, lateral subluxation and dislocation of the patella postoperatively, even in cases in which the patella was subluxed preoperatively, should not be a problem. Postoperative management of these cases is no different than the standard rehabilitation for a normal knee.

Permanent Patellar Dislocation. Cases of permanent patellar subluxation are rare but difficult to treat. The typical patient with permanent lateral dislocation of the patella presents with a long-standing history of knee dysfunction that has gradually led to valgus deformity and instability. Radiography shows the patella to be completely dislocated laterally (Fig. 8). I have seen only three such cases in the past 10 years, but such patients represent a technical challenge. In two of the three cases it was necessary to perform a medialization of the tibial tubercle. Since the tibial tubercle was in an extreme lateral position, it could not be centralized by external rotation of the tibial component and still maintain proper stability between the tibial and femoral components. Although a TTO is not commonly necessary during total knee replacement, it remains a useful adjunct for the treatment of postoperative instability of the extensor mechanism, since one of the common causes of such instability is failure to align the tibial component correctly in a rotational sense. In such cases, the alternative to medialization of the tibial tubercle is complete revision of the tibial component, which can be difficult in the presence of an intact femoral component. Therefore, if the tibial–femoral articulation is functioning satisfactorily and the tibial tubercle is displaced laterally, causing or contributing to instability of the extensor mechanism, medialization of the tibial tubercle according to the Trillat modification of the Elmslie procedure is extremely useful (5).

Tibial Tubercle Osteotomy For Medialization

In order to perform a medialization of the tibial tubercle, either at the time of total knee replacement or at any time after a total knee replacement, the standard total knee incision is extended distally for approximately 2½ inches. The muscles of the anterior compartment are dissected subperiosteally from the anterolateral crest of the tibia, exposing the crest. Using a small Steinmann pin, the distal extent of the osteotomy is delineated at 3 to 4 mm behind the crest of the tibia, 5 to 7

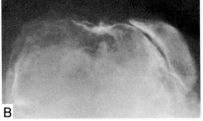

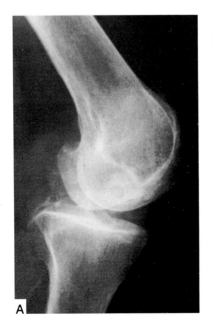

Figure 8. A: Lateral radiograph of a 60-year-old woman with severe arthritis and a completely dislocated patella, invisible on this view. **B:** "Skyline" view shows the deformed, dislocated patella (From ref. 4.)

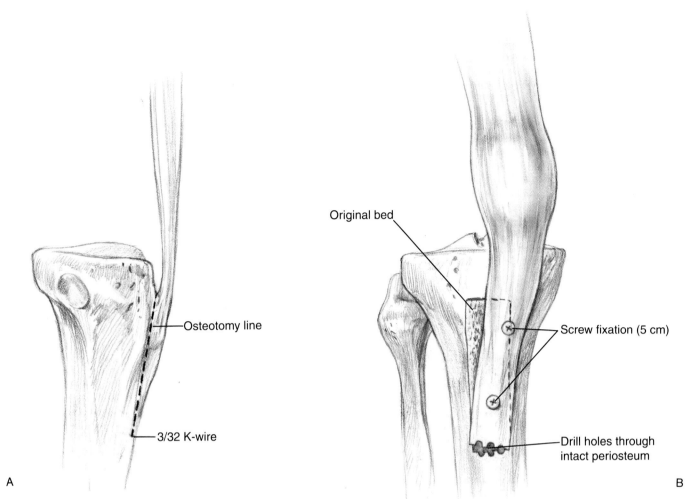

Figure 9. A: The osteotomy extends from behind the patellar tendon to a drill hole
5 to 7 cm distally. **B:** The tubercle is rotated medially to the desired degree and fixed
with two screws.

cm distal to the tibial tubercle (Fig. 9A). Using a thin oscillating saw, a coronal
osteotomy is made from the lateral side, 4 to 5 mm posterior and parallel to the
crest of the tibia and exiting just proximal to the tibial tubercle. It is usually not
necessary to elevate the periosteum on the medial side of the tibial metaphysis,
since the latter is already exposed and can be seen when the medial cortex is
penetrated by the oscillating saw. Once the osteotomy is created, the anterior
bridge of intact cortex at the level of the transverse Steinmann pin is perforated
in three places with a smooth K-wire through the intact periosteum, producing a
postage-stamp effect (Fig. 9B). The semi-isolated tibial tubercle osteotomy can
now be cracked through this postage-stamp perforation and pushed medially by
the desired amount. The osteotomy can be temporarily fixed with a K-wire to
check for appropriate tracking, and its medial displacement can be increased or
decreased to the desired level, followed by its fixation with two screws. A tibial
tubercle osteotomy done at the same time as a total knee replacement will always
be accompanied by an extensive lateral release. Likewise, a TTO done as part of
the treatment for recurring patellar dislocation would always be associated with
a complete lateral release, even if a lateral release had been done at the time of
the original total knee replacement.

Patellar Erosion

The most common cause of patellar erosion is severe permanent lateral subluxation of the knee. The patella will have been riding astride the lateral trochlea for many years and gives the appearance of wrapping around the lateral trochlear facet (Fig. 10). In truth, the lateral trochlea has burrowed into the lateral and central facets of the patella. Sometimes, in cases of inflammatory disease, the patella will be eroded to a fraction of its original thickness without subluxation. Both situations present two technical problems. First there is the problem of orientation of the patellar cut. This must be done extremely carefully, with circumferential debridement of the soft tissue, removal of osteophytes, and identification of the line of insertion of the quadriceps tendon, medial and lateral retinacula, and patellar tendon. Identifying this "equator" of soft tissue inserting into the periphery of the patella is essential to establishing the proper orientation of the cut and preserving these all-important soft-tissue attachments. The residual bone is then resected with several passes of an oscillating saw, using the same precautions outlined in the previous section.

The second problem with severe erosion is that adding a prosthesis will displace the extensor mechanism proximally. Even if the size of the femoral component of the prosthesis has been properly chosen, it is likely that in the case of severe patellar erosion, some degree of flexion will be lost when the extensor mechanism is reduced. Rarely, the patellar bone stock is so thin that it is not possible to considering resurfacing, since there is little or nothing on which to seat the prosthesis (see Illustrative Case for Technique). In such cases the patella has simply been debrided and left unresurfaced, with surprisingly good comfort and extensor function. The most common circumstance in which this is seen is the erosion associated with patellar loosening. In my experience it has been better to leave the bony remnant of the eroded patella to serve as a secure soft-tissue attachment for the quadriceps and patellar tendon than to try to excise the patella and convert the procedure to a patellectomy.

Patellar Absence

It is not uncommon for patients who have had a patellectomy to eventually present with the need for total knee replacement, and this does not usually constitute a great technical challenge. Moreover, if the proper indications for total knee replacement are present, the patient can expect a good result. However, some patients present with continued anterior knee pain following a series of various

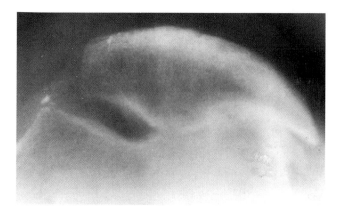

Figure 10. An example of severe patellar erosion associated with severe subluxation.

knee procedures that have been of limited success. For such patients, the "indication" for total knee replacement is as a "court of last resort." Unfortunately, the procedure is usually futile and a last act of desperation on the part of the surgeon, the patient, or both. When in such cases the only indication for total knee replacement is pain, with very little evidence of dysfunction of the tibial femoral joint, I would encourage orthopedic surgeons to resist the temptation to do a total knee replacement. In my experience, no patient with a patellectomy who has had more than three previous surgical procedures of the knee without relief, and in whom pain has been the only indication for total knee arthroplasty, has had a successful result.

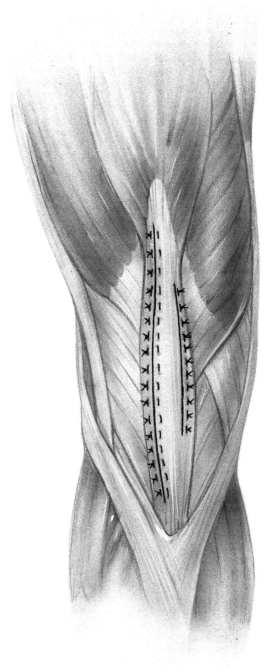

Figure 11. Repair of the quadriceps mechanism after exposure in a patient with prior patellectomy.

The typical successful candidate for total knee arthroplasty is a patient who has had a patellectomy at least one year previously, has evidence of significant tibial femoral arthrosis both clinically and radiologically, and who has had a clinically successful interval between the patellectomy and the symptoms now leading to the need for total knee replacement. In such patients the extensor mechanism is usually well centered in the trochlea. If the extensor mechanism is subluxing or dislocating laterally, all of the techniques discussed earlier in this chapter for centralizing and stabilizing the quadriceps mechanism will have to be employed.

The only special aspect of a total knee replacement in the patellectomized knee is that the incision into the quadriceps mechanism is centered on the extensor mechanism rather than on the median parapatellar region. The incision then runs from the center of the quadriceps tendon through the center of the scar tissue that occupies the former location of the patella and splits the patellar tendon. This provides good quality tissue medially and laterally, which can be repaired by a pants-over-vest suture line similar to that in the patellectomy technique of Boyd and Hawkins (1) (Fig. 11). With such an exposure and repair, the patient can be handled postoperatively in a manner identical to that for a patient who has had a standard total knee replacement, with supervised range-of-motion exercises, quadriceps' setting exercises, and straight leg raising as soon as tolerated. There is no need for postoperative splinting.

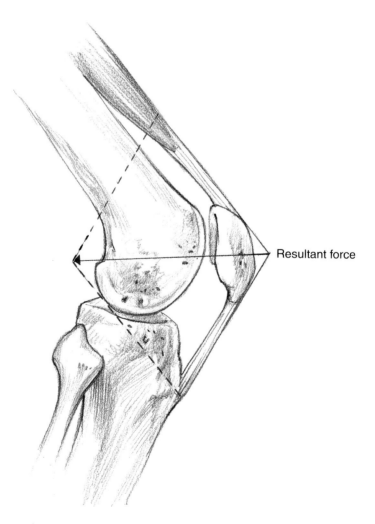

Figure 12. The patellofemoral joint reaction force stabilizes the anteroposterior plane of the tibial–femoral articulation.

The only other caveat concerning the absent patella is to remember that the reaction force in the patellofemoral joint also has an important stabilizing effect on the femur throughout the range of motion of the knee (Fig. 12). The concentration of the resultant force vector from the extensor mechanism through the patella, with a focus on the anterior femur, helps prevent the femur from subluxing anteriorly. The angle of attack of the patellar tendon on the tibial tubercle helps prevent the tibia from subluxing posteriorly. Some of this stabilizing effect has been lost in the patellectomized patient because of an altered angle of attack of the patellar tendon on the tibial tubercle, and also because of the lack of a focused patellofemoral joint reaction force on the anterior femur. Therefore, if the patella is not present, either the posterior cruciate ligament must be maintained and properly tensioned to stabilize the tibial femoral articulation in the anteroposterior plane, or a posterior-stabilized prosthesis should be used.

POSTOPERATIVE MANAGEMENT

The postoperative care of a patient who has had a total knee replacement because of patellar malposition, erosion, or absence varies with the surgical technique employed. Stable patellar tracking should be achieved in the operating theater. But if medial imbrication or tibial tubercle transposition occurs, a slower rehabilitation course, which limits flexion and increases protected weight-bearing, may be necessary. Early motion should be encouraged on a continuous passive motion (CPM) machine, but all passive and active muscle-strengthening exercises should be deferred until primary healing of the repair or tibial tubercle is achieved. The balance between early motion and aggressive muscle strengthening must be individualized.

Realization of the expectation of significant patellar function depends on the ability of the surgeon to salvage such function and centralize tracking. A total knee arthroplasty with complete absence of the patella can function very well, although not as well as a conventional knee replacement. Patients with remnants of patella that track well can also have very satisfactory results. If the patella or extensor mechanism subluxes, the overall function or results will diminish and the patient will experience weakness and discomfort. Therefore, a strong effort should be made to maintain appropriate tracking.

COMPLICATIONS

A diverse set of complications can attend arthroplasty for patellar malposition, erosion, or absence, depending on the initial problem and the results of the reconstructive surgery. These complications may include recurring subluxation or dislocation of the extensor mechanism, fracture of patellar remnants, avascular necrosis, avulsion of the patellar tendon, and extensor muscle weakness.

Recurring subluxation or dislocation of the ligament for the extensor mechanism must be recognized at the time of surgery and avoided. Careful attention should be directed to rotation of the components under the extensor mechanism. The patella should track correctly to avoid this complication. At the time of closure, the surgeon should not depend solely on soft-tissue closure to secure adequate patellar tracking.

Patellar fractures may follow extensive patellar reconstruction because the patella has eroded, become too thin, or become devascularized and necrotic. If possible, the lateral geniculate vessel should be saved and as much of the soft-tissue attachment of the patella preserved as is possible. Patellar fractures may occur late. Once they are recognized the knee must be immobilized for 6 to 8 weeks until the fracture stabilizes. Minimal displacement should not significantly compromise the overall result.

The need for extensive patellar relocation is associated with potential avulsion of the tibial tubercle. Avulsion is best avoided by recognizing its early stages and protecting the extensor mechanism from excess tension by externally rotating the tibia for more complete soft-tissue release. Some surgeons use a temporary Steinmann pin in the patellar tendon to protect against avulsion. Occasionally, avulsion is recognized late and severely compromises the result of a total knee arthroplasty.

Finally, an eroded patella may cause the quadriceps mechanism to be weakened and reduce the function of a knee replacement. Extensive rehabilitation and muscle strengthening will help reduce the risk of this problem.

ILLUSTRATIVE CASE FOR TECHNIQUE

A 28-year-old woman had long-standing pain and disability from juvenile rheumatoid arthritis with severe patellofemoral erosion. She was unable to climb or descend stairs or rise from a chair without pain. She was dependent on a walker for ambulation, and presented for knee replacement surgery.

Examination showed that she walked with a stiff knee gait, had difficulty sitting and rising from a chair, and had marked patellofemoral crepitus on motion. The range of motion was from 0° to 70°, with pain.

A preoperative lateral radiograph (Fig. 13A) showed severe patellofemoral arthritis, with a thin, eroded patella set laterally on the femoral condyle, and a diminutive femoral condyle. The patient underwent a total knee replacement with an "extra-extra small" femoral component that nevertheless projected the trochlea more anteriorly than had originally been the case. It was not possible to resur-

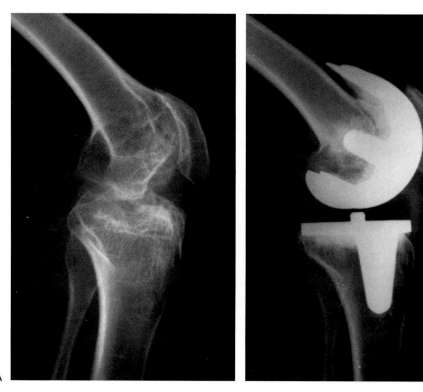

Figure 13. A: Example of a patient with severe loss of patellar bone stock. **B:** The patella was left unresurfaced. The patient has no anterior knee pain.

face the patella and still close the knee. The concave, eroded patellar surface tracked along the lateral femoral condyle, was stable, and did not dislocate.

Postoperatively the patient has done well, is comfortable, and has good extensor function. The postoperative radiograph seen in Figure 13B shows a lateral view of the prosthesis in place. The unresurfaced patella tracks securely on the lateral femoral condyle.

In summary, many of the problems referable to the patellofemoral joint in large series of total knee replacements are due to technical inadequacies that impact on the extensor mechanism. However, in patients with severe operative problems of the extensor mechanism, special techniques will have to be employed to restore patellofemoral stability and function. This chapter has detailed the author's approach to these difficult problems.

RECOMMENDED READING

1. Boyd, H. B., and Hawkins, B. L.: Patellectomy—A simplified technique. *Surg. Gynecol. Obstet.*, 86: 357, 1948.
2. Briard, J. L., and Hungerford, D. S.: Patellofemoral instability in total knee arthroplasty. *J. Arthroplasty*, 4(Suppl): S87–S97, 1989.
3. Brick, G. W., and Scott, R. D.: The patellofemoral component of total knee arthroplasty. *Clin. Orthop.*, 231: 163–178, 1988.
4. Ficat, R. P., and Hungerford, D. S.: *Disorders of the Patellofemoral Joint*. Williams & Wilkins, Baltimore, 1977.
5. Trillat, A., Dejour, H. L., and Coutelle, A.: Diagnosis and treatment of recurrent subluxation of the patella. *Rev. Chir. Orthop.*, 50: 813–824, 1964.

Master Techniques in Orthopaedic Surgery,
Knee Arthroplasty, edited by P. A. Lotke,
Raven Press, Ltd., New York © 1995.

12

Total Knee Arthroplasty After High Tibial Osteotomies

Brian P. Johnson and Lawrence D. Dorr

INDICATIONS/CONTRAINDICATIONS

High tibial osteotomy (HTO) is an acceptable surgical treatment for unicompartmental osteoarthritis, especially in the young, active patient. Initial short-term results are 80% to 90% satisfactory (2–5), but gradually worsen with time to 45% to 65% satisfactory at 7 to 10 years (2,5,10). Insall et al. have reported that 23% of HTO will require conversion to total knee arthroplasty (5). In several series the average time for the conversion to total knee arthroplasty after an HTO is approximately 6 years (1,6,10,11).

There is general agreement that an HTO does not prevent subsequent total knee arthroplasty. The latter procedure has its own unique set of intraoperative problems related to the anatomic alterations present in the proximal tibia after an HTO. Controversy exists about whether or not the results of total knee arthroplasty after HTO are comparable to those in patients without prior surgery. Our experience has been that the results of total knee arthroplasty are not compromised after HTO.

PREOPERATIVE PLANNING

The radiographs of a knee that has had an HTO usually show three major changes in anatomy. First, on anteroposterior radiographs, the tibial bone is in

B. P. Johnson, M.D.: Orthopaedic Surgery Service, Brooke Army Medical Center, HSHE-SBR, Fort Van Huston, TX 78234.

L. D. Dorr, M.D.: The Center for Arthritis & Joint Implant Surgery, USC University Hospital, Los Angeles, CA 90033-4634.

increased valgus angulation (Fig. 1). This results in a relatively increased height of the medial as compared to the lateral joint surface. This is opposite to the usual anatomy in the osteoarthritis varus knee.

Second, as seen on the lateral radiograph, there is a loss of the normal posterior slope of the proximal tibial articular surface (Fig. 2). The articulation surface has either a relative or an absolute anterior slope.

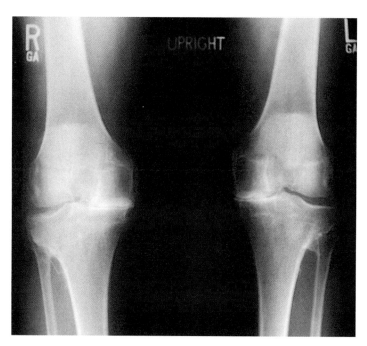

Figure 1. AP radiograph of a knee (*left*) after an HTO, showing increased valgus angulation and a relatively increased height in the medial tibial joint surface.

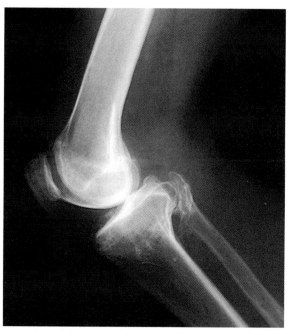

Figure 2. Lateral radiograph of a knee after an HTO, demonstrating loss of the normal posterior slope of the proximal tibia.

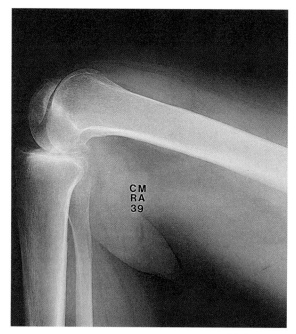

Figure 3. Lateral radiograph of a knee after an HTO in a patient with patellar baja.

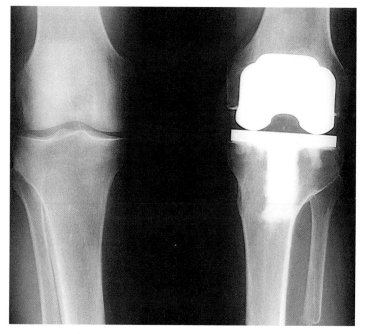

Figure 4. Thirteen year follow-up radiograph of a total knee replacement after an HTO, demonstrating the potential for impingement of a stemmed prosthesis on the sharp flare of the proximal lateral tibial cortex.

The third anatomic abnormality often present is patella infera (or baja) (Fig. 3). This may be seen in as many as 80% of patients undergoing HTO. (1,9,11).

Other, less consistent yet not less important radiographic findings that will impact on the surgical procedure include a sharp flare of the proximal lateral tibial cortex and malrotation of the articular surface (Fig. 4). Each of these anatomic changes creates technical problems that will be described in this chapter.

SURGERY

Technique

Unique exposure techniques are not needed in knees have HTO, but a few technical factors need emphasis. The skin incision used must account for previous HTO incisions (Fig. 5). Patella baja may make eversion of the extensor mechanism more difficult. If eversion is difficult, excision of a thickened fat pad and scar tissue between the patellar tendon and the proximal tibia can be helpful. The patellar tendon is often adherent by scarring to the anterior tibia, and this scarred area should be elevated. An early lateral release or elevation of the patellar tendon from the tibial tubercle by one-third of its attachment can be done (Fig. 6). Rarely is a quadriceps turndown or tubercle elevation necessary for exposure.

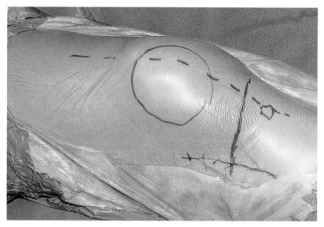

Figure 5. Standard skin incision, showing the proximity of a previous HTO scar.

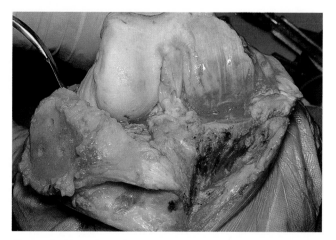

Figure 6. Eversion of the patella was facilitated by elevating scarred patellar tendon from the anterior tibia and elevating the patellar tendon from the tibial tubercle by one-third of its attachment.

The tibia should be retracted anterior to the femur. Release of the medial capsule from the anterior midline to the posterior midline will allow this to be done (Fig. 7). Fixation devices used for HTO are not routinely removed. This is done only if the fixation device interferes with the proximal tibial cut or with fixation of the tibial component (Fig. 8).

The femur usually has no adverse anatomic deformation after an HTO and standard femoral cuts (Fig. 9). After the cuts are completed and a trial femur is placed, remaining osteophytes and soft tissue are removed from the intercondylar notch. This prevents any impingement of the plastic eminence on osteophytes (Fig. 10).

We use an intramedullary cutting guide and so will illustrate the tibial cuts using this instrument. An extramedually guide can also be successfully used, and the

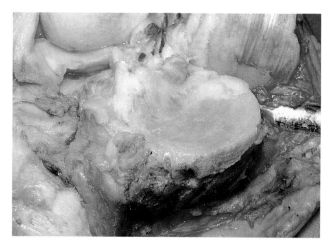

Figure 7. The tibia is retracted anterior to the femur after release of the medial capsule from anterior midline to posterior in the midline.

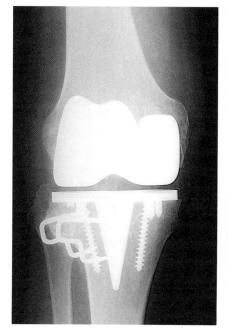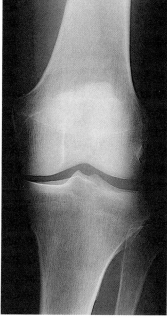

Figure 8. Postoperative AP radiograph showing previous fixation devices partially removed with a cutting bur so as not to interfere with tibial component.

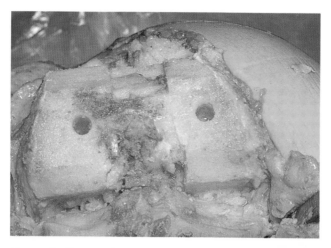

Figure 9. Femur after standard cuts have been made.

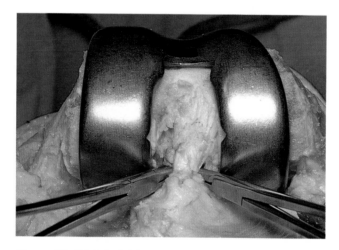

Figure 10. Distal trial femur in place, with osteophytes in the notch having been removed so that the eminence of the tibial component will not impinge on it.

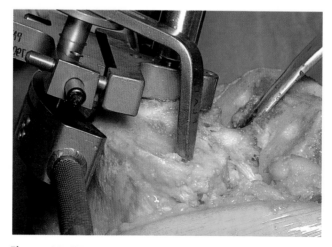

Figure 11. The tibial cutting guide has been centered over the medial side of the tibial tubercle, with the stylus on the lateral joint surface.

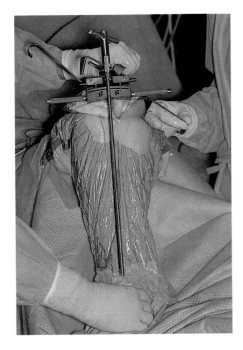

Figure 12. The extramedullary alignment rod points to the medial side of the ankle, over the anterior tibialis tendon.

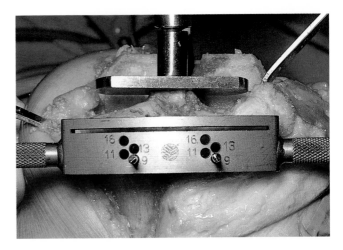

Figure 13. Proximal tibial cutting jig and intramedullary aligner, demonstrating a neutral cut.

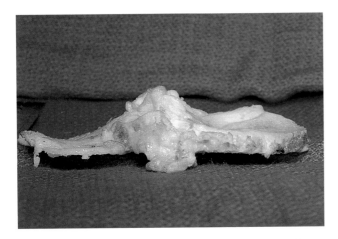

Figure 14. Postresection specimen showing greater bone resection medially than laterally.

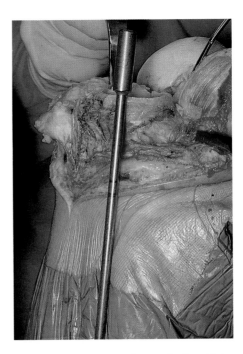

Figure 15. Lateral view of the tibia showing loss of the posterior slope after an HTO.

principles are the same. The intramedullary guide is placed and centered over the medial side of the tibial tubercle, with the stylus on the lateral joint surface (Fig. 11). The extramedullary alignment rod should point to the medial side of the ankle over the anterior tibialis tendon. This will achieve a neutral cut with regard to varus and valgus (Fig. 12). More bone will be removed medially than laterally, which is opposite to what happens in the case of a routine primary varus knee (Fig. 13). Furthermore, the cut should remove minimal bone laterally because the metaphyseal bone is of decreased thickness as a result of the previous HTO (Fig. 14). Compensation for remaining defects of the lateral condylar bone, if minimal, is made with cement, or if the defects are severe, with a bone graft or a wedged prosthesis. Please refer to Chapter 9 on bone grafts.

The second defect of the tibia is loss of the posterior slope. The posterior slope of the cut is determined by the medial rod. The anteroposterior slope can be measured with a rod that runs from the medial malleolus to the midline of the tibia (Fig. 15). The cutting guide must create at least a 90° cut and preferably a posterior slope of 5° to 8°. Our intramedullary guide provides a 7° posterior slope. Minimal or no bone is removed anteriorly; the greatest amount of bone is resected posteriorly (Fig. 16). This too is in contrast to what happens in a routine primary total knee replacement. The posterior slope can also be evaluated by an intramedullary alignment guide, which will measure the varus–valgus and anterior–posterior angles (Fig. 17).

After HTO, the intramedullary canal is displaced from its ordinary position, with an overhanging lateral condyle. If a stemmed tibial component is to be used, as is done with almost all cemented tibias, a preoperative template should be

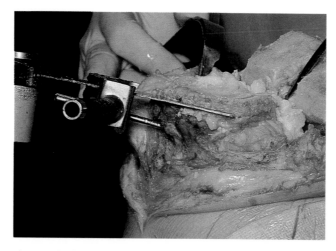

Figure 16. Lateral view of the tibia showing minimal bone removal anteriorly and greater removal posteriorly in order to restore the normal posterior slope.

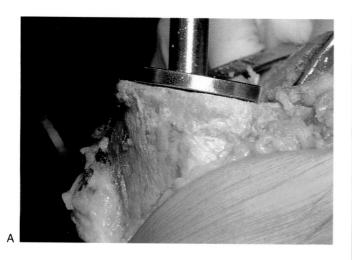

A

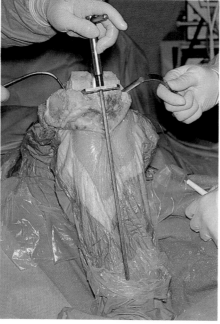

B

Figure 17. A: Lateral view of the proximal tibia after cut, showing restoration of the posterior slope. **B:** Anterior view of the tibia with an intramedullary guide and extramedullary alignment rod, demonstrating a neutral varus/valgus cut as the rod points to the anterior tibialis tendon.

placed on the anteroposterior radiograph to insure that the stem will go into the bone correctly (Fig. 18). If the tibial canal is offset so much medially that the stem does not fit into the canal, a different tibial component is required. Either a custom component with an offset stem or a stemless component is needed. To place the stem into the canal, the tibial template for the stem hole should be placed as far medially as possible without overhang. The tibial template used to make the stem hole must be positioned correctly both medially and rotationally (Fig. 19). The template handle is placed so that the external guide rod points to the anterior tibialis tendon (Fig. 20). We put a methylene blue mark on the anterior tibia for future reference in centering the tibial component (Fig. 21). In knees undergoing routine primary arthroplasty the correct rotational position aligns the tibial eminence to the medial side of the tibial tubercle. This landmark may not be correct after HTO, since the tubercle may be malaligned.

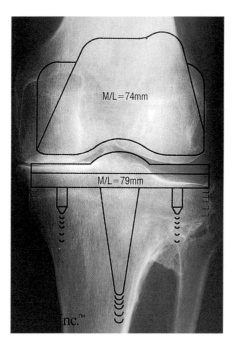

Figure 18. Preoperative AP radiograph with a template overlying the proximal tibia to ensure stem fit.

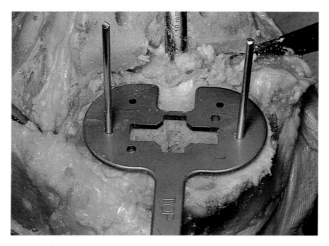

Figure 19. The proximal tibial template is positioned as medially as possible without overhang.

Fixation devices may prevent correct stem placement. If so, the fixation device is partially or completely removed. Partial removal is done by cutting the metal with a metal-cutting bur (Fig. 8).

Prior to trial reduction, posterior osteophytes are removed. A lamina spreader is used for exposure and a curved osteotome is used to remove excess bone (Fig. 22). Capsular release for a tight posterior capsule (with a flexion contracture) can also be done with this exposure (Fig. 23).

A trial reduction is performed, alignment is assessed, and medial–lateral stability is tested through a full range of motion. Adjustments of the tibial component thickness and routine soft-tissue releases are usually adequate to balance the soft tissues. In an overcorrected HTO with a valgus deformity exceeding 20° a complex ligamentous reconstruction as described by Krackow (7) or a more constrained prosthesis may be necessary.

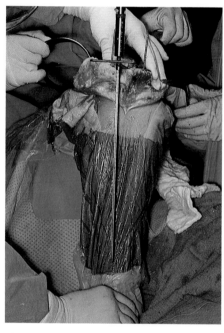

Figure 20. The tibial template handle is placed so that the external alignment rod points to the anterior tibialis tendon in order to achieve correct rotation.

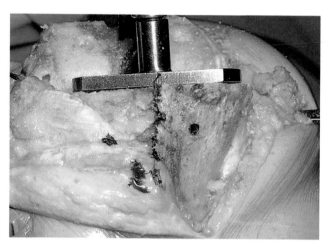

Figure 21. A methylene blue mark has been placed on the anterior tibia for future reference in centering the tibial component.

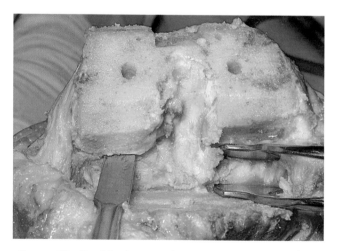

Figure 22. Residual osteophytes are removed using a lamina spreader and curved osteotome.

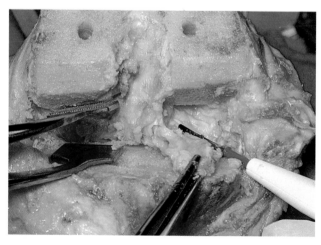

Figure 23. Excess capsule is being removed in a similar fashion.

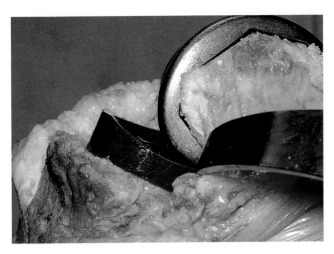

Figure 24. Lateral view of the knee demonstrating that the tibial component is anterior to the distal femur.

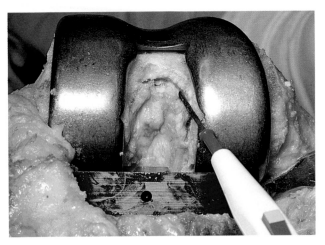

Figure 25. A partial PCL recession off the femur is performed.

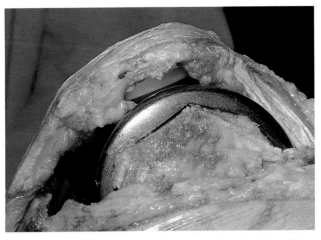

Figure 26. Lateral view of the knee showing the tibia properly seated under the femur, with the patellar tendon reduced.

At 90° flexion, when viewed from the side, the tibial component should seat under the femoral component such that the articular surface of the femoral component is seated just posterior to central in the plastic of the tibial component and the distal femoral surface overlays the anterior third of the tibial surface. This is best judged with the patella reduced, because an everted patella can displace the tibia anteriorly. If the tibial component is largely anterior to the distal femur, and the femoral articulating surface is seated on the posterior edge of the plastic, a recession of the posterior cruciate ligament from its femoral attachment is done until the correct relationship is achieved (Figs. 24–27) (8).

The third problem present with previous HTO is patella baja. It is difficult to compensate for this. The simplest maneuver is to use a smaller patella component.

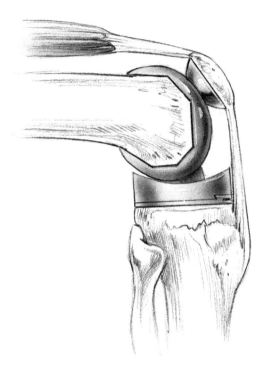
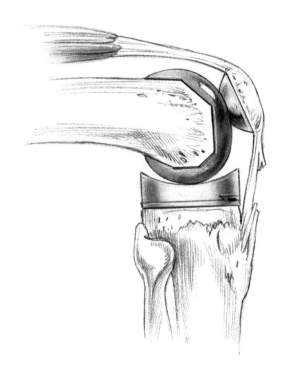

Figure 27. Lateral view of the knee after a partial PCL recession showing the tibial component centered and seated properly under the femoral component.

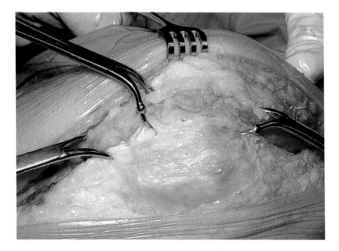

Figure 28. Anterior view of the knee in extension, with the medial retinaculum reapproximated with three towel clips.

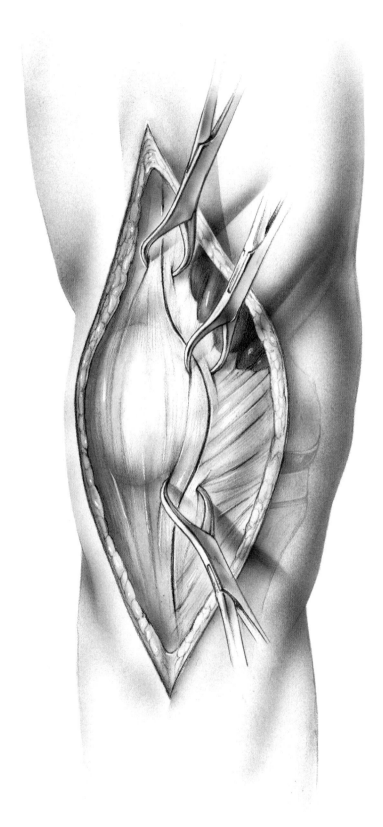

Figure 29. Anterior view of the knee in extension with the medial retinaculum reapproximated with three towel clips.

Figure 30. Anterior view of the knee in flexion with
good patellar tracking, no tilt, and no gapping of reti-
naculur reapproximation. In this case a lateral release
is not indicated.

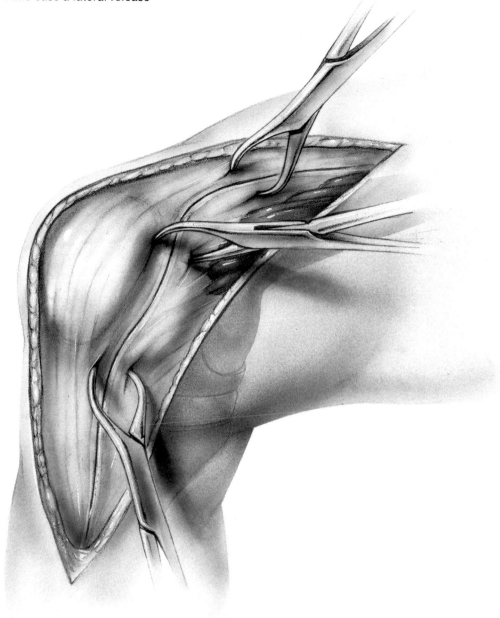

Additionally, the tibia can be cut up to 5 mm deeper, with little removal of the
bone from the femur to lower the joint line or at least insure that the joint line is
not elevated.

To assess patellar tracking, the "no thumbs" test, as described by Scott, has
been the traditional test and not truly accurate when active muscle contraction is
present. We test tracking dynamically through a full range of motion, with the
medial retinaculum reapproximated with three towel clips (Figs. 28 and 29). If the
patella tracks centrally through a full range of motion with tilt or excessive tension
on the medial retinaculum, then a lateral release is not indicated (Fig. 30). If not,
a lateral release is performed (Fig. 31). The wounds are closed in routine fashion.

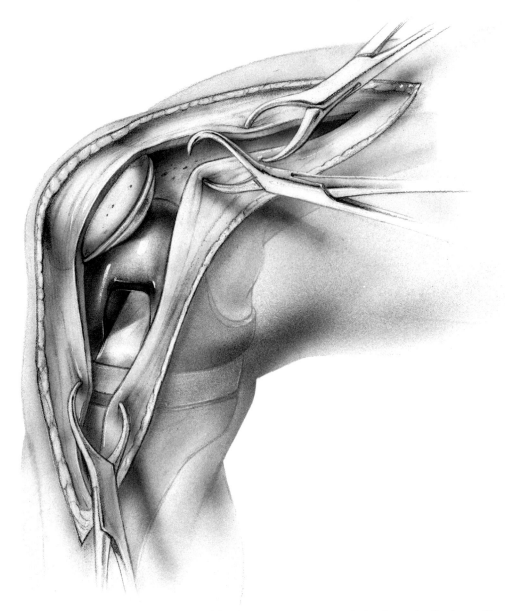

Figure 31. Anterior view of the knee in flexion with poor patellar tracking, patellar tilt, and gapping of the retinacular reapproximation. In this case a lateral release is indicated.

POSTOPERATIVE MANAGEMENT

Standard protocols for postoperative rehabilitation are followed after an HTO. Cemented total knee arthroplasties are allowed to bear full weight and the patients rapidly progressed to walking with a cane in 5 to 7 days. Noncemented total knee arthroplasties are subjected to partial weight bearing for 4 weeks (Fig. 32). If bone grafts are used, caution is extended for longer periods to allow biologic incorporation. The larger graft will require longer protection, even for as long as one year.

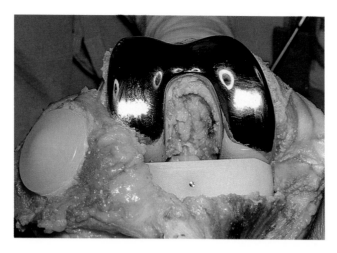

Figure 32. Postoperative anterior view with a cemented Apollo Knee (Intermedics Orthopedics Inc., Austin, TX) in place.

Our expectations after a total knee replacement following a previous tibial osteotomy are for an excellent result. The overall results are not compromised when compared with those of a primary total knee replacement.

COMPLICATIONS

The complications of total knee replacement after tibial osteotomy are the same as those to be anticipated after any total knee arthroplasty. However, there are some complications that may be more likely to occur after tibial osteotomy than with a primary total knee replacement. These would include: (i) Rupture of the patellar tendon in association with patella baja and the difficulty of surgical exposure. (ii) Limitation of motion associated with patella baja and potential impingement of the inferior pole of the patella against the anterior flange of the tibial component. (iii) A bone defect in the posterior lateral corner, which may require augmentation with bone grafts or wedges, and may therefore create the problems of compensating for this defect. (iv) Ligament balancing may be a problem with excessive overcorrection of the previous tibial osteotomy. Recognition of the soft-tissue sleeve deformity will help prevent this problem. (v) The potential for malalignment of the extremity is increased because of the prior osteotomy and valgus alignment of the tibia. Care must be taken to carefully align the tibial osteotomy cut in order to prevent a malalignment.

ILLUSTRATIVE CASE FOR TECHNIQUE

A 68-year-old male is 8 years past a proximal tibial osteotomy for medial femoral osteoarthritis. He had obtained good relief of his symptoms for the first 5 years, but during the past 3 years has had increasing difficulty that has become unresponsive to conservative therapy. A total knee replacement was advised, in recognition of a significant deformity in the proximal tibia and the surgical technique and dissection will be more difficult (Fig. 33).

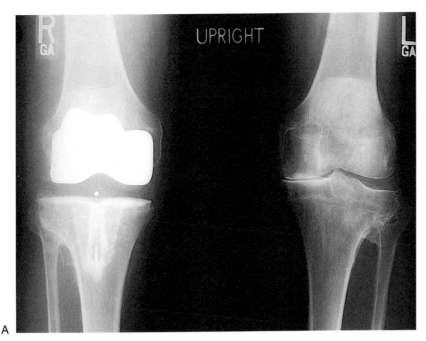
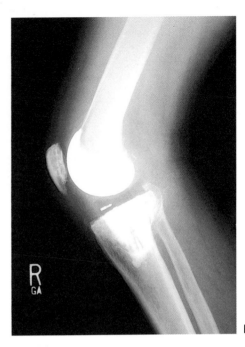

A
B

Figure 33. A: This patient has a total knee replacement on the right, which is functioning satisfactorily, and a left knee on which a proximal tibial osteotomy was done 8 years previously. **B:** Postoperative lateral radiograph demonstrating good position of the total knee replacement and a relatively normal anatomic position of the patella.

RECOMMENDED READING

1. Annuniato, A., Roraveck, C. H., Bourne, R. B., and Abyan, P. M.: Total knee arthroplasty following high tibial osteotomy for osteoarthritis. *J. Arthroplasty* (Suppl 4): S11–S17, 1989.
2. Coventry, M. B.: Upper tibial osteotomy for gonarthrosis. The evolution of the operation in the last 18 years and long-term results. *Orthop. Clin. North Am.* 10: 191–210, 1979.
3. Coventry, M. B.: Current Concepts: Upper Tibial Osteotomy for Osteoarthritis. *J. Bone Joint Surg.* 67A: 1136–1140, 1985.
4. Herningou, P. H., Medevielle, D., Debeyre, J., and Goutallier, D.: Proximal tibial osteotomy for osteoarthritis with varus deformity. *J. Bone Joint Surg.* 69A: 332–354, 1987.
5. Insall, J. N., Joseph, P. H., and Msika, C.: High tibial osteotomy for varus gonarthrosis. A long-term follow-up study. *J. Bone Joint Surg.* 66A: 1040–1048, 1984.
6. Katz, M. D., Hungerford, D. S., Krackow, K. A., and Lennox, P. W.: Results of total knee arthroplasty after failed proximal tibial osteotomy for osteoarthritis. *J. Bone Joint Surg.* 69A: 225–233, 1987.
7. Krackow, K. A., and Holtgrewe, J. L.: Experience with a new technique for managing severely overcorrected valgus high tibial osteotomy at total knee arthroplasty. *Clin. Orthop.* 258:213–224, 1990.
8. Ritter, M. A., Faris, P. M., and Keating, E. M.: Posterior cruciate ligament balancing during total knee arthroplasty. *J. Arthop.* 3(4): 323–326, 1988.
9. Scuderi, G. R., Windsor, R. E., and Insall, J. N.: Observations on patellar height after proximal tibial osteotomy. *J Bone Joint Surg.* 71A: 245–248, 1989.
10. Staeheli, J. W., Cass, J. R., and Morrey, B. F.: Condylar total knee arthroplasty after failed proximal tibial osteotomy. *J. Bone Joint Surg.* 69A: 28–31, 1987.
11. Windsor, R. E., Insall, J. N., and Vince, K. G.: Technical considerations of total knee arthroplasty after proximal tibial osteotomy. *J. Bone Joint Surg.* 70A: 547–554, 1988.

PART III

Revision Total Knee Arthroplasty

Master Techniques in Orthopaedic Surgery,
KNEE ARTHROPLASTY, edited by P. A. Lotke,
Raven Press, Ltd., New York © 1995.

13

Revision Total Knee Arthroplasty for Aseptic Loosening

James A. Rand

INDICATIONS/CONTRAINDICATIONS

Aseptic loosening of a total knee arthroplasty has been the most frequent mode of failure of early designs of such arthroplasies (12) (Fig. 1). Failure of current condylar knee arthroplasties occurs much less frequently than that of older hinged or resurfacing prostheses (16) (Fig. 2). The 10-year survivorship of total condylar-type prostheses has been in the range of 90% or better (14,16). The mechanical reasons for failure of early implant designs, caused by overstressing of the bone–cement interface, are largely resolved with current implant designs. At present, failure of total knee arthroplasty by aseptic loosening occurs with uncemented implants, through failure of bone ingrowth and persistent pain, or in both cemented and cementless knees in relation to biologic factors resulting from particulate wear debris, usually from polyethylene (Fig. 3). Particulate debris elicits a marked foreign-body response, with secondary resorption of bone and loosening of the implant (Fig. 4). Such biologic mechanisms of failure are being recognized with increasing frequency.

Failure of total knee arthroplasty can result from one of three basic mechanisms: poor implant design, improper patient selection, or incorrect surgical technique. Poor implant design is less often seen with current condylar knee arthroplasties than with older designs. Problems remain with cementless implants providing inadequate fixation on the tibial plateau (Fig. 5). The addition of auxiliary fixation mechanisms, such as screws, has provided the potential for polyethylene wear

J. A. Rand, M.D.: Division of Orthopedic Surgery, Mayo Clinic Scottsdale, Scottsdale, AZ 85259.

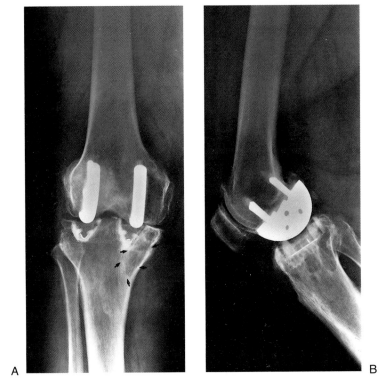

Figure 1. AP **(A)** and lateral **(B)** radiographs of loose polycentric total knee arthroplasty. *Arrows* indicate area of osteolysis.

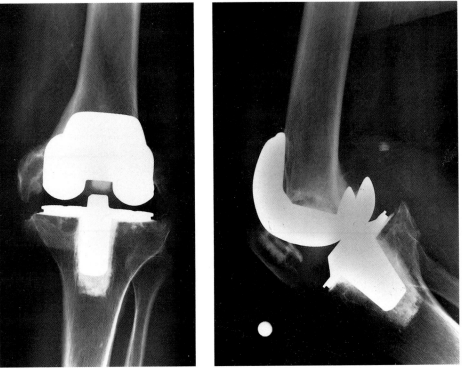

Figure 2. AP **(A)** and lateral **(B)** radiographs of a loose Insall–Burstein total knee arthroplasty.

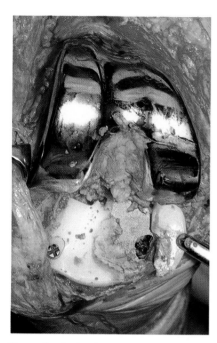

Figure 3. Polyethylene wear of metal backing of the tibial component of porous-coated anatomic total knee arthroplasty.

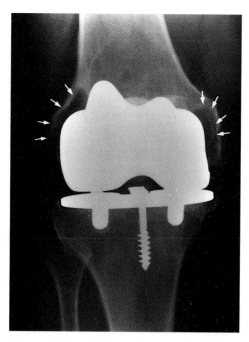

Figure 4. Osteolysis of femur *(arrows)* from polyethylene debris following porous-coated anatomic total knee arthroplasty.

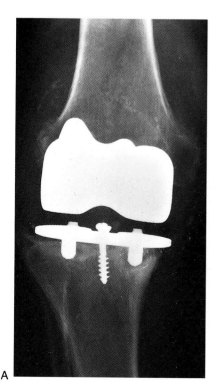

A

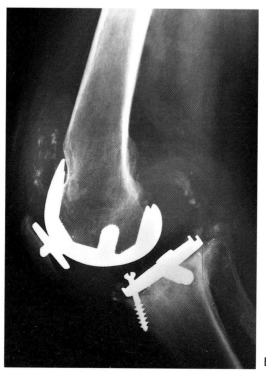

B

Figure 5. AP **(A)** and lateral **(B)** radiographs of subsidence of cementless porous-coated anatomic prosthesis.

debris to gain access to the interfaces between bone and the components of the arthroplasty, which may cause biologic loosening as a long-term consequence (3). Inadequate polyethylene thickness has led to significant delamination and wear in some designs, such as the Porous-Coated Anatomic knee, and has resulted in both biologic and mechanical failure. In the absence of technical errors, mechanical loosening of the tibial component of current cemented knee arthroplasties occurs infrequently, as an isolated event. Mechanical failure results from inappropriate application of the implant. Loosening may occur from arthroplasty fixation to an area of deficient bone. The young athletic individual who is selected for knee arthroplasty and who returns to a high level of activity will overstress the knee, causing the arthroplasty to loosen. The patient with massive obesity may put excessive stress on the implant, resulting in mechanical failure or loosening of the device.

The most frequent mechanism of failure of a knee arthroplasty relates to incorrect surgical technique. Failure to correct overall limb alignment and obtain proper component position, soft-tissue balance, and adequate range of motion will result in a suboptimal result for the patient. Malalignment has been correlated with mechanical loosening of the implant in many different designs (2,4,6,9,15). Clearly, a combination of these three basic mechanisms may be operative, as in the poorly performed arthroplasty in the incorrectly selected patient. When confronted with the patient with a loose total knee prosthesis, it is essential to determine the reason or reasons for failure so as not to repeat the causative errors at the time of the revision procedure.

PREOPERATIVE PLANNING

Evaluation of the patient with a failed total knee arthroplasty should begin with a detailed history and physical examination, seeking potential reasons for the failure. The history must include all prior surgical procedures and any operative complications that occurred in association with the prior arthroplasty. The physical examination must include a detailed evaluation of the soft tissues about the knee. Many of these patients will have had multiple prior incisions. Therefore, incision placement and quality of the underlying skin must be carefully assessed (Fig. 6). In cases of multiple prior surgical incisions that criss-cross over the anterior aspect of the knee, or patients with deficient soft tissues that have been skingrafted, it is wise to have plastic surgical consultation preoperatively in order to

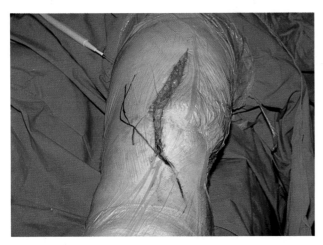

Figure 6. In the knee with multiple prior incisions, usually the most lateral anterior incision should be utilized to preserve the blood supply of the skin.

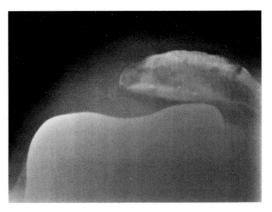

Figure 7. Merchant radiograph of dislocated patella following total knee arthroplasty.

plan for the exposure and for management of any soft-tissue deficiencies that may occur following surgery. The status of the extensor mechanism must be carefully reviewed. If the patella is subluxed or dislocated and the extensor mechanism is poorly functioning, the patient will not have a satisfactory result following the revision procedure (Fig. 7). Plans will be needed to realign the extensor mechanism at the time of surgical revision. The patient who has sustained a patellar tendon rupture presents a very difficult problem for salvage, and revision surgery may be fraught with a high failure rate in this group of patients (11). The status of the collateral and cruciate ligaments must be carefully assessed on the basis of a careful physical examination, since the presence or absence of these ligaments will influence the choice of the revision prosthesis.

When planning for revision surgery it is essential to have appropriate radiographs. True anteroposterior and lateral radiographs of the knee with radiographic markers for magnification are very helpful in assessing bone size for a subsequent revision prosthesis (Fig. 8). A full length radiograph of the lower extremity is helpful in determining overall limb alignment, and is valuable in the patient with

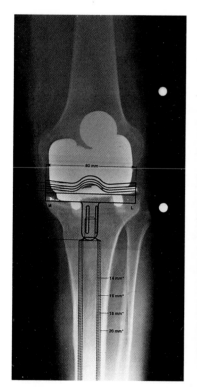
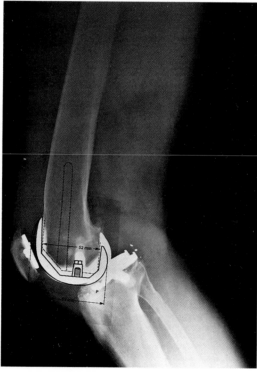
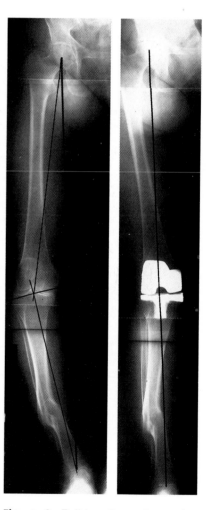

Figure 8. AP **(left)** and lateral **(right)** radiographs with magnification markers for preoperative templating.

Figure 9. Full-length radiographs of the lower extremity are useful in planning for the patient with a prior fracture deformity in the tibia or femur. **Left:** AP radiograph of medial compartment osteoarthritis and varus malunion of tibia. **Right:** AP radiograph after total knee arthroplasty.

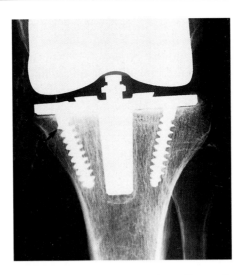

Figure 10. AP fluoroscopic radiograph of interface adjacent to loose, cementless tibial component of AMK (DuPuy, Warsaw, IN) total knee arthroplasty. There is fracture of the medial screw *(arrow)*.

bowing of the femur or tibia or who has had a prior fracture deformity in the femoral or tibial shaft (Fig. 9). A true lateral radiograph of the opposite knee if it has not undergone arthroplasty is helpful in sizing for the revision prosthesis. The revision prosthesis should be of a size that restores the normal anterior and posterior dimensions of the femur as well as the joint line. This results in restoration of normal collateral ligament kinematics and knee function. Restoration of femoral size may necessitate the use of or planning for augmented implants to deal with bone deficiency. In the case of the prosthesis with subtle loosening, fluoroscopically positioned radiographs of the interfaces can be very helpful in defining radiolucent lines that may not otherwise be visualized on routine radiographs (Fig. 10) (7). Aseptic loosening must always be differentiated from that of low-grade infection, and differential technetium-99 and indium-111 bone scans can be useful in this determination, with 82% accuracy (8).

It is necessary to carefully assess the amount of remaining bone stock. Bone loss often involves the distal and posterior aspect of the femur, and can vary in extent in both locations as well as from medial to lateral. Tibial bone loss can be either central, peripheral, or combined, and may need to be corrected. Patellar bone loss should not be ignored. Bone loss in the patella can be substantial to the point at which patellar resurfacing is not feasible. Generally, if there is less than 12 mm of bone remaining on the patella, placement of another patellar prosthesis is unlikely to be successful and poses the risk of patellar fracture. In these instances the alternatives of patelloplasty or patellectomy should be considered. In planning for the revision prosthesis, one must also consider the degree of constraint that is necessary, as in the case of posterior stabilization in a posterior-cruciate-deficient knee or a constrained condylar device in the case of an absent collateral ligament. The choice of prosthesis will have to take into consideration the bone loss and need for augmentation on the femoral or tibial side. Finally, one must decide whether an intramedullary stem will be required. With modular designs, the alternative of adding a stem to the implant is possible, with the choice of either press-fitting the stem or cementing the stem (Fig. 11). An extended intramedullary stem should be utilized to relieve stress on deficient metaphyseal bone. If the stem is cemented, the entire metaphysis is stress-shielded for the length of the cemented stem (1). Therefore, some surgeons use press-fit stems in an attempt to relieve the stress-shielding. Whether or not cemented or cementless stems

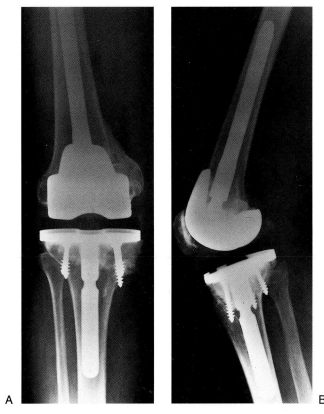

Figure 11. AP **(A)** and lateral **(B)** radiographs of revision total knee arthroplasty with the Genesis prosthesis, using a press-fit femoral and tibial stem.

should be used in revision surgery is unclear at present, and awaits a randomized prospective study.

I prefer to use an uncemented long stem for fixation of deficient bone. A long stem would be utilized if more than 50% of the tibial or femoral condyle requires bone grafting or if there is a peripheral deficiency that requires filling with bone graft or an augmentation wedge. A stem will be selected at surgery that will provide a press-fit into the medullary canal and will extend past any potential stress risers in the cortex. In general, a stem length of approximately 100 mm on the tibia and 100 to 150 mm on the femur will be adequate. Stems are selected for cementing primarily in elderly patients or if an adequate press-fit cannot be achieved because of extreme osteoporosis or poor bone quality. A stem would also be considered for cement fixation if massive allografting of the distal femur or proximal tibia were required, or for rotational stability of the stem within the medullary canal.

SURGERY

The technique of revision consists of four basic steps. (i) Exposure of the prosthesis; (ii) removal of the old implant; (iii) preparation of the bone; and (iv) insertion of a new, revision prosthesis. Exposure of the total knee arthroplasty for revision can be difficult. An anteromedial longitudinal incision over the knee is preferred. This approach should be followed by an anteromedial arthrotomy. There are no indications for a subvastus approach or anterolateral approach in the revision of a knee replacement. A great deal of scar tissue is usually present, and these alternative exposures will be most difficult and should be avoided. The problem in selecting the approach to the revision of a knee replacement relates to prior surgical incisions. Often the patient will have more than one prior surgical incision, which makes the choice of the exposure more difficult. In general, the most lateral anterior longitudinal incision that will allow exposure of the knee is the safest to utilize.

Technique

An anterolateral longitudinal incision through the skin and subcutaneous tissue can be followed by elevation of a full-thickness flap of skin and subcutaneous tissue to maintain its blood supply. This exposure can then be followed by an anteromedial arthrotomy incision, and wound healing can be expected. It must

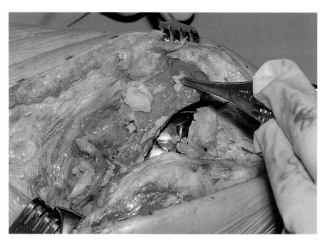

Figure 12. Hypertrophic synovium and scar encountered in revision of total knee arthroplasty.

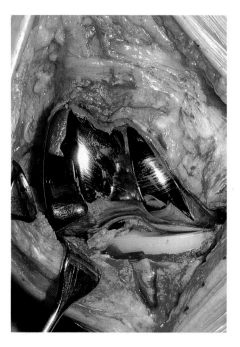

Figure 13. Excision of scar begins in the suprapatellar pouch, followed by the medial and lateral gutters.

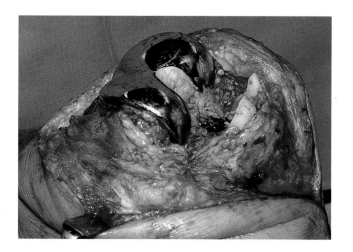

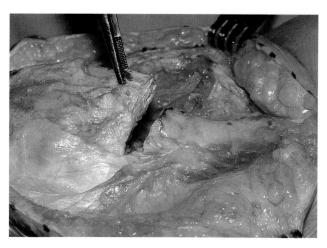

Figure 14. Medial soft-tissue release from the tibia allows external rotation of the tibia and decreases tension on the extensor mechanism.

Figure 15. V-Y quadricepsplasty for exposure of the stiff knee.

be emphasized that if a flap is elevated it must be full-thickness skin and subcutaneous tissue without undermining of the skin, or skin sloughing will occur.

The proper level of dissection is the level of the junction of the superficial and deep fascia. Once an anteromedial arthrotomy has been made, there will be extensive scar tissue within the joint (Fig. 12). The scar tissue must be thoroughly excised in order to gain soft-tissue mobility and motion of the knee for the revision procedure. A systematic approach of sharp dissection with excision of hypertrophic synovium and scar tissue from the suprapatellar pouch and medial and lateral gutters should be employed (Fig. 13). Often, a lateral retinacular release will assist in gaining exposure for the revision and decreasing tension on the extensor mechanism. An attempt should be made to preserve the superior lateral geniculate vessels. A medial soft-tissue release from the tibia can be performed to improve exposure. The release consists of a dissection of the soft tissues from the tibia, releasing the superficial and deep portions of the medial collateral ligament and pes anserinus tendons as a sleeve (Fig. 14). The release done for exposure of the knee in revision surgery is similar to the release done for a knee with severe varus. The soft-tissue release will allow external rotation of the tibia in reference to the femur, and allow subluxation of the extensor mechanism laterally to expose the joint. This exposure has not resulted in postoperative instability after revision once the soft-tissue sleeve has been closed.

Dissection at the attachment of the patellar tendon to the tibia should be minimal. A patellar tendon avulsion presents a tremendous problem in terms of salvage and is best avoided (11). In the stiff knee that does not allow flexion, it may be necessary to perform either a long tibial tuberosity osteotomy (17) or a V-Y quadricepsplasty with proximal turndown of the extensor mechanism (Fig. 15) (13). However, it must be emphasized that neither of these approaches is often required, and that most knees can be dealt with by the exposure techniques described above. Once the knee has been adequately exposed, the prosthesis will need to be removed. With most current designs the tibial polyethylene is modular and can be removed from the metal-backed tibial component, allowing improved exposure of the knee.

Dissection will have to be performed at the interface between the prosthesis and cement or prosthesis and bone on the femoral component. Removal of the femoral component is done first, since it will provide better exposure for the tibia, which is harder to mobilize. Dissection should be performed adjacent to the femoral component in order to minimize any loss of bone from the distal femur.

A thin, flexible osteotome placed into this interface has proven to be quite useful in freeing the femoral component with minimal loss of bone (Fig. 16). Alternative techniques would include the use of a high-speed cutting instrument, such as a Midas-Rex bur, or the use of a Gigli saw to free the interfaces (Fig. 17). Angled osteotomes are also quite useful in freeing around the condylar portion of the femoral component (Fig. 18). Once all the interfaces have been freed, the femoral component can usually be tapped loose from the underlying bone with minimal loss of bone stock (Fig. 19).

Attention is next directed toward the tibial component. If the tibial component is not loose, then a similar technique is utilized for removal of the tibia as for the femur. Flexible osteotomes are used at the interface on the medial side of the plateau. On the lateral side, exposure can be more difficult. A Gigli saw placed over the posterolateral corner of the tibial component and worked back toward the central stem will often free the condylar portion of the metal-backed component (Fig. 20). Once this is freed the tibial component can often be extracted. If the tibial component still cannot be freed, it may be necessary to section the metallic tibial plateau adjacent to the stem with a diamond saw so as to allow access to free the stem. This would most likely be necessary in the case of a porous stem that had been cemented and was securely fixed about the central cement. If the tibial component is all polyethylene it can be mobilized in a similar

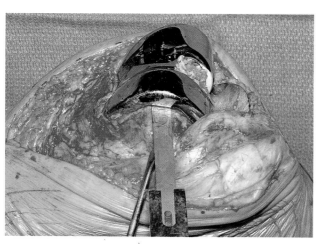

Figure 16. Flexible osteotome is used to dissect at the implant–bone interface of the femoral component.

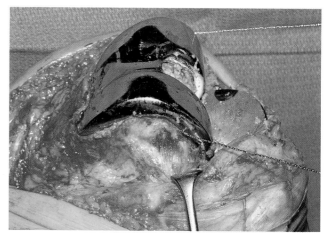

Figure 17. A Gigli saw can be used to free the prosthesis–bone interface.

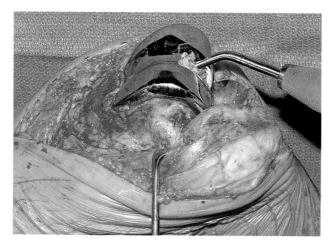

Figure 18. An angled osteotome is useful for reaching the distal interface of the femoral component.

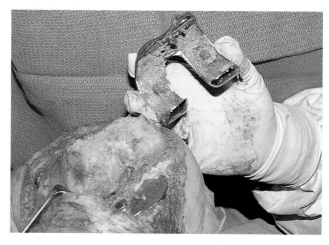

Figure 19. Removed porous-coated femoral component with minimal loss of bone.

manner under the plateau, and the central peg can be sectioned with an osteotome (Fig. 21). This allows easy access to the central peg for removal. It must be emphasized that the goal is not only removal of the implants but preservation of remaining bone stock. Once the implants have been removed, attention will be directed toward the patella. If the patellar implant is a domed design and it is securely fixed, it should usually be left, since this design will generally articulate with most other femoral designs. If the patellar component must be removed, great care must be taken to avoid loss of patellar bone stock. In the case of a metal-backed patellar component with secure ingrowth, it may be necessary to section the porous pegs with a diamond saw to remove the metal plate and allow access to the underlying pegs.

Once the implants have been removed, some cement will remain fixed to bone. The cement can be easily removed with osteotomes or a rongeur. A high-speed drill, such as a Midas-Rex bur, can be quite useful in removing cement around the fixation lugs of a femoral component, the central stem of a tibial component, and the central peg of a patellar component without risking additional loss of bone. Once the implant and cement have been removed there will remain a fibrous tissue membrane on the bone surfaces. This membrane can best be identified after a high-speed pulsating lavage of the bone surfaces (Fig. 22). The fibrous membrane can then be removed with a small bur. A meticulous debridement back to healthy

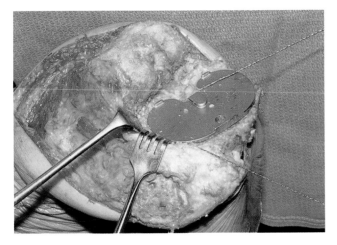

Figure 20. A Gigli saw is used to free the lateral aspect of the tibial component.

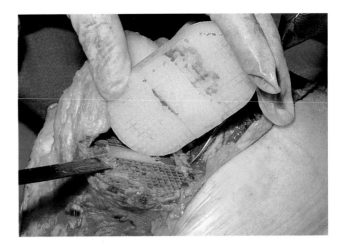

Figure 21. The central peg of an all polyethylene component can be cut with an osteotome to allow removal.

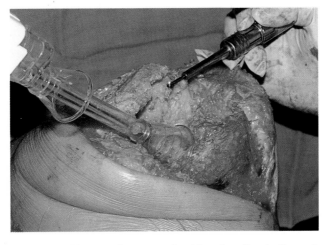

Figure 22. Fibrous tissue can best be visualized after pulsatile lavage, allowing its removal with a small bur.

bone is essential in order to have good bone into which to fix the revision prosthesis.

There often remains thickened capsule and synovium with scarring in the posterior aspect of the knee. This will need to be excised back to flexible tissue (Fig. 23). If this thickened scar tissue is not excised, the knee will tend to hinge on the posterior scar tissue, resulting in abnormal kinematics. Clearly, both the collateral ligaments and neurovascular structures must be carefully preserved during this dissection. Once all scar tissue has been excised and the bone surfaces cleaned, planning can be done for the revision prosthesis (Fig. 24).

The objective of fitting a revision prosthesis should be to restore the joint line, provide equal flexion–extension spaces, and permit at least 90 degrees of knee flexion. The femoral component in its interior dimension should fit the remaining femoral bone. With modular-implant designs, the potential exists for augmenting the implant intraoperatively to fit the remaining bone and yet fill the soft-tissue spaces.

Two basic bone cuts are universal for most knee arthroplasty prostheses: (i) the distal femoral and (ii) the proximal tibial cuts. The proximal tibia should be cut at a 90-degree coronal orientation, with the degree of posterior slope depending upon the revision prosthesis selected. The femoral cut will usually have to be made at a valgus angulation of 7 degrees to accommodate the stems of most revision implants. However, there are some femoral revision components that have 5- or 9-degree angled stems, and the implant selected will determine the angle of cut on the distal femur. If no femoral stem will be utilized, then an overall assessment of the mechanical and anatomic axis of the femur can be used to determine the angle of femoral resection, as in the case of primary arthroplasty. The surgeon must remember that the bone cuts performed at the prior arthroplasty may be incorrect, making it essential to check all of the cut surfaces. The distal femur is usually assessed first. Since most total-knee-arthroplasty instrumentation systems rely on the posterior femoral condyles for rotational alignment, the first problem the surgeon will recognize is the absence of these landmarks. The femoral epicondyles provide a good secondary reference point for overall prosthetic alignment (Fig. 25). These should be identified and the medial and lateral epicondyles marked with a Kocher clamp. The lateral femoral epicondyle lies slightly posterior to the medial femoral epicondyle. The epicondyles also provide a useful reference for joint-line positioning with the joint line lying approximately 2.5 cm distal to the femoral epicondyles. An initial drill hole is made to open the medullary canal of the distal femur, and the intramedullary alignment jig should then be placed,

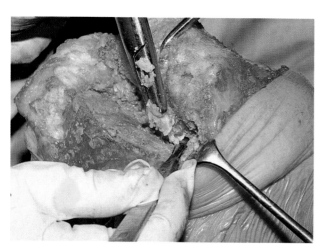

Figure 23. Thickened scar must be removed from the posterior capsule to allow soft-tissue gliding.

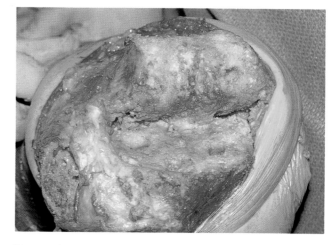

Figure 24. Bone reappearance after thorough debridement.

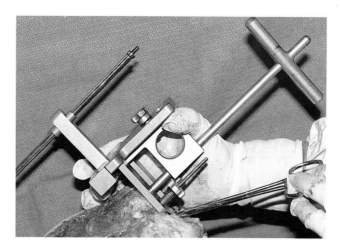

Figure 25. Use of femoral epicondyles (marked by clamps) for rotational alignment of the femoral cutting jig. The lateral femoral epicondyle lies slightly posterior to the medial femoral epicondyle.

Figure 26. Sagittal view of femoral alignment guide, using extramedullary and intramedullary alignment.

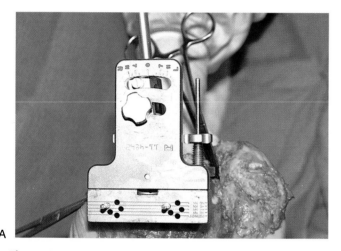

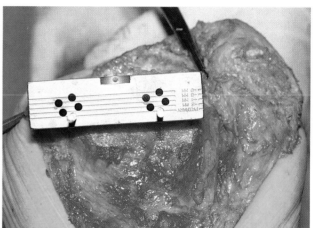

A   B

Figure 27. A: The distal femoral cutting block is fixed so that it can be moved distally, allowing a minimal bone resection. **B:** Block moved distally.

using the epicondylar references for rotational alignment. The degree of valgus selected will depend upon the implant design (Fig. 26). It is important not to resect any more bone from the distal femur than is necessary to provide a flat, level surface upon which to seat subsequent jigs and the implant. Therefore, the cutting block is not secured through the normal level for primary resection, but is instead secured through one of the more distal holes (Fig. 27). The block can then be moved distally, resulting in minimal bone resection from the distal femur. Once the femoral resection has been performed, the tibia will need to be recut. Again, the objective is minimal bone removal. If a long-stemmed tibial component is selected, an intramedullary tibial alignment guide should be utilized. If a short-stemmed tibial component will be used, then an extramedullary alignment guide may be used at the surgeon's discretion (Fig. 28).

Once the femoral and tibial surfaces have been prepared, it will be necessary to measure the flexion and extension spaces. The extension space is measured with the knee in full extension and distracted, and should be equal on the medial

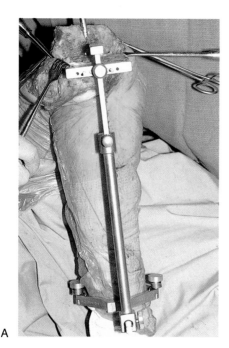

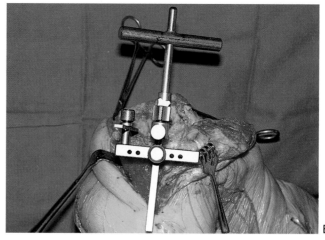

B

Figure 28. Extramedullary **(A)**, and intramedullary **(B)** cutting guide for the tibia.

A

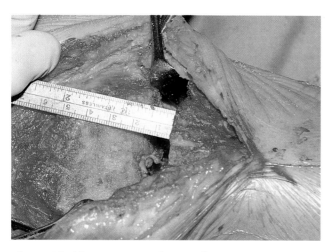

Figure 29. Measurement of extension space.

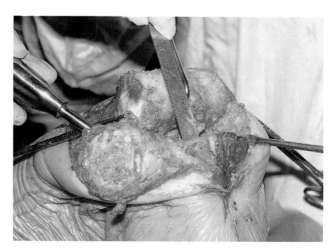

Figure 30. Measurement of flexion space at 90 degrees.

and lateral sides (Fig. 29). If the extension space is not even, then appropriate soft-tissue releases for varus or valgus deformity will have to be made to equalize the space. The knee is then flexed 90 degrees and again distracted, and the flexion space is measured (Fig. 30). If there is a differential in size between the flexion and extension spaces, implant augmentation will be necessary on either the distal or posterior aspect of the femur in order to restore an even tension between the flexion and extension gaps. The remaining bone dimensions of the femur and tibia will need to be measured. A calliper is very useful for measuring the remaining femoral and tibial bone in both the anteroposterior and medial–lateral dimensions (Fig. 31). Using the information about the flexion–extension spaces and the remaining femoral bone, the femoral component will be selected and selectively augmented so that its interior dimension matches the remaining femoral bone and its exterior dimensions fill the flexion–extension spaces. It must be remembered that the distal thickness of the femoral component determines the extension space, while the posterior thickness of the femoral component determines the flexion space. The thickness of the tibial component will affect both the flexion and extension spaces. It is also important to try and restore the joint line as closely as possible to normal. This will influence the augmentation and choice of the femoral component as well.

An additional element in the selection of a femoral component is the status of the ligaments. If a posterior-stabilized mechanism will be required, the femur will have to be prepared for the components of this mechanism. If a collateral-ligament-substituting prosthesis will be used, an appropriate housing will have to be cut on the distal femur to accommodate this design. If there is deficient bone on the femur or proximal tibia, it may be necessary to add augmentation wedges or bone grafts to deal with some of the deficiency. Additionally, intramedullary stems may be selected to relieve stress on deficient metaphyseal bone.

The preceding descriptions of exposure and bone preparation are generic for all total knee arthroplasty designs. The following description of instrumentation technique pertains to the instrumentation used for revision using the Genesis total-knee-arthroplasty system, which has proven helpful in preparing the femur for meeting the goals previously discussed. An initial guide is utilized to make the drill hole in the distal femur at the appropriate level to accommodate an intramedullary stem (Fig. 32). The choice of cutting block will be determined by the size of the implant that will be necessary for the femur. The handles of the cutting block are aligned with the epicondylar reference points on the femur, while the anterior

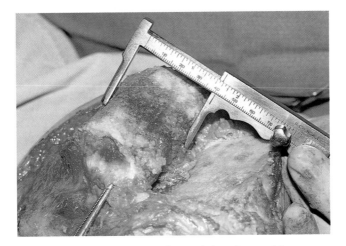

Figure 31. Measurement of remaining femoral bone.

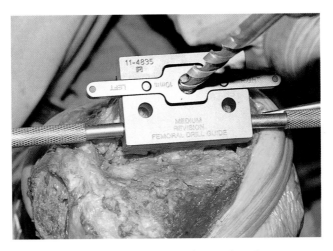

Figure 32. Drill guide for femoral stem location.

ledge of this guide lies on the anterior surface of the femur. The intramedullary canal is reamed successively using intramedullary reamers until there is a tight fit of the reamer within the canal. Drill holes are then made through the two drill holes in the block to accommodate the lugs for the subsequent cutting blocks as well as the pegs on the femoral component (Fig. 33). A revision anteroposterior cutting block can then be placed over the intramedullary reamer, which is left in place within the medullary canal (Fig. 34). The anterior and posterior surfaces of the femur can then be cut at the appropriate level to fit the prosthesis. Slots are available in the revision cutting block that permit cutting of the posterior femur to allow placement of posterior augmentation wedges of either 4 or 8 mm. The chamfers can also be cut through the revision block. If a posterior stabilized design will be utilized, then a central housing hole will need to be cut on the distal femur using the posterior stabilized instrumentation.

The modular components are then assembled and the trial reduction performed. With an appropriate trial reduction the knee should be stable and have at least 90 degrees of flexion, and there should be restoration of the correct joint line (Fig. 35). There also must be correct limb alignment and proper patellar tracking. If

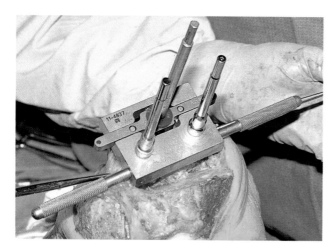

Figure 33. Reamer in femoral medullary canal and drilling of holes in the distal femur for the cutting block.

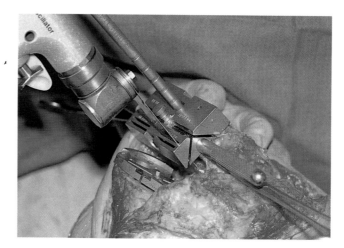

Figure 34. Revision cutting block for the anteroposterior and chamfer cuts. The intramedullary reamer provides a point of fixation.

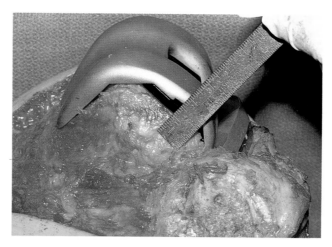

Figure 35. Trial component with augmentation. The joint line has been restored to its correct level 2.5 cm distal to the lateral femoral epicondyle.

these goals have been achieved, then the knee will be ready for fixation of the implant. In most instances a cemented revision arthroplasty will be performed. If the stems are going to be press-fit, then the stem of the same diameter as the last reamer used on the femur is selected. If an extended stem is going to be press-fit on the tibia, then the tibia will also need to be reamed to the appropriate diameter for the press-fit stem. Again, a stem of the same diameter as the last reamer is selected. A trial reduction of the stem should be performed in the medullary canals to be sure that they are going to fit appropriately but not impact. If modular augmentation is going to be added to the tibial or femoral component, it should be added at this time. Distal wedges should be fixed to the femoral component with lug nuts rather than being cemented. Posterior wedges on the femoral component are cemented, as are wedges on the tibial side (Fig. 36). These should be cemented and the cement allowed to harden before attempting to place the augmented implants into the patient. A second cementing will then be used to fix the implants to bone. In order to have adequate bone surfaces upon which to seat the implant, it is important to thoroughly lavage the bone with a water pick. Areas of sclerotic bone can be drilled to improve cement penetration (Fig. 37). Once the bone surfaces are adequately prepared, the implants can be cemented into place. If the stems are going to be press-fit, cement should be put only on the condylar portion of the femoral and tibial components and onto the femoral condyles and tibial plateau. If the stems are to be cemented, techniques similar to those for total hip arthroplasty should be used, with plugging of the medullary canal and pulsatile lavage. Once the femoral and tibial components are securely fixed, the real polyethylene can be inserted and the knee should again be tested for range of motion, stability, and patellar tracking.

In revision arthroplasty, it has been the author's preference to release the tourniquet prior to insertion of the real polyethylene. This allows access to the posterior soft tissues, in which bleeding vessels are often encountered. A careful search should be made for the medial inferior geniculate and lateral inferior and lateral superior geniculate vessels, which are the major sources of bleeding after surgery. Once hemostasis has been obtained, careful attention must be directed toward wound closure. If there are problems with patellar tracking it may be necessary to advance the vastus medialis and perform additional lateral release in order to assure proper balance of the extensor mechanism. Nonabsorbable suture material should be used for repair of the fascia. If the vastus medialis is being advanced, a heavier suture should be used to secure it firmly in place, and a double layer

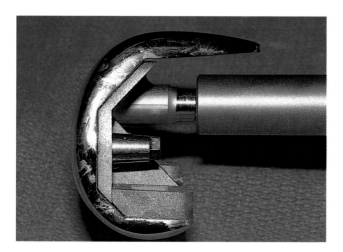

Figure 36. Femoral component with modular augmentation distally and posteriorly.

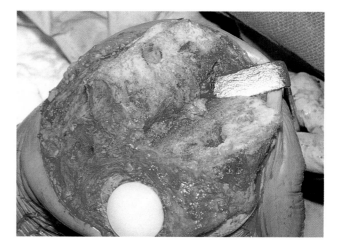

Figure 37. Bone surfaces prepared for implantation.

of sutures can be helpful in these circumstances. The most difficult area to close is at the distal portion of the fascia and the patellar tendon. Often the soft tissue here is deficient, especially with release and correction of a varus deformity. Multiple sutures should be placed at this level and a very thorough subcutaneous closure performed. The author's preference is to use a running suture in the skin distally combined with a xeroform gauze to help seal the area more thoroughly than can be accomplished with interrupted sutures or staples.

POSTOPERATIVE MANAGEMENT

Suction drains are routinely used after revision surgery, and are removed when the drainage diminishes, usually over the ensuing 12 to 24 hours. A bulky Robert–Jones dressing is used to immobilize the knee for the first 24 hours so as to minimize swelling, after which motion can be initiated in a continuous passive-motion machine and physical therapy begun.

The overall results of revision of a total knee arthroplasty will depend on the severity of the patient's problem, the quality of the soft tissues, and the extent of bone loss. In general, the results of revision are not equivalent to those of primary arthroplasty, and the patient should be informed of this prior to surgery. Good or excellent results can be anticipated in 50% to 80% of revision procedures. An increased complication rate of 15% to 30% can also be anticipated. It should also be remembered that the durability of revision surgery is not the same as that of primary arthroplasty, with only a 72% survivorship in 1,131 revisions, as compared to an 81% survivorship in 8,069 primary arthroplasties ($p < 0.0001$) at 10 years in one study (10).

REHABILITATION

Physical therapy following the revision of a total knee replacement should emphasize range of motion of the knee and gait training. If there has been any violation of the extensor mechanism by V-Y quadricepsplasty or tibial tuberosity osteotomy, the knee is protected from active extension for 6 weeks but passive extension is allowed. During this rehabilitation period, a brace can be useful for protecting the extensor mechanism. Weight bearing is performed with hinges locked and unlocked to allow range of motion; it is allowed to progress as tolerated in most instances. A period of protected weight bearing should be utilized only if there has been a cementless revision or if extensive structural bone grafting has been performed. In these circumstances weight bearing is limited until graft incorporation is visualized radiographically.

COMPLICATIONS

The most frequent complications of revision surgery are problems of extensor mechanism maltracking and of distal wound drainage or hematoma. Extensor mechanism tracking should be assessed and, if necessary, a tube realignment procedure (5) should be performed. Wound drainage distally can be minimized by careful attention to wound closure and protecting motion until wound healing occurs. It must always be remembered that wound healing takes priority over motion. Postoperative hematoma can largely be avoided by careful hemostasis at the time of surgery and by the placement of postoperative drains. A postoperative hematoma will delay rehabilitation of the patient, and if it drains spontaneously, opens the potential for contamination of the knee and subsequent deep infection.

Less common problems that can occur with revision surgery are wound sloughing and problems with wound healing. These can be largely avoided by careful attention to exposure. Any problems with delayed healing or skin sloughing should be treated early and aggressively by achieving soft tissue coverage with skin grafts, gastrocnemius flaps, or free muscle flaps. A plastic surgeon is very useful in dealing with these problems. Deep infection is a major complication after revision surgery. In some instances it may stem from a low-grade infection that existed when the revision of an arthroplasty was done for supposed aseptic loosening. However, most postoperative infections result either from wound contamination at the time of surgery or from the postoperative failure of wound healing and secondary infection of the knee. It has been the author's preference to use antibiotic-impregnated cement for most revisions. Since Palacos gentamicin cement has not been readily available in the United States, either tobramycin or vancomycin powder has been added to the cement. Generally, 600 mg of tobramycin powder is added to 40 g of cement, or 500 mg of vancomycin powder is added to 40 g of cement. The antibiotic cement is supplemented with intravenous antibiotics until cultures obtained at the time of revision surgery are reported as negative, usually at 5 days.

ILLUSTRATIVE CASE FOR TECHNIQUE

This 63-year-old man presented 5 years after the revision of a failed unicompartmental arthroplasty to a Kinematic condylar arthroplasty (Howmedica, Rutherford, NJ) with complaints of pain, effusion, and a squeak within the knee (Figs. 38–48).

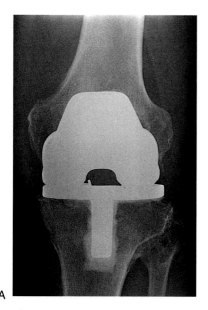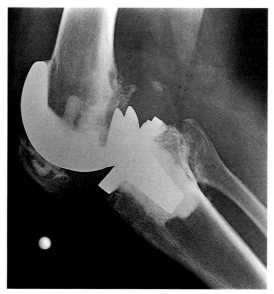

A   B

Figure 38. Following **(A)** AP and **(B)** lateral radiography, a diagnosis of polyethylene wear on the tibial component was made.

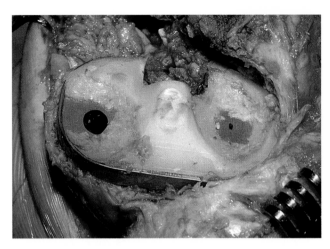

Figure 39. At the time of surgical exploration, complete wearing through of the polyethylene to the metal-backed tray was identified.

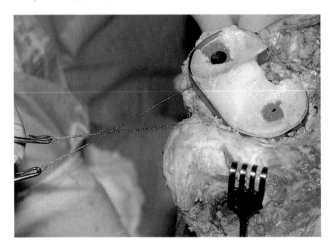

Figure 40. The tibial tray was extracted after freeing the undersurface with a Gigli saw.

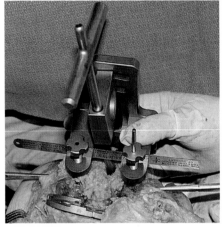

Figure 41. The proximal tibia was then recut at 90 degrees in the coronal and sagittal plane. The distal femur was recut at a 7-degree valgus angulation to accommodate the stem of the revision femoral component, using the epicondyles as a guide for rotational alignment.

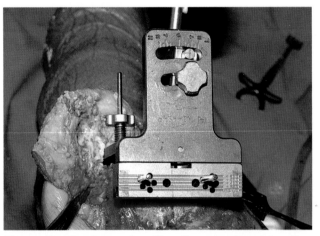

Figure 42. The femoral cutting jig was placed to allow displacement of the cutting surface distally so as to remove a minimal amount of bone from the femur.

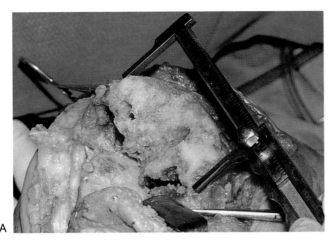
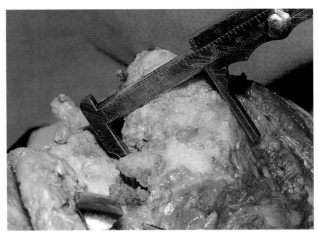

A   B

Figure 43. After preparation of the distal femoral and proximal tibial cuts, the **(A)** medial lateral dimensions and **(B)** anterior-posterior dimensions of the femur were measured.

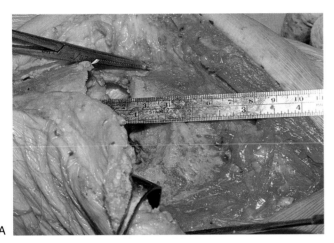
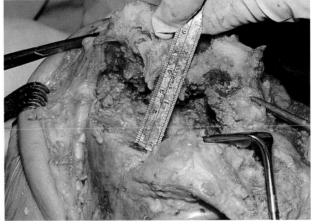

A   B

Figure 44. The extension space **(A)** and flexion space **(B)** were measured.

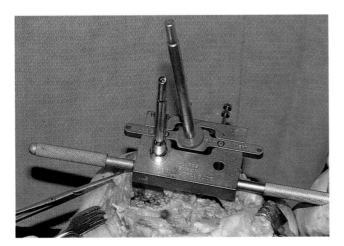
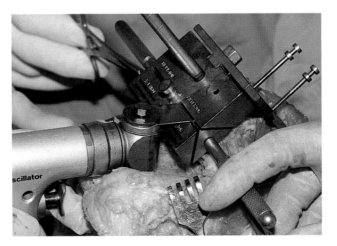

Figure 45. A revision femoral component was selected that matched the remaining bone in its interior dimension, restored the joint line, and filled the flexion and extension spaces. The distal femur was reamed with an intramedullary reamer to allow press fitting of an intramedullary stem.

Figure 46. A revision cutting block was used to prepare the femur.

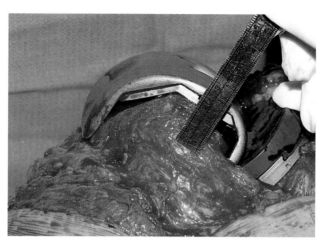

Figure 47. Trial reduction was performed. Measurements were noted to confirm that the joint line was reproduced 25 mm distal to the femoral epicondyles.

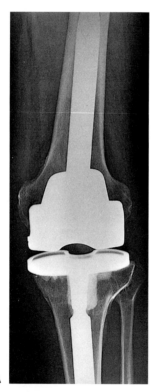
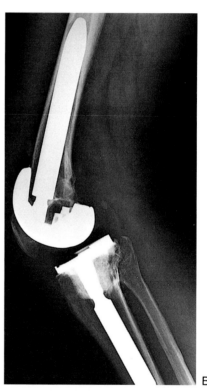

A   B

Figure 48. The patient had a satisfactory result following revision arthroplasty, although there was inadequate bone on the patella to allow patellar resurfacing. The long intramedullary stems were press-fit, with only the condylar portion of the prosthesis cemented. **A:** AP; **B:** lateral radiographs.

RECOMMENDED READING

1. Bourne, R. B., and Finlay, J. B.: The influence of tibial component intramedullary stems and implant-cortex contact on the strain distribution of the proximal tibia following total knee arthroplasty. *Clin. Orthop.*, 208: 95–99, 1986.
2. Dorr, L. D., Conaty, J. P., Schreiber, R., Mehne, D. K., and Hull, D.: Technical factors that influence mechanical loosening of total knee arthroplasty. In: *The Knee:* Papers of the First Scientific Meeting of the Knee Society. pp. 121–135. University Park Press, Baltimore, 1985.

3. Engh, G. A., Dwyer, K. A., and Hanes, C. K.: Polyethylene wear of metal-backed tibial components in total and unicompartmental knee prostheses. *J. Bone Joint Surg.,* 74B: 9–17, 1992.

4. Ewald, F. C., Jacobs, M. A., Miegel, R. E., Walker, P. S., Poss, R., and Sledge, C. B.: Kinematic total knee replacement. *J. Bone Joint Surg.,* 66A: 1032–1040, 1984.

5. Insall, J. N., Bullough, P. G., and Burstein, A. H.: Proximal tube realignment of the patella for chondromalacia patellae. *Clin. Orthop.,* 144: 63–69, 1979.

6. Lotke, P. A., and Ecker, M. L.: Influence of positioning of prosthesis in total knee arthroplasty. *J. Bone Joint Surg.,* 59A: 77–79, 1977.

7. Mintz, A. D., Pilkington, C. A. J., and Howie, D. W.: A comparison of plain and fluoroscopically guided radiographs in the assessment of arthroplasty of the knee. *J. Bone Joint Surg.,* 71A: 1343–1347, 1989.

8. Rand, J. A., and Brown, M. L.: The value of indium-111 leukocyte scanning in the evaluation of painful or infected total knee arthroplasties. *Clin. Orthop.* 259: 179–182, 1990.

9. Rand, J. A., and Coventry, M. B.: Stress fractures after total knee arthroplasty. *J. Bone Joint Surg.* 62A: 226–233, 1980.

10. Rand, J. A., and Ilstrup, D. M.: Survivorship analysis of total knee arthroplasty. *J. Bone Joint Surg.* 73A: 397–409, 1991.

11. Rand, J. A., Morrey, B. F., and Bryan, R. S.: Patellar tendon rupture after total knee arthroplasty. *Clin. Orthop.* 244: 233–238, 1989.

12. Rand, J. A., Peterson, L. F. A., Bryan, R. S., and Ilstrup, D. M.: Revision total knee arthroplasty. *Instructional Course Lectures* 35: 305–318, 1986.

13. Scott, R. D., and Siliski, J. M.: The use of a modified V-Y quadricepsplasty during total knee replacement to gain exposure and improve flexion in the ankylosed knee. *Orthopedics* 8:45–48, 1985.

14. Scuderi, G. R., Insall, J. N., Windsor, R. E., and Moran, M. C.: Survivorship of Cemented Knee Replacements. *J. Bone Joint Surg.* 71B: 798–803, 1989.

15. Tew, M., and Waugh, W.: Tibiofemoral alignment and the results of knee replacement. *J. Bone Joint Surg.* 67B: 551–556, 1985.

16. Vince, K. G., Insall, J. N., and Kelly, M. A.: The total condylar prosthesis: 10- to 12-year results of a cemented knee replacement. *J. Bone Joint Surg.* 71B: 793–797, 1989.

17. Whitesides, L. A., and Ohl, M. D.: Tibial tubercle osteotomy for exposure of the difficult total knee arthroplasty. *Clin. Orthop.* 260:6–9, 1990.

Master Techniques in Orthopaedic Surgery,
KNEE ARTHROPLASTY, edited by P. A. Lotke,
Raven Press, Ltd., New York © 1995.

14

Extensor Mechanism Failure
Treatment of Patella Fracture, Dislocation, and Ligament Rupture

Patellar Tendon Rupture Following Total Knee Arthroplasty

INDICATIONS/CONTRAINDICATIONS

Patellar tendon rupture following or during total knee arthroplasty is a rare (0.17%) but serious complication, and carries with it a generally poor prognosis for recovery of full active extension with normal strength. However, such rupture may occur under a variety of circumstances, and there may be differences among them in terms of prognosis and optimal treatment alternatives.

The most common cause of patellar tendon rupture is intraoperative avulsion during revision surgery or primary arthroplasty in a stiff or ankylosed knee. Scarring of the lateral gutter renders it shallow and effectively binds the lateral retinaculum to the distal femur. This, combined with collateral ligament shortening and entrapment, results in excessive tension on the patellar tendon when the patella is everted and the knee is flexed during exposure. To prevent rupture of the tendon, extensive debridement of the lateral gutter, including a lateral release, excision of the thickened tissue surrounding the patella, and possibly subperiosteal release of the femoral attachments of the collateral ligaments should be done before everting the patella and flexing the knee. Medial release is also desirable because it allows the tibia to rotate laterally, reducing the tension on the extensor

N. A. Johanson, M.D.: Department of Orthopaedic Surgery, Temple University School of Medicine, Philadelphia, PA 19140.

mechanism during knee flexion. After thorough release of the medial and lateral structures, there may be situations that require turndown of the quadriceps tendon. Alternatively, the tibial tubercle may be osteotomized. Tibial tubercle osteotomy has been associated with a high rate of nonunion and proximal migration of the tubercle, and the turndown procedure may fail because of devascularization of the distal quadriceps tendon.

Intraoperative patellar tendon avulsions should be repaired by a suturing technique with or without augmentation with a semitendinosus autograft. The distinction between partial and complete avulsion is often subtle, in that the tendon may not translate superiorly because of a small remaining lateral tendinous attachment and/or lateral retinacular attachment to the proximal tibia. Even with a substantial amount of tendon avulsed from the tubercle, normal knee function can be obtained without any formal repair of the patellar tendon if a secure closure between the patellar tendon and the medial tibial periosteum is achieved and the remaining lateral attachments are preserved.

Patellar tendon ruptures that occur outside of the operating room, following total knee arthroplasty, usually occur during the first 6 months postoperatively, but may occur more than 3 years after surgery. The rupture may be associated with overly aggressive postoperative physical therapy, manipulation, or activities such as climbing or descending stairs or getting up from a chair. Acute ruptures should be explored and repaired unless there is a high risk of wound problems or general medical complications. A relative contraindication to the surgical repair of a patellar tendon rupture occurs in active rheumatoid arthritis, which naturally leads to tendon attrition (see Illustrative Case for Technique: Case 1). In this situation the rupture is usually found in the midsubstance of the tendon. The tendon should be sutured and the repair augmented by an autogenous semitendinosus tendon, unless the medial hamstring tendons have undergone a similar degree of attrition. Nonsurgical treatment is usually recommended in active severe rheumatoid arthritis, in which the risk of infection and mechanical failure is substantial.

PREOPERATIVE PLANNING

Ruptures of the patellar tendon present with localized pain, a palpable loss of patellar tendon tension during active knee extension, and an extensor lag. An incipient postoperative flexion contracture may obscure the diagnosis because of the difficulty in appreciating an extensor lag. The patella alta that is associated with patellar tendon rupture is often accentuated when the patient is in the supine position with both quadriceps contracted, and can be identified in this way. There is often an associated hemarthrosis, and this may obscure the diagnosis.

Anteroposterior (AP) and lateral radiographs should be obtained and compared with either immediate postoperative or preoperative films. To establish the diagnosis and surgical indication of complete rupture of the patellar tendon, a significant patella alta should be demonstrated by comparison with earlier studies. In addition, patellar fracture should be ruled out, since it may occur simultaneously with tendon rupture (see Fig. 3A).

SURGERY

The surgical approach to a postoperative patellar tendon rupture is through the inferior half of the pre-existing scar, using the same type of preparation, draping, and considerations for anesthesia as for a primary total knee arthroplasty. The tissue medial to the tendon is incised longitudinally and the patellar tendon is mobilized to identify the site of the tear. Depending on the chronicity of the injury, a variable amount of scar tissue is lysed to prepare the tendon for repair. The joint should also be drained of any hematoma and irrigated using pulsatile lavage. The method of repair of the patellar tendon varies with the location of the rupture (tendon insertion versus midsubstance) and the condition of the tendon.

Midsubstance tears should be repaired with a Kessler suture, using a braided, nonabsorbable suture material (No. 2 Ty-Cron) proximally and distally to oppose the torn ends of the tendon, and completing the repair by suturing the torn ends with slowly absorbable suture (2-0 Vicryl). Augmentation of the repair with a semitendinosus tendon autograft should be performed if the repair is not of adequate strength. This procedure is performed by dissecting medially to locate the pes anserinus tendons and identifying the semitendinosus insertion. A separate posteromedial incision is made to locate the musculotendinous junction and to divide the tendon as far proximally as possible (Fig. 1). The tendon is passed out anteriorly through the main incision. The tendon graft should measure 20 to 25 cm long. A ¼-inch drill is used to transversely drill through the distal pole of the patella, taking care not to interfere with the prosthetic interface of the patellar component of the knee. If there is inadequate bone in the distal patella, the tendon graft should be woven through the distal quadriceps tendon. The distal portion of the patella should be stabilized by suturing the tendinous stump to the tendon graft. The tension of the graft should be adjusted to maintain a length of the infrapatellar tendon that is approximately equal to the length of the patella. However, the height of the patella may have to be adjusted to provide optimal articula-

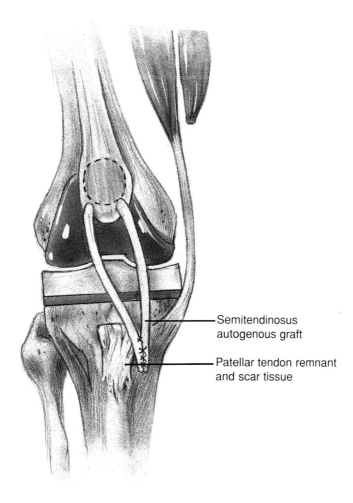

Semitendinosus
autogenous graft

Patellar tendon remnant
and scar tissue

Figure 1. Augmentation of patellar tendon repair using a semitendinosus tendon graft.

tion with the femoral component of the knee if the joint line had been altered during the total knee arthroplasty. The semitendinosus graft is doubled back on itself and sutured with a slowly absorbable suture material.

Repairing an avulsion of the patellar tendon from either the tibial tubercle or the patella requires the use of a suture placed through a drill hole in the bone (either the patella or tibial tubercle). The most common site of tendon avulsion is from the tibial tubercle. The suturing technique can be used in repairing a complete avulsion or as a safety measure when a partial avulsion is recognized intraoperatively (Fig. 2). The tendon is exposed in its entire width proximally, and using No. 2 Ty-Cron suture and Keith needles, a Kessler suture is passed first transversely across the proximal tendon and then longitudinally in the substance of the tendon medially and laterally, down to the point of attachment to the tibial tubercle (Figs. 2B, C). If a medial parapatellar incision has been made, the lateral Keith needle will be in the subcutaneous tissue of the lateral skin flap, and can be located through a separate incision (Fig. 2D). A $\frac{7}{64}$-inch drill hole is made transversely through the base of the tibial tubercle. A 1 cm incision should be made overlying the point where the drill bit and the tip of the lateral Keith needle meet. The drill is then removed and a Keith needle is inserted in a retrograde manner through the drill hole, after which the lateral suture is threaded through the needle and pulled medially. The two ends of the suture are then tied in such a way that the distal end of the tendon is reapposed to the tubercle while maintaining the original effective length of the tendon (Figs. 2E, F). Closure is then performed in the usual fashion, with care taken to suture the medial tibial periosteal tissue to the tendon. If this tissue is incised sharply during the initial incision, and elevated off the tibia without weakening or disrupting its continuity (buttonholing or distally tearing it medially to create a flap), it can be used to augment the repair by suturing it directly to the tendon during closure.

POSTOPERATIVE MANAGEMENT

In complete tendon ruptures the patient should be managed postoperatively with a hinged long leg brace locked in full extension or a cylinder cast for 6 weeks.

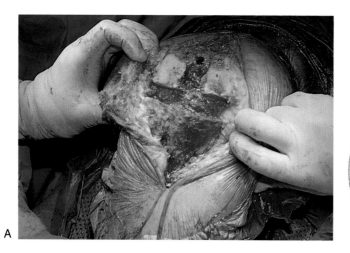

A

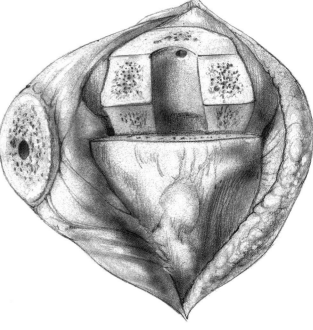

A'

Figure 2. A,A': Anterior view of the right knee following bone cuts performed during a revision. The patellar tendon has been avulsed from the tibial tubercle.

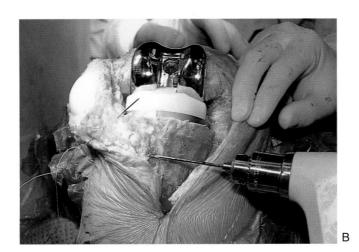

B

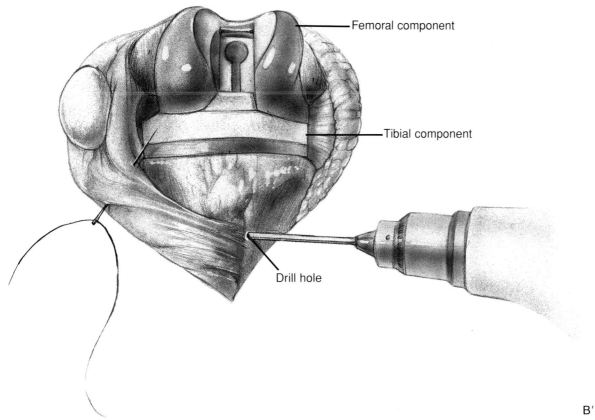

Femoral component

Tibial component

Drill hole

B'

Figure 2. (*Continued.*) **B,B':** A medial-to-lateral transverse drill hole has been placed at the base of the tibial tubercle, and a transverse suture is being placed in the proximal patellar tendon.

Text continues on page 228.

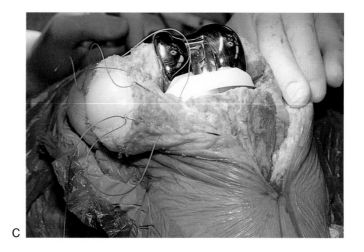

C

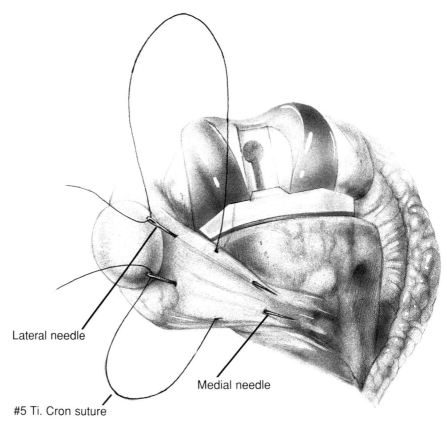

Lateral needle

Medial needle

#5 Ti. Cron suture

C′

Figure 2. (*Continued.*) **C,C′:** The patellar tendon suture is passed distally through the medial and lateral substance of the tendon.

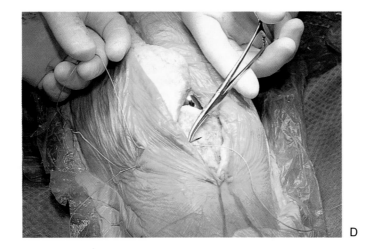

D

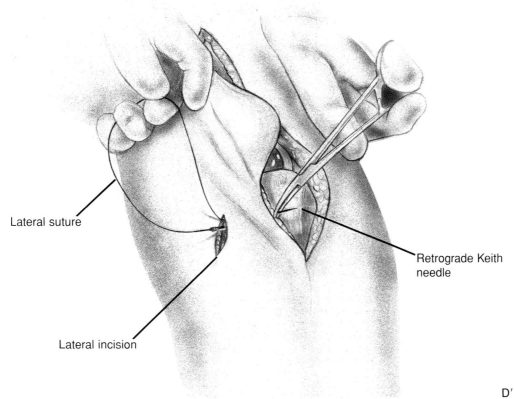

Lateral suture

Lateral incision

Retrograde Keith
needle

D'

Figure 2. (*Continued.*) **D,D'**: The lateral patellar tendon suture is passed out through
a separate incision and threaded onto a retrograde Keith needle.

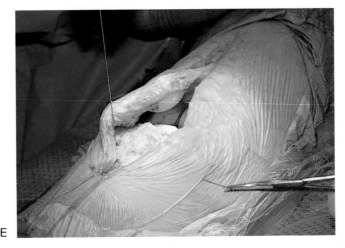

E

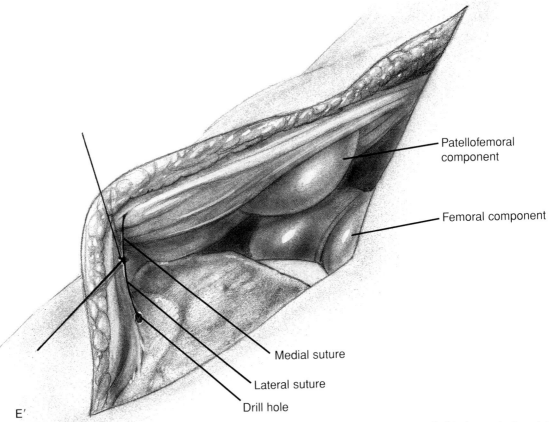

Patellofemoral
component

Femoral component

Medial suture

Lateral suture

Drill hole

E′

Figure 2. (*Continued.*) **E,E′:** The lateral suture is passed medially through the drill hole and tied to the medial end of the suture.

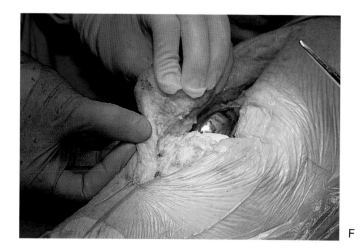

F

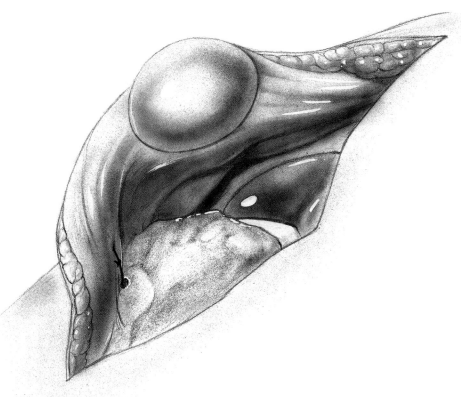

F′

Figure 2. (*Continued.*) **F,F′:** The repair is completed by adjusting the tension on the suture, with care taken to maintain the original length of the patellar tendon.

A suction drain should be placed in the knee for 12 to 24 hours and the patient should be kept in the hospital overnight with an ice pack on the knee and the leg elevated. Twenty-four hours of treatment with an intravenously administered, broad-spectrum antibiotic should be used for prophylaxis against infection. The drain may be removed the following day, and if pain can be managed with oral analgesia, the patient should be discharged. The patient may walk full weight-bearing status with crutches. Isometric quadriceps exercises are performed along with straight-leg raising throughout the initial recovery period. The sutures or skin staples are removed at 2 weeks after surgery. If lateral knee radiographs at 6 weeks demonstrate the repair to be intact (without proximal migration of the patella), 60 degrees of flexion with gravity is permitted, but the hinged brace should be locked in extension for walking, and no active knee-extension exercises should be initiated until 3 months postoperatively. Progressive strengthening exercises are initiated at 3 months.

In patients who have undergone repair of partial patellar tendon avulsions, motion can be initiated in the immediate postoperative period. A hinged long-leg brace is used to protect the knee against sudden excessive flexion. Continuous passive motion (CPM) may also be utilized.

If full passive extension is preserved during the healing period, and radiographs show no proximal migration of the patella, the patient may be expected to walk well, but may be left with a significant extensor lag and have persistent difficulty with stairs. The results are not as good in the setting of a flexion contracture or with late recognition of a patellar tendon rupture.

COMPLICATIONS

The most common complication of patellar tendon rupture, whether treated surgically or not, is extensor lag and flexion contracture. The primary preventive measure for this complication, regardless of the treatment plan, used for the rupture, is maintaining the knee in full extension throughout the treatment period, even after knee flexion exercises are allowed. Patellofemoral pain as well as disability, particularly on stairs and while getting out of a chair, is the most important complaint resulting from the gait disturbance caused by a chronic flexion contracture. Re-rupture of the repaired tendon, either acutely or subacutely from stretching, will leave the patient with a result that is similar to a nonsurgically treated rupture. Again, the key to preventing disaster is the prevention of flexion contracture.

Infection of a surgical repair is the most feared complication of surgical treatment for rupture of the patellar tendon because it will almost certainly lead to a result that is inferior to nonsurgical treatment. Infection may arise from intraoperative contamination or from superficial wound necrosis that becomes secondarily infected and extends to the deep tissues. Early recognition of wound problems, and treatment with debridement and antibiotics, may prevent their deep extension. Removal of a prosthesis for the treatment of deep infection should be accompanied by a primary knee arthrodesis. It is unlikely that reimplantation of the prosthesis after eradication of the infection would be successful, because of the severely compromised status of the extensor mechanism.

ILLUSTRATIVE CASE FOR TECHNIQUE

CASE 1. A 66-year-old man with polyarticular rheumatoid arthritis treated for over 10 years with 10 to 15 mg per day of prednisone sustained bilateral patellar tendon ruptures 1 year after staged bilateral total knee arthroplasties. Figure 3A, an AP radiograph of both knees, demonstrates the characteristic patella alta. The

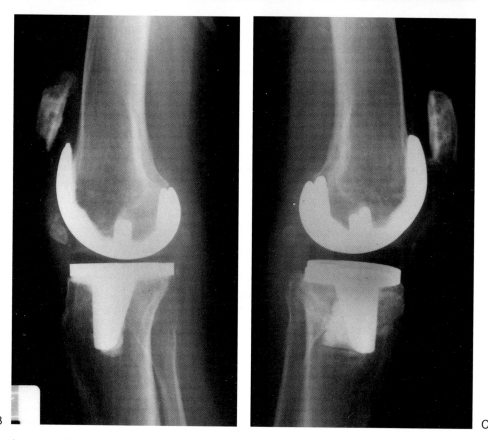

Figure 3. (Case 1.) **A:** AP radiograph demonstrating characteristic patella alta seen in patellar tendon rupture. The left patella also has a minimally displaced superior pole fracture. **B:** Lateral projection of the left knee 4 months after attempted tendon repair, demonstrating failure. **C:** Lateral projection of the right knee 3 months after patellar tendon rupture.

left patella also has a minimally displaced superior pole fracture in addition to the tendon rupture. An attempt was made to repair the tendon with augmentation, using the medial hamstring tendons. The tissue quality of the tendons, however, was found to be too poor for their use, and the remnant of the patellar tendon that had avulsed from the inferior pole of the patella was therefore sutured to the patella. Figure 3B is a lateral projection of the left knee 4 months after attempted repair and 6 weeks of immobilization. The superior pole fracture had healed, but the inferior pole of the patella had avulsed with the tendon repair. The patient had no active extension of his left knee. Shortly after his left patellar tendon ruptured, the patellar tendon on the right side ruptured spontaneously and nearly painlessly. Because of the poor outcome of the surgical treatment of the patient's left knee, the right knee was not opened. Figure 3C shows a lateral projection of the right knee 3 months after tendon rupture. The patient had essentially no knee pain, but was confined to bed and was not ambulatory. In addition to his knee problems, he had a mild cervical myelopathy.

Patellar Subluxation and Dislocation Following Total Knee Arthroplasty

INDICATIONS/CONTRAINDICATIONS

Patellar tracking problems following total knee arthroplasty have been reported to occur with an incidence of as high as 29%. The symptoms reported vary over a broad spectrum from intermittent anterior knee pain to frank dislocation and giving way of the knee that constitutes a danger to the safety of the patient, especially on stairs and while crossing busy streets.

The causes of patellofemoral instability are multifactorial, and it is therefore often difficult to accurately rank their importance and identify them in any given case. Soft-tissue imbalance, usually because of excessively tight lateral retinacular structures, is a common causative factor. This situation often arises in the setting of a preoperative valgus knee deformity or in chronic lateral subluxation of the patella (see Illustrative Case for Technique: Case 2). Postoperative patellar instability can be exacerbated by undersizing or internally rotating the femoral component of a prosthesis, internally rotating the tibial component (functional external tibial rotation leading to an increased Q angle), laterally tilting the patellar bone cut, laterally placing the patellar component, or performing a weak closure of the medial arthrotomy that can tear during physical therapy.

In most cases, patellar subluxation that causes intermittent symptoms and is not disabling tends to improve during the first 12 to 18 months after arthroplasty, as the retinacular scar tissue matures and contracts. Frank dislocation that causes giving way of the knee and actual stumbling or falling should be addressed surgically with soft-tissue realignment or, in severe cases of malalignment or malrotation of a prosthesis, by component revision.

PREOPERATIVE PLANNING

A patient with patellofemoral instability characteristically complains of catching or giving way of the knee when it is moving from full extension to flexion while the quadriceps muscle is contracting (as in going down stairs, stepping off a curb, or walking vigorously). Physical examination often reveals laxity of the retinacular structures (particularly medially) when the knee is in full extension. Active quadriceps contraction may cause the patella to deviate laterally. This will be accentuated in the setting of patella alta, in which case the patella rides at or above the superior margin of the femoral prosthesis. In severe cases, quick passive flexion of the knee will actually cause subluxation or dislocation of the patella. Otherwise, the patient will have to be observed while performing those activities that cause the problem.

Radiographic evaluation of a total knee arthroplasty consists of standard AP, lateral, and "skyline" or Merchant views. The alignment of the knee is checked for excessive valgus, and the patellofemoral view may demonstrate a lateral tilt or frank subluxation. A radiographic evaluation for component rotation is difficult to accomplish with plain films because of the contribution of femoral neck anteversion to overall femoral rotation. A computed tomographic (CT) scan that includes the femoral neck as a reference is useful for detecting problems associated with gross malrotation of a prosthesis, but even this study may miss more subtle cases in which the malrotation merely exacerbates a primary soft-tissue imbalance.

SURGERY

When performing surgery for patellar tracking problems, a hierarchy of procedures should be kept in mind, each being more aggressive and having the potential for more complications and more prolonged rehabilitation than its predecessor. This sequence starts with a simple lateral release and progresses to medial plication, distal realignment, and, in the case of gross malrotation of a component, revision of a femoral and/or tibial component. It is rare to have to revise the patella in the case of tracking problems that are not accompanied by mechanical loosening or failure of the patellar component of a prosthesis.

The knee is prepped and draped in a manner similar to that for a primary total knee arthroplasty. If possible, the incision is made through the scar of the primary incision and the knee is exposed and brought up into flexion so that rotation of the femoral component can be checked in relation to the epicondyles of the femur and the rotation of the tibial component can be checked in relation to the tibial tubercle. After malrotation is ruled out, the knee is brought back into extension and attention is turned to the lateral patellar retinaculum.

A lateral release is performed from inside out, using electrocautery extending from the joint line (including transection of the remnant of the lateral meniscus) proximally, and passing approximately 2 cm lateral to the lateral margin of the patella (Fig. 4). The release extends through the synovium and capsule, exposing the inner surface of the iliotibial band. The superior lateral geniculate vessels are identified and preserved. The proximal portion of the release curves medially into the tendinous portion of the vastus lateralis. Releasing this tendon eliminates the dynamic lateral force that subluxes the patella. The release stops at the vastus lateralis, with care taken not to interfere with the integrity of the quadriceps tendon. Overzealous lateral releases have been associated with quadriceps tendon ruptures.

With each successive stage of the lateral release, patellar tracking is tested to determine the amount of improvement achieved. The adequacy of the lateral release should be finally checked with the placement of one or two medial reefing sutures just proximal to the patella. If the patella tracks well, the medial closure is completed after irrigation with pulsatile lavage and the placement of tubing for suction drainage. During closure, the tendon of the vastus medialis is advanced 1 to 2 cm distally, and imbricated over to the central portion of the quadriceps tendon. The secure closure, with medial reefing, is continued down to the joint line.

Proximal realignment is adequate treatment for most patellar tracking problems. Distal realignment by medially translocating the tibial tubercle results in a significant risk of nonunion and mechanical failure, and should therefore be avoided. If the tracking problem is severe enough to warrant more than a proximal realign-

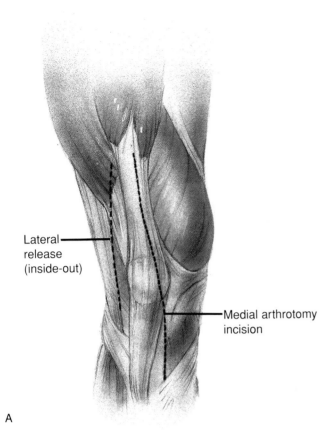

Lateral release (inside-out)

Medial arthrotomy incision

A

Figure 4. A: Proximal realignment for patellar maltracking. Dotted lines represent medial parapatellar arthrotomy incision and the line of the inside-out lateral retinacular release. **B:** Arthrotomy and lateral release have been performed. **C:** Reefing of the medial retinaculum on the quadriceps tendon has been performed.

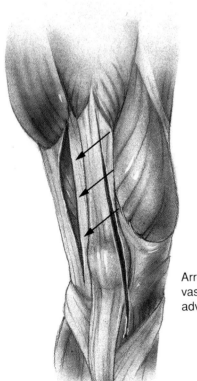

Arrows demonstrate vastus medialis advancement

B

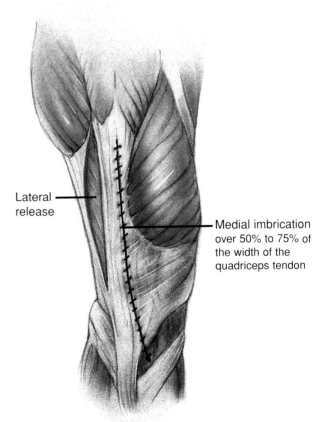

Lateral release

Medial imbrication over 50% to 75% of the width of the quadriceps tendon

C

ment, a revision should be considered. Revision surgery, particularly on the femoral side, is technically challenging, in that derotating the femoral component of a prosthesis requires recutting anteriorly and posteriorly and utilizing posterior augmentation to fill the resulting lateral gap. Care must also be taken not to notch the anterior femoral cortex during recutting.

POSTOPERATIVE MANAGEMENT

A suction drain is placed in the knee and kept there for 12 to 24 hours postoperatively, and routine prophylactic antibiotics should be employed in the same manner as for a primary procedure. The patient is placed in a postoperative hinged brace with full extension and a flexion stop of 40 degrees. The patient should be hospitalized at least overnight for intravenous antibiotics and pain control. The leg should be elevated and an ice pack placed on the knee. Recently developed, continuous cold water flow systems incorporated into the knee dressing are especially helpful for preventing swelling and controlling pain. Many of these systems are brought home by the patient and used until the postoperative dressing is removed for suture or staple removal at 2 weeks after surgery. During the first 6 weeks of recovery, a CPM machine is helpful for promoting motion while minimizing potentially disruptive active muscular contraction (primarily to protect the medial reefing). Quadriceps setting exercises are begun early so as to prevent excessive atrophy. The flexion stop is gradually increased to 90 degrees over the first 4 weeks postoperatively. When the patient is comfortable, antigravity exercises are initiated. At 6 weeks, aggressive range of motion (ROM) exercises and strengthening are initiated, and the brace may be removed.

More than 90% of patients who have patellar tracking problems following total knee arthroplasty treated with proximal realignment can be expected to have a satisfactory result. Decreased pain, improved patellar stability, and decreased apprehension and giving way can be expected within the first 6 months to 1 year postoperatively, although improvement in symptoms may actually extend over a 2 year period (see Illustrative Case for Technique: Case 2).

COMPLICATIONS

The most common problem following proximal realignment of the patella is early loss of flexion. This occurs as a result of overtightening of the medial patellar retinaculum and binding of the patella during flexion, combined with the lack of aggressive postoperative physical therapy for fear of tearing out the medial repair. Motion is expected to return to or near the preoperative range over a 3- to 6-month period. Extension lag following this procedure has been reported, but is rare. Other less common complications include persistent, disabling anterior knee pain and clicking because of chronic patellar maltracking. The most important preventive measure for this constellation of complications is adequate release of the capsular structures down to the joint line, complete release of the vastus lateralis tendon, a secure medial reefing that will enable the patient to perform early ROM and strengthening exercises, and the recognition of important malrotation problems in either the tibial or femoral components of the prosthesis.

ILLUSTRATIVE CASE FOR TECHNIQUE

CASE 2. A 69-year-old man with severe bilateral varus osteoarthritis and lateral tibial subluxation underwent bilateral total knee replacements. The patient had a moderate lateral thrust and medial instability. His preoperative ROM was from 0 to 120°. Figure 5A is a preoperative standing AP radiograph of the patient's left knee. Note the lateral subluxation of the patella on the femur, which has been translated medially on the tibia. Figure 5B is a lateral projection of the left knee, showing mild degenerative changes in the patellofemoral articulation. The preoperative radiographs of the right knee were similar in appearance to those of the

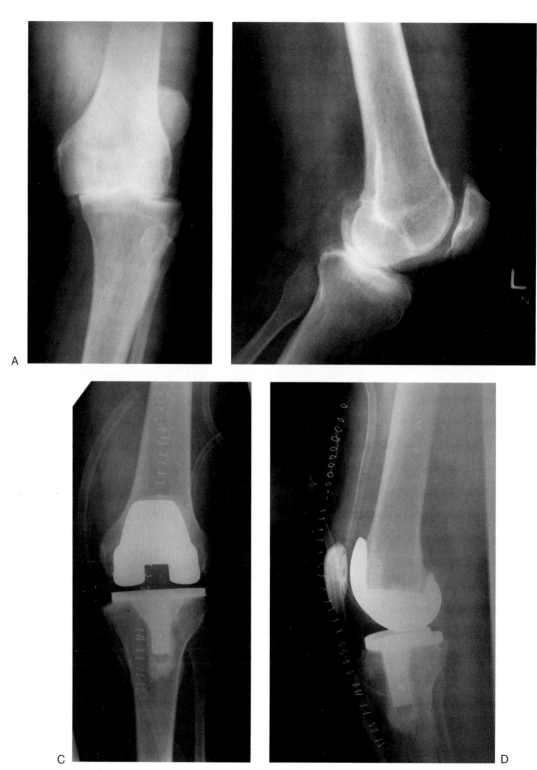

Figure 5. (Case 2) **A:** Preoperative AP radiograph of the left knee. **B:** Preoperative lateral radiograph of the left knee. **C:** Postoperative AP radiograph of the left knee. **D:** Postoperative lateral radiograph of the left knee.

left knee. Intraoperatively, after the components of the patient's prosthesis had been cemented, the patellae were thought to be tracking adequately in both knees, and therefore no lateral release was performed. Figures 5C and D are postoperative AP and lateral radiographs of the left knee, demonstrating the correction of the varus deformity and re-establishment of the normal patellofemoral relationship on the AP projection. After an uneventful recovery the patient returned for his 6-week follow-up visit with complaints of the left patella "popping out" when he descended stairs. On physical examination the right patella was found to track normally, but the left patella subluxed laterally with active knee extension, and actually dislocated laterally when the knee was quickly flexed (as in going down stairs). The vastus lateralis tendon was prominent, but there was no evidence of a fixed lateral retinacular tightness. After unsuccessful attempts at taping and bracing the knee to prevent subluxation, an open lateral release and medial reefing procedure was performed. The tendon of the vastus lateralis was completely released during this procedure. Postoperatively the patient was immobilized for 2 weeks and then gradually advanced in physical therapy. He continued to have problems with subluxation for the first 18 months postoperatively, but the problem slowly became less frequent and less severe. Two years after undergoing proximal realignment, the patient was asymptomatic, with excellent active motion (0 to 115 degrees).

Patellar Fractures Following Total Knee Replacement

INDICATIONS/CONTRAINDICATIONS

Patellar fracture following total knee arthroplasty using prostheses of contemporary design and current techniques occurs in fewer than 5% of cases, and is often asymptomatic. Earlier reports noted patellar fracture in as many as 20% of cases. The causes of patellar fracture have been thought to be related to certain design features of the femoral implant, or to maltracking of the patella, both of which have been associated with excessive concentrations of patellar stress. Over-resection or under-resection of patellar bone have been thought to be additional factors predisposing to fracture. The integrity of the bone and its capacity for the repair of microtrauma may also be compromised by devascularization of the patella during lateral release, resection of the fat pad, or aggressive stripping of soft tissue from around the patella.

As in patellar fractures in knees that have not had arthroplasty, the need for surgical intervention is contingent upon the degree of disruption of the medial and lateral retinacula, as well as on the disruption of prosthetic fixation. A nondisplaced or minimally displaced fracture (less than 2 mm) is treated in a knee immobilizer for 3 to 4 weeks with the expectation of little residual deformity or disability. Displaced fractures, however, require surgical repair for the prevention of significant dysfunction of the extensor mechanism. Fractures that disrupt the fixation of the patellar component of a prosthesis also require surgical treatment for removal or revision of the prosthesis. Revision surgery in this difficult situation should be undertaken only if there is sufficient bone to assure adequate fixation, and if the revision will not interfere with fracture healing, which is the highest priority of treatment in cases of fracture. Removal of the patellar component and, if necessary, internal fixation of the fracture can lead to an acceptable result, provided that the fracture heals without complication. Patellectomy should be reserved as a salvage procedure.

PREOPERATIVE PLANNING

Fractures that require surgical treatment present with severe pain and swelling, and are usually associated with a traumatic injury. A displaced fracture is actually palpable, with an accompanying extensor lag and painful knee motion. There is usually a large hemarthrosis of the knee that can be aspirated under sterile conditions.

Plain radiographs (AP, lateral, and "skyline" or Merchant views) should be obtained for preoperative evaluation. The orientation (horizontal, vertical) and location of the fracture(s) should be evaluated in relation to the patellar component. Evidence of loosening or wear of the prosthesis is most clear on Merchant or "skyline" views. Even with an all-polyethylene component and an intact cement mantle, the patellar component may dislodge from the cement. In an acute fracture with blood in the joint, the "shadow" of the displaced polyethylene dome can be detected by its differing density from the surrounding blood.

Any loosening or displacement of the patellar component of a prosthesis represents an indication for surgery, the primary reason being prevention of catastrophic wear. If the patella is loose but the fracture is displaced by less than 5 mm, and the extension lag is not greater than 15 degrees, the fracture can be treated with immobilization until healing, after which a delayed arthrotomy is performed either for removal of the patellar component or for revision. Revision surgery should be performed only if there is sufficient bone stock. Otherwise the bone should be smoothed and ROM exercises started as soon as possible.

In the case of fracture displacement by more than 5 mm and an extension lag of more than 20 degrees, the fracture should be treated with open reduction and internal fixation, using a K-wire and tension band technique (see Fig. 6). This procedure should be performed within the first 2 weeks after the fracture. After this period the fracture becomes progressively harder to reduce without medial and lateral resection of retinacular scar tissue, a procedure that will further devascularize the patella.

In the case of dislodgment of a patellar component and a displaced fracture, priority should be given to fracture fixation, with patellar revision undertaken only if there is sufficient bone stock and if cementing will not interfere with fracture healing.

SURGERY

The leg is prepped and draped using the same technique as for a primary knee arthroplasty, with the same considerations for anesthesia. The knee should be approached through the pre-existing surgical scar. The undermining of skin flaps should be minimized throughout the procedure so as to minimize the occurrence of marginal wound necrosis that can seriously compromise the end result. The joint is opened through the patellar fracture and retinacular tears (Fig. 6A, B). If possible, no new arthrotomy incision should be made unless necessitated by revision of a patellar component during the same procedure. If the patellar component has been dislodged, it is removed along with any loose fragments of cement, polyethylene, or bone. The joint should be thoroughly irrigated with pulsatile lavage, and the fracture surfaces defined and debrided of hematoma and devascularized bone. If the patellar component is well fixed, it is left in place and the reduction and fixation proceeds with care taken to avoid disrupting the interface with the fixation devices.

After the fracture surfaces are defined, the fragments are reduced and held in place with a circlage wire or heavy suture. To fix a horizontal fracture, two K-wires are passed through the bone longitudinally on either side of the patellar component (Fig. 6C, D). A figure-eight tension band is passed around the ends

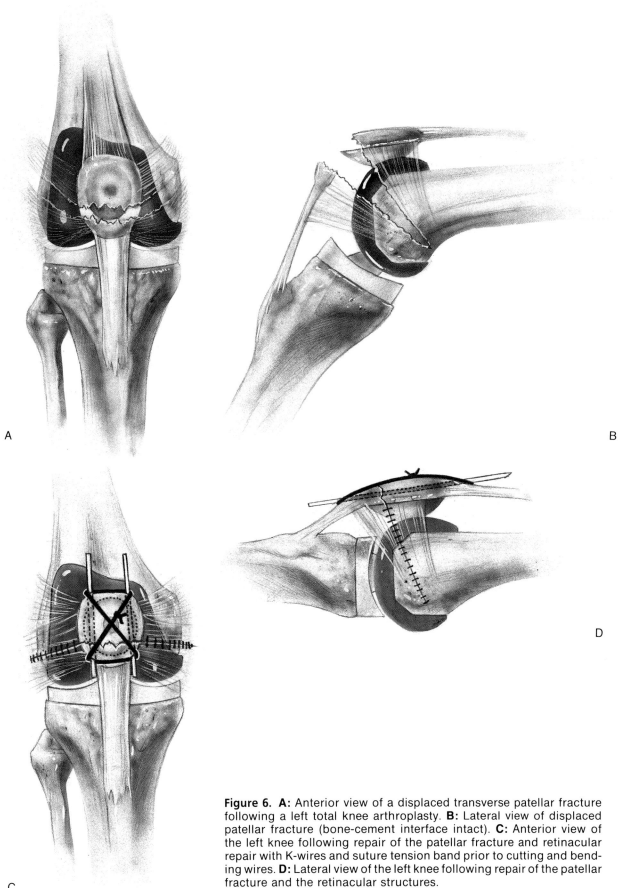

A

B

C

D

Figure 6. A: Anterior view of a displaced transverse patellar fracture following a left total knee arthroplasty. **B:** Lateral view of displaced patellar fracture (bone-cement interface intact). **C:** Anterior view of the left knee following repair of the patellar fracture and retinacular repair with K-wires and suture tension band prior to cutting and bending wires. **D:** Lateral view of the left knee following repair of the patellar fracture and the retinacular structures.

of the K-wires using either heavy suture material or wire (Fig. 6C, D). The author prefers heavy suture (No. 5 Ty-cron) because of its superior conformity with the anterior surfaces of the patella. The ends of the K-wires are then bent posteriorly to avoid pressure on the overlying skin.

A suction drain should be placed in the knee prior to repair of the retinacular tears. The medial and lateral retinacular tears are then repaired with interrupted sutures made with a slowly absorbable material (0 Vicryl). Subcutaneous tissue and skin are closed in a routine fashion. If extensive dissection has resulted in large skin flaps and there is concern about substantial deadspace postoperatively, a separate drain should be placed in the subcutaneous tissue overlying the patella and retinacular structures.

POSTOPERATIVE MANAGEMENT

The suction drain(s) is maintained for at least 24 hours after surgery to assure that no important hematoma will form around the repair. Prophylactic antibiotics should be used for at least 24 hours. The knee is immobilized in a postoperative hinged knee brace with its flexion/extension stops locked initially at zero. Elevation of the treated limb and the application of ice are important during the first postoperative day. Hospitalization is usually required for 2 to 3 days for pain management, wound observation, and drain management. The drains may be removed when there is less than 50 cc of drainage per 8 hours from the knee joint and less than 25 cc per 8 hours from the subcutaneous tissues. When comfortable, the patient may begin ambulation, with weight bearing as tolerated. The sutures or skin staples are removed after 2 weeks. The wound should be observed frequently until healing is complete, and any subcutaneous collections of fluid should be aspirated and cultured. The knee is held locked in extension for at least 4 weeks before CPM is initiated, and then only under the following optimal conditions: (a) wound healing without subcutaneous collections, (b) anatomic reduction, (c) optimal fixation and (d) no evidence of subcutaneous pin pressure. If any of these potential sources of risk are present, immobilization should be continued for another 2 weeks or until there has been radiographic evidence of early fracture healing.

As motion is liberalized, the patient first has passively and actively assisted flexion, followed by antigravity knee extension exercises. At 2 months more aggressive strengthening can begin. The knee brace locked in extension should be continued for walking activities during the first 6 weeks so as to save the knee from sudden buckling and injury to the repair.

COMPLICATIONS

Infection is the most serious postoperative complication of patellar fracture repair after total knee arthroplasty, and is unfortunately not uncommon. The extensive dissection and potential devascularization of peripatellar tissue, along with the proximity of the tips of the fixation wires to the skin, may be factors predisposing to infection. Infection will almost always result in removal of the components of a prosthesis and either arthrodesis or pseudarthrosis of the knee. Meticulous soft-tissue technique, thorough irrigation, and proper wound drainage are preventive measures for this disastrous complication.

Loss of fixation and delayed union or nonunion may occur in cases of patellar fracture following arthroplasty. This underscores the need for judgment about the actual possibility of improving the outcome with surgical treatment. Because part of the patella has already been resected during primary knee arthroplasty, there is relatively less bone surface at the fracture for secure healing. Less surface area at the fracture site also compromises the tension band effect, or compression created at the fracture surface remote from the tension band. The result is often nonunion because of excessive bending motion during the healing process.

A painful subcutaneous wire is a frequent late complication of the tension band technique. A preventive measure is cutting the ends of the K-wires, close to the bone and bending the end posteriorly. The wires should routinely be removed within 18 months of the fracture.

ILLUSTRATIVE CASES FOR TECHNIQUE

CASE 3.   A 70-year-old woman reported mild to moderate left knee pain 6 months after total knee arthroplasty. Examination revealed tenderness around the patella but no extension lag or loss of muscle strength. Figure 7A is a lateral radiograph of the left knee shortly after the patient's symptoms began. She was kept under observation and 6 weeks later her symptoms subsided. Figure 7B demonstrates partial healing but retraction of the inferior pole fragment. The patient was not functionally impaired and had no extension lag.

CASE 4.   A 79-year-old woman had acute left knee pain 8 months after a total knee arthroplasty. Examination revealed patella alta with a palpable infrapatellar defect. The patient had a 45-degree extension lag. Figure 8A is a lateral projection of the left knee during the patient's symptoms, demonstrating an avulsion fracture of the inferior pole of the patella. An attempt was made to repair the fracture surgically using a suture technique. Postoperatively the patient was immobilized in a cylinder cast. Two weeks later a radiograph in the cast demonstrated redisplacement of the patella superiorly (Fig. 8B). The patient was left in the cast for an additional 4 weeks and then mobilized. She developed a chronic extension lag of 35 degrees, but was ambulatory with a brace.

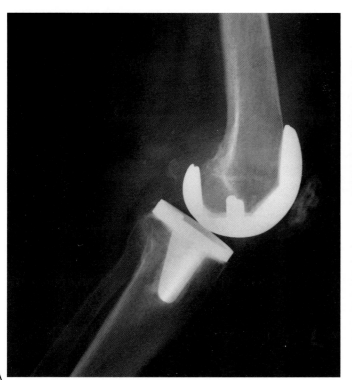 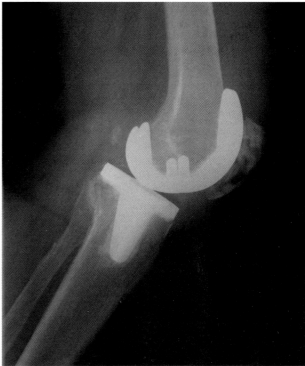

A   B

Figure 7. (Case 3) **A:** Lateral radiograph of the left knee. **B:** Lateral radiograph demonstrating displacement of the inferior pole of the patella after 6 weeks of observation. The patient had no functional impairment and no extension lag.

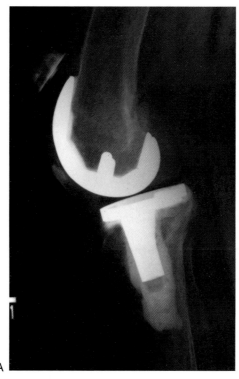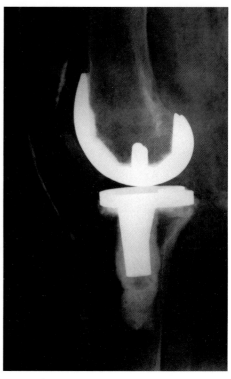

A   B

Figure 8. (Case 4) **A:** Lateral radiograph of the left knee demonstrating a displaced fracture. **B:** Lateral radiograph of the left knee 2 weeks after attempted repair of the fracture with a suture technique. After failure of the repair, the patient was mobilized. She subsequently developed an extensor lag.

RECOMMENDED READING

1. Cacambi, A. C., and Engh, G. A.: Use of a semitendinosus tendon autogenous graft for rupture of the patellar ligament after total knee arthroplasty. *J. Bone Joint Surg.*, 74-A: 974–979, 1992.
2. Clayton, M., and Thirupathi, R.: Patellar complications after total-condylar arthroplasty. *Clin. Orthop.*, 170: 152–155, 1982.
3. Figgie, H. E. III, Goldberg, V. M., Figgie, M. P., Inglis, A. E., Kelly, M., and Sobel, M.: The effect of alignment of the implant on fractures of the patella after condylar total knee arthroplasty. *J. Bone Joint Surg.*, 71-A: 1031–1039, 1989.
4. Goldberg, V. M., Figgie, H. E. III, Inglis, A. E., Figgie, M. P., Sobel, M., Kelly, M., and Kraay, M.: Patellar fracture type and prognosis in condylar total knee arthroplasty. *Clin. Orthop.*, 236: 115–122, 1988.
5. Leblanc, J. M.: Patellar complications in total knee arthroplasty. A literature review. *Orthop. Rev.*, 18(3): 296–304, 1989.
6. Lynch, A. F., Rorabeck, C. H., and Bourne, R. B.: Extensor mechanism complications following total knee arthroplasty. *J. Arthroplasty*, 2: 135–140, 1987.
7. Merkow, R. L., Soudry, M., and Insall, J. N.: Patellar dislocation following total knee replacement. *J. Bone Joint Surg.*, 67-A: 1321–1327, 1985.
8. Mochizuki, R. M., and Schurman, D. J.: Patellar complications following total knee arthroplasty. *J. Bone Joint Surg.*, 61-A: 879–883, 1979.
9. Ranawat, C. S.: The patellofemoral joint in total condylar knee arthroplasty. *Clin. Orthop.*, 205: 93–99, 1986.
10. Rand, J. A., Morrey, B. F., and Bryan, R. S.: Patellar tendon rupture after total knee arthroplasty. *Clin. Orthop.*, 244: 233–238, 1989.
11. Scott, R. D., and Siliski, J. M.: The use of a modified V-Y quadricepsplasty during total knee replacement to gain exposure and improve flexion in the ankylosed knee. *Orthopedics*, 8: 45–48, 1985.

Master Techniques in Orthopaedic Surgery,
Knee Arthroplasty, edited by P. A. Lotke,
Raven Press, Ltd., New York © 1995.

15

The Management of Skin Necrosis

Don LaRossa

INDICATIONS/CONTRAINDICATIONS

Although it is infrequent, postoperative necrosis of skin overlying a total knee arthroplasty can threaten the success of the procedure. It is most commonly seen in patients who have had repeated surgeries causing extensive scarring of the anterior skin. The necrosis should be viewed as serious and treated promptly rather than expectantly. Once wound dehiscence, exposure of the prosthesis, or bacterial contamination occurs, the chance for salvage is drastically reduced (1). The seemingly radical approach of prompt wound excision and reconstruction with a muscle flap is in fact the conservative approach. We have successfully used the medial and/or lateral heads of the gastrocnemius muscle to salvage threatened total knee arthroplasties. Since reconstruction with gastrocnemius muscle flaps is such an important tool in this salvage, it should probably not be used when an obvious joint exposure and/or documented infection exists; the chance for salvage in such cases is so remote that the muscles should be saved for a secondary arthroplasty if that is part of the treatment plan.

Other contraindications to wound reconstruction with gastrocnemius muscle flaps are the same as for any major surgical intervention.

PREOPERATIVE EVALUATION

The area of suspected necrosis is usually discovered at the first dressing change. The skin is commonly ecchymotic and may have blistering (epidermolysis). Epi-

---

D. LaRossa, M.D.: Department of Surgery, Hospital University of Pennsylvania, Philadelphia, PA 19104.

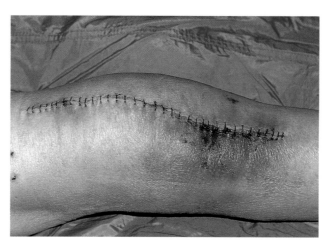

Figure 1. Typical appearance of knee wound at first dressing change. Areas of deep ecchymosis indicate full-thickness loss, as does epidermolysis.

dermolysis almost always indicates deep necrosis, since the blood supply to the skin comes primarily through the underlying fat. Epidermal death can be confirmed by peeling off the blistered skin and, within hours, observing a dry eschar that indicates a full-thickness injury (Fig. 1; see also Figs. 16 and 19). If the zone of injury is minimal and involves only a few millimeters of skin at the margins of the skin incision, nonsurgical therapy can be considered. However, even in this instance a deep tract down to the prosthesis can develop, particularly when the skin incision line directly overlies the knee-joint incision. Certainly, when a greater area of necrosis exists, wound excision and reconstruction should be undertaken.

SURGERY

The patient is put in the supine position under either general or spinal anesthesia (Fig. 2). A tourniquet applied to the ipsilateral thigh will facilitate a bloodless dissection. Skin-graft donor sites can be on the ipsilateral leg above or below the tourniquet. The leg is fully exposed during draping, so as to permit its full visualization. The midline of the calf from the popliteal fossa to the Achilles tendon is marked as an aid to the surgeon during dissection. Appropriate intravenous antibiotics are given in the perioperative period.

Following a sterile preparation of the skin, the area of skin necrosis is outlined and a small margin of viable-looking skin is included to facilitate adequate debridement of necrotic tissue (Fig. 3). As an aid to determining the extent of necrosis, intravenous fluorescein can be used at a dose of 5 mg/kg in Caucasians and 10 mg/kg in darkly pigmented individuals, given slowly over a 5- to 10-minute period, and the skin examined with a Woods lamp 20 minutes after the injection. Necrotic areas will fail to fluoresce and will appear deep blue, while perfused skin will appear yellow-green (2).

The sutures in the involved skin are removed while those in healed, unaffected skin are left in place. Sharp excision of the wound is done until a bleeding wound margin is encountered. The wound is then explored. The prosthesis need not be exposed unnecessarily. However, if the prosthesis is encountered, which occurs commonly, the joint cavity and wound are irrigated with antibiotic solutions, using the Jet Irrigator (Bard Access Systems/Davol Inc., Cranston, RI) (Fig. 4). If a portion of the closure of the internal joint capsule has been opened, it may be reclosed, although the muscle flap will cover the exposed prosthesis.

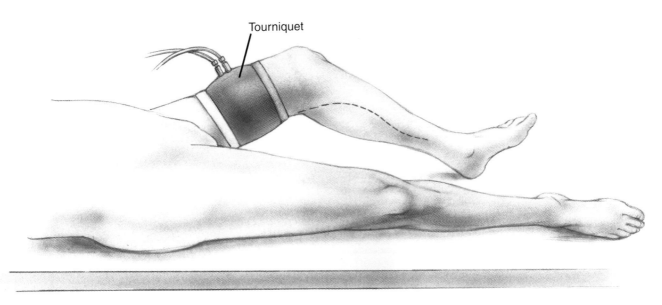

Figure 2. The patient is put in the supine position. A tourniquet is placed on the thigh and all other areas of the leg and buttocks are prepped, providing maximum exposure for muscle and skin-graft harvesting, as well as exposure of the knee.

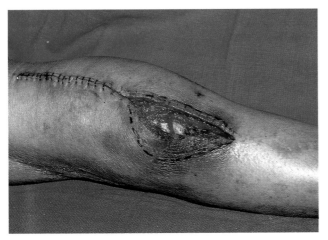

Figure 3. The area of suspected necrosis is outlined on the skin. A narrow margin of normal-appearing skin is included to assure complete removal of necrotic tissue.

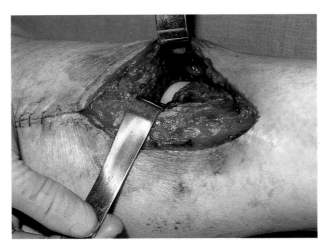

Figure 4. Exposed knee prosthesis in the depths of the wound following debridement.

At this point the surgeon can determine which muscle head of the gastrocnemius (or both) is to be used to cover the wound. The medial head of the gastrocnemius is the larger of the two and can frequently be used to cover defects that extend more laterally in addition to ones located medially. The lateral head is used for laterally placed defects (see Figs. 16 and 19). Both muscles can be used for extensive skin loss.

To harvest the muscle, an incision is outlined on the calf (see Fig. 2). For harvest of the medial or lateral head, the incision is planned where one palpates the separation between the bellies of the gastrocnemius and soleus muscles. The cephalad end of the incision can be curved toward the posterior midline to facilitate dissection of the proximal end of the muscle.

The leg is elevated and/or an Eschmark bandage is applied to exsanguinate the leg. The tourniquet is inflated for the muscle dissection.

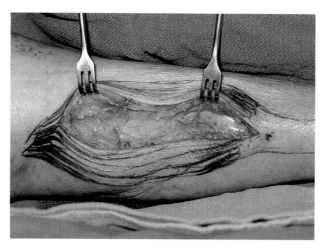

Figure 5. Under tourniquet control, an incision is made through the skin and subcutaneous tissue to the underlying muscle fascia.

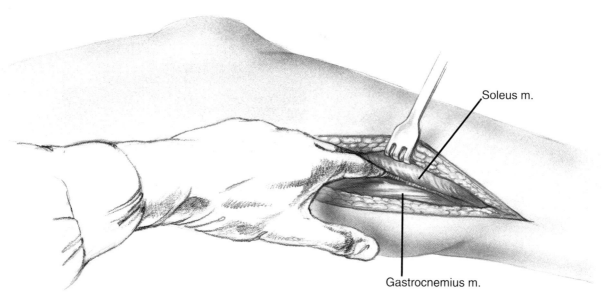

Soleus m.

Gastrocnemius m.

Figure 6. After division of the investing muscle fascia, the plane between the gastrocnemius and soleus muscles is easily and safely opened with finger dissection.

The incision is made and deepened to the muscle fascia, which is divided longitudinally (Fig. 5). This exposes the plane between the gastrocnemius and soleus muscles. This plane is essentially avascular and is easily opened with finger dissection toward the popliteal space and distally to the insertion of the gastrocnemius into the Achilles tendon (Fig. 6).

Using finger dissection, the plane between the muscle, its external fascia, and the overlying skin is opened until the median raphe is encountered. A large perforating vessel is encountered coming from the muscle into the overlying skin near the midpoint of the muscle belly (Fig. 7). It supplies the fasciocutaneous unit overlying the gastrocnemius muscle and is the basis of the gastrocnemius fasciocutaneous unit. The vessel can be divided at this time.

Lying adjacent to the midline raphe are the sural nerve and lesser saphenous vein, which should be preserved if possible (Fig. 8).

Release of the muscle is accomplished by cutting the dense fascia on the deep surface of the muscle as it attaches to the Achilles tendon (Fig. 9). Preserving a small edge of fascia is helpful in the inset of the muscle flap at the recipient site. The incision is carried to the midline raphe, where it is directed cephalad toward the popliteal fossa. The muscle fibers interdigitate in this region and so have to

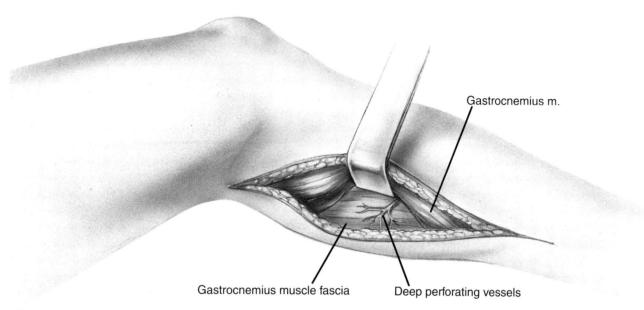

Figure 7. A large perforating vessel, which supplies the fasciocutaneous territory overlying the gastrocnemius muscles, is encountered. It can be divided unless a skin-muscle flap or fasciocutaneous flap is planned.

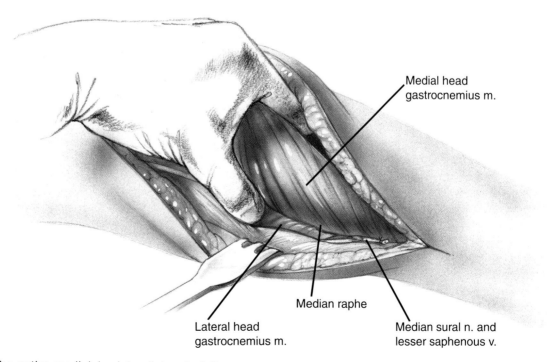

Figure 8. The entire medial (or lateral) head of the gastrocnemius muscle can be grasped and rotated to expose the median raphe, sural nerve, and lesser saphenous vein. The nerve should be preserved if possible.

be cut. Often, small vessels are encountered crossing the midline, and must be dealt with. Care is exercised to avoid injury to the sural nerve.

Once the upper edge of the raphe is divided, the muscle belly will become freely mobile, being attached only by its insertion (Fig. 10). Additional length can be achieved by further dissection toward the insertion, although one should exercise care to avoid injury to the sural vessels, which enter the deep medial surface of the muscle belly, where they are well protected.

Dissection of the lateral head of the gastrocnemius is essentially the same as that of the medial head, except for the presence of the common peroneal nerve as it becomes superficial and winds around the head of the fibula.

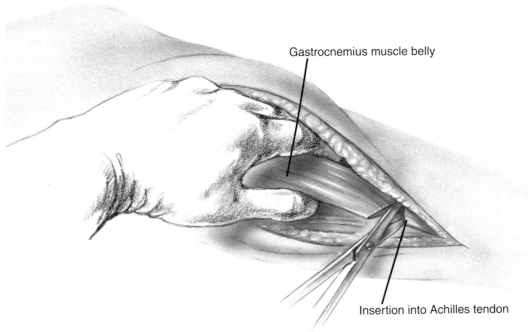

Gastrocnemius muscle belly

Insertion into Achilles tendon

Figure 9. With the muscle belly being grasped, the fibrous insertion into the Achilles tendon is divided to the median raphe. Preservation of the distal centimeter of gastrocnemius tendon will aid in attaching the muscle at its new location.

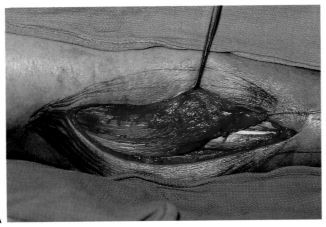
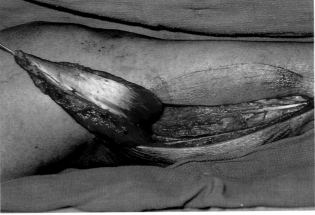

Figure 10. Once the muscle insertion has been detached **(A)** and the median raphe completely divided, the muscle becomes freely mobile **(B)**.

The tourniquet can be released at this point and hemostasis obtained in the donor site.

A subcutaneous tunnel is dissected to connect the knee wound with the muscle donor site. It should be external to the ligamentous capsule of the knee joint and extensive enough to permit easy transfer of the muscle through it (Fig. 11). Compression of the muscle by a narrow tunnel may cause necrosis of the muscle.

The muscle can be transferred into the wound with either its external or internal surface exposed. Turning it over does not impair the blood supply. Crosshatching or removal of the deep fascia can facilitate further advancement of the muscle and does not impair the blood supply (Fig. 12); it also provides a better bed for the eventual skin-graft cover.

The muscle flap is inset by securing it beneath the margins of the wound with mattress sutures of 2-0 Prolene (Ethicon, Raritan, NJ) tied over bolsters (Fig. 13). The muscle will endure a great deal of tension without compromise of its blood supply. Furthermore, insetting pulls the wound margin toward the muscle, reduc-

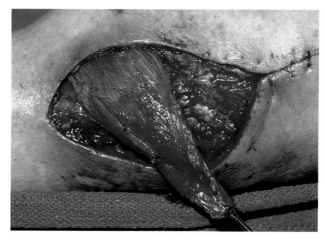

Figure 11. The muscle belly should pass easily through the subcutaneous tunnel into the knee wound site.

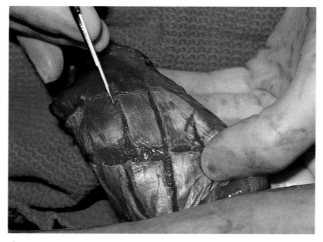

Figure 12. The deep fascia can be stripped or crosshatched (author's preference) to increase the available muscle length and breadth. Stripping or crosshatching also aids in skin-graft take by providing a more vascularized bed.

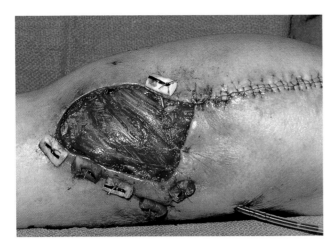

Figure 13. Sutures of 2–0 Prolene tied over bolsters secure the muscle beneath the undermined wound margin.

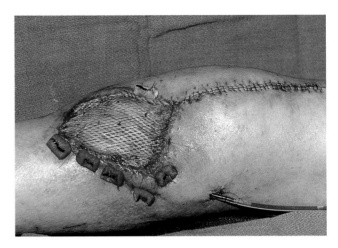

Figure 14. The muscle surface is grafted with expanded or unexpanded skin. A tie-over dressing is commonly used, although care must be exercised to avoid excessive compression of the muscle when tying down over the tie-over dressing.

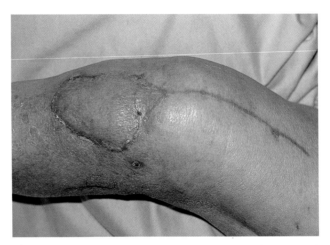

Figure 15. Closed knee wound approximately 1 month postoperatively.

ing both the size of the wound and the tension on the muscle. The margin proximate to the muscle tunnel is closed with suture of 3-0 or 4-0 Vicryl (Ethicon, Raritan, NJ) between the muscle surface and overlying subcutaneous tissue.

A skin graft, meshed at 1:1.5 or unmeshed, is applied to the recipient site (Fig. 14). A tie-over dressing is gently applied to maintain compression on the graft.

The donor site is closed in layers over a suction drain and the leg is dressed. A knee immobilizer is carefully applied to avoid compression of the reconstructed site (Fig. 15).

POSTOPERATIVE MANAGEMENT

The patient is maintained on bed rest with the knee immobilized for one week. Gently graded mobilization is then begun, increasing the angulation by 5 to 10 degrees each subsequent day. Ambulation is begun on the tenth postoperative day.

The skin graft is inspected by removal of the tie-over dressing on postoperative day 4. Topical antibiotic ointment and nonadherent gauze are applied and changed daily. The skin-graft donor site dressing is also removed. The original dressing is antibiotic ointment on Telfa (The Kendall Company, Boston, MA), sealed with Tegaderm (3M/Medical-Surgical Division, St. Paul, MN). After removal of the original dressing, the donor site is re-dressed with Telfa and antibiotic ointment, and the dressing is changed daily.

COMPLICATIONS

Complications of wound reconstruction with gastrocnemius flaps are rare. No instances of complete flap loss have been encountered. Minor areas of skin graft loss have been seen, and for these the treatment consists of topical antibiotics and protective dressings until healing is complete. Skin-graft donor-site problems can occur and may delay healing. They are usually treated with topical antibiotics, though systemic antibiotics are occasionally needed when a cellulitis occurs.

The most important nonlethal complication of reconstruction is the recurrence or persistence of an infection in the prosthetic knee. This generally requires removal of the prosthesis. A second procedure, using the remaining head of the gastrocnemius (if it has not been used) should not be undertaken in this situation, so as to preserve the muscle for later reconstructive efforts.

ILLUSTRATIVE CASES FOR TECHNIQUE

Case 1. A 72-year-old woman had a total knee arthroplasty. Blistered skin was noted at the time of dressing removal 1 week postoperatively. Within hours of removal of the blister, a dry eschar was noted, indicating full-thickness skin loss

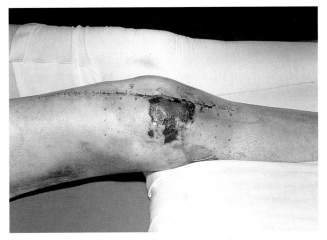

Figure 16. Within hours of removal of blistered skin, desiccation of the dermis occurs, leaving a dry eschar indicating full-thickness loss. Skin loss is lateral to the knee incision in this 72-year-old patient at 1 week after a total knee arthroplasty.

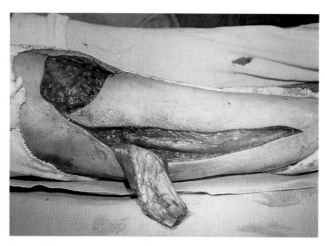

Figure 17. Lateral head of the gastrocnemius muscle dissected and knee wound excised in the patient in Figure 16.

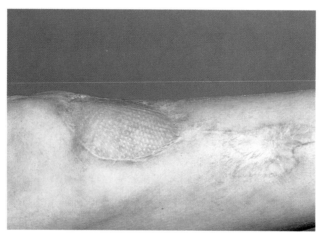

Figure 18. Appearance following successful coverage and healing in the patient in Figures 16 and 17.

(Fig. 16). The affected skin was excised and the lateral head of the gastrocnemius muscle was mobilized for coverage of the exposed knee prosthesis (Fig. 17). A meshed split-thickness skin graft was used to resurface the exposed portion of the muscle flap. Uneventful healing took place (Fig. 18).

Case 2. This 57-year-old woman had multiple knee surgeries following a severe knee injury at age 9. The resultant scars produced ischemic zones of skin following total knee arthroplasty. Extensive full-thickness skin loss was noted, threatening the prosthesis (Fig. 19). Debridement of the involved soft-tissue cover was done with exposure of the knee prosthesis (Fig. 20). The extensive defect required the use of both the medial and lateral gastrocnemius muscles for secure coverage. A meshed split-thickness skin graft completed the closure and eventuated in uneventful healing (Fig. 21).

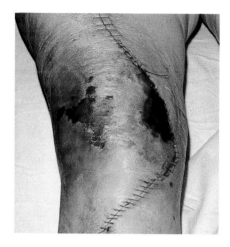

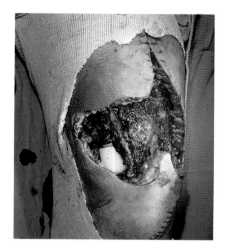

◄Figure 19. Extensive skin necrosis in a 57-year-old woman with multiple previous knee surgeries following a childhood injury.

►Figure 20. Extensive wound and exposed prosthesis following excision in the patient illustrated in Figure 19.

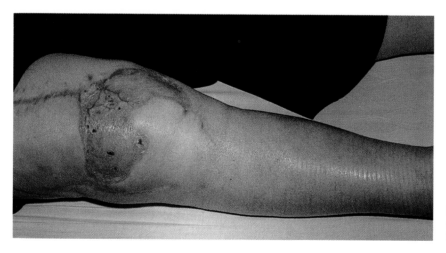

Figure 21. Appearance following successful coverage and healing in the patient depicted in Figures 19 and 20.

Acknowledgment.   Special thanks to Dr. David Low for photographing his patient's operative procedure (Figs. 1, 3–5, and 10–15).

RECOMMENDED READING

1. Greenberg, B., LaRossa, D., Lotke, P. A., Murphy, J. B., and Noone, R. B.: Salvage of jeopardized total knee prostheses—The role of the gastrocnemius muscle flap. *Plast. Reconstr. Surg.,* 79: 959–965, 1987.
2. Silverman, D., LaRossa, D., Barlow, C., Bering, T., Popky, L., and Smith, T.: Quantification of tissue fluorescein delivery and prediction of flap viability with the fiberoptic dermofluorometer. *Plast. Reconstr. Surg.,* 66: 545–553, 1980.
3. Boileau Grant, J. C., editor: *Grant's Atlas of Anatomy.* Williams and Wilkins, Baltimore, 1991.
4. McCraw and Arnold's Atlas of Muscle and Musculocutaneous Flaps. pp. 491–443. Hampton Press Publishing Company, Norfolk, Virginia, 1986.

Master Techniques in Orthopaedic Surgery,
KNEE ARTHROPLASTY, edited by P. A. Lotke,
Raven Press, Ltd., New York © 1995.

16

Delayed Exchange Reimplantation for Infected Total Knee Arthroplasty

Thomas S. Thornhill

INDICATIONS/CONTRAINDICATIONS

The diagnosis of an infected total knee arthroplasty is suspected on the basis of clinical grounds and confirmed by arthrocentesis, cell count, and culture of joint fluid. It is critical to differentiate superficial infection from deep sepsis. Moreover, it is helpful to consider both acute perioperative infections (within 3 weeks after surgery) and late infections. Late infections may originate from an acute hematogenous source, by direct invasion, or as indolent, chronic low-grade sepsis. Table 1 lists the surgical options available for treatment of an infected total knee arthroplasty.

Patients with acute superficial cellulitis following total knee arthroplasty can usually be treated with intravenous antibiotics and prosthesis retention. If there is an established deep infection with a highly susceptible streptococcal organism, the joint can be aspirated and intravenous antibiotics administered. The joint may require repeated aspiration, and it is critical that a boggy synovitis not persist following aspiration. Within 24 hours, the patient must respond with a decrease in the white cell count, symptomatic improvement, and negative cultures (4). Antibiotics are continued for a minimum of 3 weeks, with monitoring in conjunction with an infectious disease consultant. Aspiration and antibiotics alone have little or no role in the treatment of late infection. Bengston et al. reported only a 15% success rate in 225 knees treated with antibiotics without open debridement. (1).

T. S. Thornhill, M.D.: Department of Orthopedics, Harvard Medical School, Brigham and Women's Hospital, New England Baptist Hospital, Boston, MA 02115.

TABLE 1. *Surgical options for treatment of the infected TKR*

Arthroscopic debridement
Open debridement
Immediate exchange
Delayed exchange
Arthrodesis
Resection arthroplasty
Amputation

In acute perioperative deep infection with organisms other than *Streptococcus,* in cases in which there is an associated synovitis, and in those patients who fail to respond to intravenous antibiotics and aspiration, open debridement may be indicated. The role of arthroscopic lavage and debridement is unclear. Limited experience has shown that arthroscopic lavage may be helpful in cases with marginal indications for aspiration alone and in whom open debridement may be considered too aggressive.

Patients undergoing open debridement with prosthesis retention should have a synovectomy and copious lavage (5 L) with an antibiotic irrigant. If a metal-backed modular tibia is in place, the polyethylene should be removed, the tibial tray thoroughly irrigated, and a new insert implanted. Frequently the new insert is 2 mm thicker than the original polyethylene insert in order to correct the added laxity caused by reopening the soft-tissue envelope. The knee is closed over a drain and intravenous antibiotics are administered for 3 to 6 weeks.

The treatment of late established infection (occurring more than 3 weeks following surgery) with open debridement and prosthesis retention is indicated in highly selected patients. Radiographs must show no evidence of prosthesis loosening or bone erosion. The organism must be a *Streptococcus* or other highly susceptible organism sensitive to an antibiotic program tolerated by the host. The host defense mechanisms must be intact. The prosthesis must be well aligned, with no evidence of mechanical problems (polyethylene wear, component breakage, malrotation). The presentation must be acute and the infection recognized within the first 48 to 72 hours. The radiographs must show no evidence of loosening, osteolysis, or periosteal reaction. The skin, soft tissues, and extensor mechanism must be suitable for retention of the implant. The presence of a sinus tract indicates a chronic infection and requires delayed exchange.

In our institution, immediate exchange is indicated in patients with a highly susceptible organism, adequate soft tissue, an adequate host response, and radiographs demonstrating a need for revision other than infection. There must be no bony reaction suggesting osteomyelitis, and the infection must be diagnosed early. The revision should be straightforward, without requiring significant restoration of bone stock (8).

Delayed exchange is the predominant treatment for established deep infection in total knee arthroplasty. A variety of options exist in the protocol for such exchange, including the interval to reimplantation, length of intravenous antibiotic treatment, and use of cement spacers with immobilization versus early mobilization during the resection period. Delayed exchange is contraindicated in patients with skin and soft tissues unsuitable for reconstruction, patients in whom multiple previous exchanges have failed, and patients with an incompetent extensor mechanism. In these cases, arthrodesis or resection arthroplasty should be considered. Amputation is reserved for those patients with life-threatening infections due to gas-forming organisms or in end-stage refractory situations unsuitable for other treatment options (8).

The results of open debridement with prosthesis retention are not comparable to those of exchange operations. Borden reported a 55% failure rate in 11 infected total knees treated by open debridement with prosthesis retention (3). Wilson, Kelley, and Thornhill reported a 45% recrudescent infection rate in 42 infected total knee replacements, and that knees with *Staphylococcus aureus* infection had a much higher failure rate than originally suspected (12). Schoifet and Morrey found a 77% recurrence rate in 31 infected knees (mean follow-up 8.8 years) treated by open debridement with prosthesis retention (5). In this series there was a 58% failure rate when *S. aureus* was the infecting organism (5). Bengston reported a 24% success rate in 150 knees treated by soft-tissue surgery alone, without prosthesis removal (1).

The role of immediate exchange in the treatment of the infected total knee is unclear. Bengston reported a 75% success rate in eradicating infection in 107 knees treated by exchange surgery (1). In this study there was no difference between one- and two-stage exchange. Von Foerster examined 104 infected total knee arthroplasties (5- to 15-year follow-up) treated by immediate exchange and antibiotic-impregnated cement (10). In this series there was a 73% cure rate with a single exchange and an overall 84% cure rate with a second exchange (10).

Windsor and Insall and their associates reported an 89.5% success rate in 38 infected total knees treated by delayed exchange (13,14). Wilson, Kelley, and Thornhill showed similar data, with an 80% success rate in 24 infected knees treated by delayed exchange (12). Borden (3) presented a 91% success rate in 11 knees, while Teeny and colleagues (7) had 100% success rate in 9 infected knees treated by delayed exchange.

PREOPERATIVE PLANNING

Once the diagnosis of an infected total knee arthroplasty is confirmed and delayed exchange is considered the appropriate treatment, the surgeon must choose from a variety of options within the delayed exchange protocol. In consultation with the infectious disease specialist, an appropriate initial antibiotic program is established. Superficial wound cultures and even aspirates may be misleading. Unless a definitive single organism is identified by aspiration or biopsy, it is preferable to withhold antibiotics until deep cultures of synovial fluid, synovium, and bone are obtained. Oral antibiotic suppression or preoperative parenteral antibiotics should be discontinued unless the organism is known or unless they are medically necessary to control systemic symptoms of sepsis. It may be necessary to stop oral suppressive antibiotics from 7 to 14 days prior to culture, to avoid false-negative readings. Cultures should be taken directly to the laboratory and placed on both aerobic and anaerobic media.

The delayed exchange protocol and protocol options are listed in Table 2. Among the several protocol options from which the surgeon must choose are the

TABLE 2. *Delayed exchange protocol*

Removal of components and cement
Debridement of necrotic and devitalized tissue
Thorough irrigation with antibiotic solution
Measurement of remaining bony surfaces
Estimation of bone deficit
Establishing/maintaining joint space during resection interval
   Cement spacer
   Primary closure with early mobilization/CPM
Parenteral antibiotics with measurement of antibiotic levels
Re-evaluation prior to reimplantation
   Interval aspiration/biopsy
   Evaluation of systemic signs/symptoms
Reimplantation
   Intraoperative culture, gram stain, frozen section
   Careful joint inspection
   Decision to reimplant
   Reimplantation
Postoperative management
   Parenteral antibiotics until intraoperative antibiotics return
   Modified physical therapy protocol

length of antibiotic treatment and the time before reimplantation, the use of a cement spacer or continuous passive motion (CPM) with early mobilization, and the need for an interval biopsy prior to reimplantation.

SURGERY

It is preferable that the infected implant be removed by the surgeon who will be performing the reimplantation. This allows the surgeon to identify areas of bone loss, prevent excessive debridement, and plan for the subsequent revision arthroplasty. Once the decision for delayed exchange is made, the surgeon must carefully plan the initial implant removal to optimize eventual revision arthroplasty.

Patients with infected total knee replacements are more likely than others to have undergone previous surgery and have multiple skin incisions. In general, previous skin incisions should be utilized in the exchange procedure if they allow adequate exposure. If the patient has had a previous medial and lateral incision, it is generally preferable to honor the lateral incision. Care should be taken to avoid undermining skin flaps and to be certain that all dissection is beneath the deep investing fascia. If there is a single incision from the index arthroplasty, it should be utilized. Dissection should go directly to the capsular tissues and the capsule should be opened in a median parapatellar fashion.

Patients with an infected total knee arthroplasty are more prone to avulsion of the infrapatellar tendon, owing to soft-tissue adhesion or scarring of the quadriceps mechanism. Prior to eversion of the patellar tendon, it is beneficial to excise the inflamed synovium and granulation tissue and perform a lateral retinacular release. If the quadriceps mechanism cannot be everted and the knee flexed, a proximal turndown or tibial tubercle osteotomy (TTO) is necessary. In most cases a proximal soft-tissue turndown is preferred to a TTO in order to avoid exposure of the cancellous bone of the proximal tibia to the infecting organism. The turndown, as shown in Figure 1, is frequently a short modified V, as previously described by Scott and Siliski (6). A short oblique release of the proximal quadriceps is usually sufficient to relax the tight medial edge of the quadriceps mechanism and allow flexion without avulsion of the infrapatellar tendon (Fig. 2).

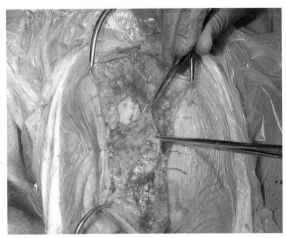

Figure 1. Short turndown of quadriceps tendon, allowing eversion of the quadriceps mechanism without risking avulsion of the infrapatellar tendon.

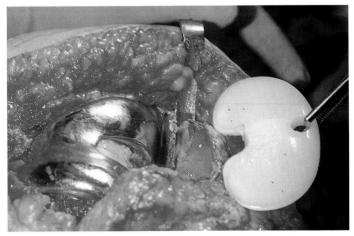

Figure 2. Following eversion of the quadriceps mechanism, the knee is flexed and the polyethylene tibial insert removed.

Soft-Tissue Debridement

A synovectomy is routinely performed to debride the infected soft tissue, mobilize the soft tissues, and facilitate tissue balancing. A lateral patellar retinacular release is frequently necessary to mobilize the tight lateral structures. This release is performed from inside the joint after first identifying the edge of the vastus lateralis. The supralateral geniculate vessel should be identified and spared if present, and the release performed distally to the tibia and curving anteriorly in its proximal arm toward but not into the vastus lateralis muscles. The knee is now flexed.

Component Removal

In cases of deep sepsis, both components of the existing prosthesis are frequently loose and can be removed easily. At times, a well-fixed component will require disruption of the interface to permit component removal. On the femoral side, removal of a fixed implant is best performed using osteotomes that disrupt the interface between the cement and implant or at the implant–bone interface in uncemented designs (Fig. 3). Care should be taken to carefully disrupt the interface so that the component can be removed by hand and not require forcible extraction. Alternatively a Gigli saw can be used to disrupt the anterior half of the interface. When the Gigli saw is used it is necessary to use an osteotome to disrupt the interface posterior to the fixation lugs.

Removal of a well-fixed all-polyethylene tibial component is best performed by amputating the tibial component at the junction of the plateau and the stem. The polyethylene stem can then be removed by use of a corkscrew, osteotomes, or both. In modular tibial designs the polyethylene insert is removed and thin osteotomes are used to disrupt the interface at the tibial plateaus (Fig. 3). A tibial extractor may facilitate removal of the tibial component.

The patellar component is removed with either sharp osteotomes or a saw. It is frequently necessary to use a high-speed drill to remove the remaining cement from the patellar lugs.

At this point all remaining cement is removed and multiple specimens are taken for aerobic and anaerobic culture. The tourniquet is then deflated and a broad-spectrum antibiotic, directed toward the presumptive pathogen, is administered.

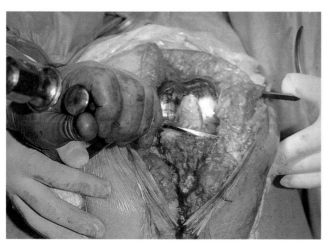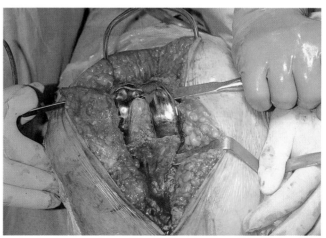

A   B

Figure 3. A,B: Osteotomes are used to carefully define the interface between the implant and cement or adjacent bone. This interface is thoroughly developed to allow the components to be extracted by hand.

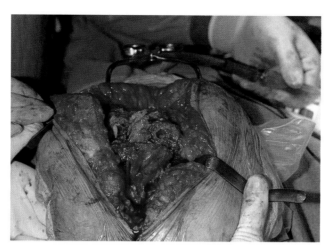

Figure 4. The components are removed and cultures of periprosthetic bone are obtained. Broad-spectrum intravenous antibiotics are then administered and the knee thoroughly irrigated with antibiotic irrigant. The surfaces are measured for sizing of the subsequent component, and estimates are made of areas of bone loss. Prior to closure of the knee, an antibiotic-impregnated cement prosthetic analogue for the femoral and tibial components is fashioned. The wound is closed over suction drainage.

Careful hemostasis is achieved. The wound, bony surfaces, and soft tissues are then thoroughly irrigated with antibiotic solution (minimum 5 L). Five minutes after antibiotic instillation, and after careful hemostasis is achieved, the tourniquet may be reinflated for closure (Fig. 4).

Estimation of Bony Defects

The anteroposterior (AP) and lateral dimensions of the tibia and femoral surfaces are measured and recorded. Estimated bone loss is carefully recorded to plan for subsequent revision. The flexion and extension gaps are measured in order to estimate soft-tissue balance at the time of revision.

Use of Cement Spacers

Prior to closure of the wound, the surgeon may elect to use an antibiotic-impregnated cement spacer (2). The advantage of the cement spacer is that it will deliver a pulse of antibiotic at the implant–bone interface, where remaining organisms may reside. Second, the cement spacer will maintain a soft-tissue space to facilitate subsequent revision. Additionally, the spacer will confer stability to the extremity during the interval prior to reimplantation. Several techniques are available for the fabrication of cement spacers. Antibiotics can be mixed at twice the dose usually used when the cement is intended for fixation of an implant. A common mixture is 1200 mg of powdered tobramycin per 40 g of methacrylate (Simplex). It is important to extend the cement spacer anteriorly to maintain the space of the patellofemoral joint, and also posteriorly when possible. Care should be taken not to overdistract the extension space, since this will stretch the collateral ligaments and necessitate extension augmentation at the time of reimplantation.

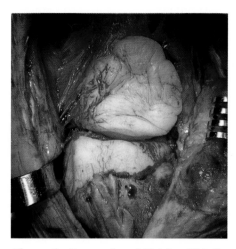

Figure 5. Femoral and tibial antibiotic-impregnated methacrylate spacer in place prior to revision arthroplasty.

Figure 5 shows a cement spacer exposed at the time of reimplantation. When removed, the defect left by the spacer will create a joint space to facilitate reimplantation.

An alternative treatment plan is to close the wound without use of a cement spacer and use external immobilization prior to reimplantation. Advocates of this technique prefer the ability to use CPM to maintain the soft-tissue envelope of the joint as well as to prevent adhesions. Moreover, this technique precludes use of another foreign body. In cases of poor healing or medical illness, reimplantation may be significantly delayed or postponed, necessitating a separate procedure to remove the cement spacer to permit a permanent resection arthroplasty.

Closure of the Wound

The wound should be closed primarily, except in cases of severe sepsis with gas-forming organisms. Suction drains are utilized and are preferable to suction irrigation systems. The capsule is closed with absorbable sutures to prevent a permanent focus of chronic infection. The skin is closed with interrupted sutures with stay sutures necessary in some wounds. A pressure dressing is applied and the patient placed in a knee immobilizer.

Interval Prior to Reimplantation

If a cement spacer is utilized, the leg is immobilized either with a Velcro immobilizer or a cylinder cast. In some cases a short flexion arc is possible, but care must be taken to prevent destruction of bone by the methacrylate cement spacer. If a spacer is not used, the knee is placed in a CPM machine at day 4 and flexed from 0° to 30°. The flexion may be increased gradually as tolerated. The knee is immobilized in a Velcro dressing between therapy sessions, and the patient is allowed a touch-down weight-bearing gait.

Parenteral antibiotics are administered after discussion with the infectious disease specialist. The length of antibiotic treatment depends upon the virulence of the infecting organism, the status of the soft tissues, and the patient's host-defense mechanisms (8). In general, a minimum of 4 to 6 weeks of parenteral antibiotics is preferred. This surgeon may choose to discontinue antibiotic therapy and perform an interval biopsy prior to reimplantation.

The patient is maintained on a touch-down weight-bearing gait, using a walker or axillary crutches. General conditioning exercises and a balanced nutritional program are continued during this period.

Reimplantation

The decision to undertake reimplantation is made in consultation with the infectious disease specialist, measurement of acute-phase reactants, and evaluation of the wound. If persistent swelling and erythema are present, an interval biopsy with fluid aspiration and tissue analysis is indicated. If, at the time of revision, purulent material or active inflammation is present, the surgeon may choose to perform a further debridement without reimplantation.

Reimplantation/Patient Positioning/Exposure

The patient is placed in a supine position with a roll behind the ipsilateral trochanter to neutrally rotate the leg. A second roll affixed to the operating table at the midcalf level will allow support of the foot when the knee is flexed. The incision used for component removal is reopened, with care being taken to avoid large tissue dissection. The antibiotic-impregnated cement spacer, if utilized, is removed and the joint debrided. It may be necessary to revisit the lateral retinacular release and even perform a proximal quadriceps turndown to mobilize the quadriceps mechanism. Fluid is sent for a stat cell count and gram stain, a frozen section is made of any suspicious soft tissue, and the joint is thoroughly inspected. In cases with a high white blood cell count (greater than 5000 mm^3), if organisms are seen or there is evidence of an acute active inflammation on frozen section, the surgeon may choose to further debride the wound and delay reimplantation.

Estimation of Proper Joint Line

It is often difficult to determine the original joint line of the knee, but an estimation can be made from the index radiograph and by noting the distal femoral thickness of the original implant. On radiography, the fibular head and inferior pole of the patella may be helpful guidelines (the inferior pole of the patella should be above the joint line in full extension, and the fibular head below the tibial plateau). At operative inspection, the normal joint line is normally 14 to 16 mm distal to the origin of the posterior cruciate ligament and approximately 40 to 45 mm distal to the medial epicondylar eminence. In some cases a radiograph of the opposite knee may be superimposed on the affected side to estimate the joint line. In virtually every case of delayed exchange the posterior cruciate ligament is absent or nonfunctional, and a cruciate-substituting implant is indicated. Cruciate substituting/sacrificing designs are less sensitive to joint-line elevation than cruciate-sparing implants.

Estimation of the Soft-Tissue Gap and Bone Deficiency

After thorough debridement and careful lavage, the flexion and extension gaps are measured with spacer blocks. Moreover, bone deficiencies are noted to evaluate the need for bone or metal augmentation and the necessity for stemmed implants. Figure 6A and B shows a spacer block used to assess the flexion and

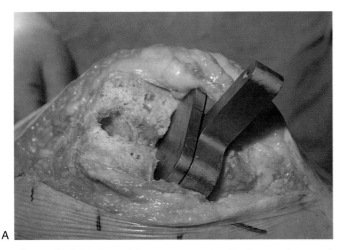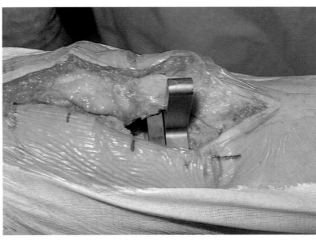

A   B

Figure 6. A,B: At revision surgery, the flexion and extension gaps are measured with appropriate spacers. If the flexion gap is greater than the extension gap, the difference is corrected by addition of a posterior femoral wedge. If the extension gap is greater than the flexion gap, distal femoral augmentation is preferred.

extension gaps. If the extension gap is greater than the flexion gap, it is necessary to augment the distal femur in order to approximate the normal joint line and balance the flexion and extension gaps. If the flexion gap is greater than the extension gap it is necessary to use posterior femoral augmentation and/or a larger femoral component. Tensioning of the soft-tissue envelope by increasing the thickness of the tibial component independently of the normal joint line will frequently produce an unacceptable patella infera and distort the kinematics of the collateral ligaments (Fig. 7A,B).

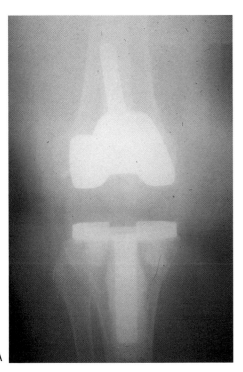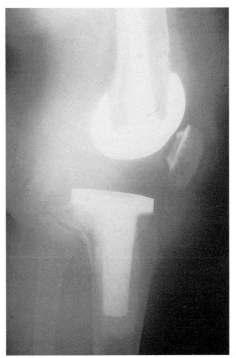

A   B

Figure 7. A,B: Anteroposterior and lateral radiograph of a revision case in which excessive tibial thickness was used to balance the soft tissues. This resulted in a markedly elevated joint line, abnormal kinematics, and marked patella infera.

Femoral Preparation

Removal of the index arthroplasty and debridement of the infected knee will usually obliterate the standard landmarks for femoral preparation. The true joint line is determined as stated above, the valgus orientation determined by a femoral intramedullary guide, and the femoral rotation determined after tibial preparation.

The femoral canal is entered with a 1/4-inch drill bit. The entry point is anterior and slightly medial to the top of the intercondylar notch. A series of hand reamers are used to expand the distal intramedullary opening until endosteal contact with the diaphysis of the femur is achieved (Fig. 8). It is important to establish a common endosteal diameter well into the diaphysis rather than wedging the tip of the reamer against the cortex at a single point (see Fig. 8B,C). This will determine the final inside diameter of the fluted press-fit stem of the femoral component. Moreover, it will determine the diameter of the sleeve guide to be fitted on the intramedullary (I.M.) rod. The appropriate sleeve is fitted onto the rod and advanced distally to a locked position (Fig. 9A). The bayonette mounting is such that the sleeve cannot be disengaged from the proximal end of the rod. The sleeve/

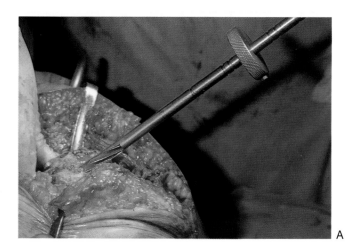

Figure 8. **A–C:** The femoral canal is sequentially reamed by hand to the minimum diameter that engages the endosteal cortex of the femur. The preferred reaming engages side contact (**B**) rather than tip contact (**C**) with the reamer.

A

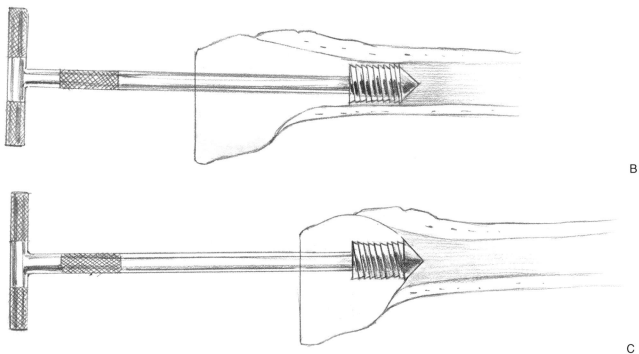

B

C

I.M. rod assembly is carefully advanced into the intramedullary canal to achieve side contact between the sleeve and the prepared endosteal cortex. By rotating the handle of the assembly by 90°, the I.M. rod can be advanced carefully to achieve rigid fixation within the intramedullary shaft of the femur. The handle is now removed, leaving a rigid fixed assembly that can be the template for femoral preparation (Fig. 9B).

The distal femoral cutting guide is advanced and pinned in place, and the distal femur is resected (Fig. 10). Distal femoral resection may be minimal and involve only a single condyle. The level of resection and determination the need for distal femoral augmentation are based on an estimation of the femoral joint line and the difference between the flexion and extension gaps (see above).

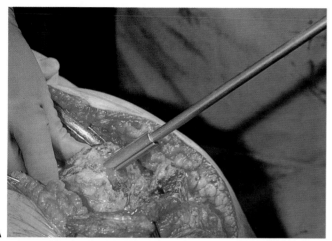
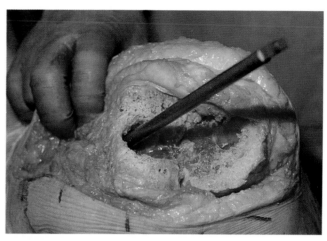

A   B

Figure 9. A,B: The intramedullary rod is assembled with the appropriate sleeve (corresponding to the diameter of the last reamer). The sleeve is assembled from the handle end of the I.M. rod, and locked distally for insertion. By rotation, the I.M. rod can be advanced once the sleeve is in place. A distal bullet prevents dissociation between the sleeve and I.M. rod, and eliminates the risk of retention of the sleeve in the diaphysis of the femur. The I.M. rod is advanced through the sleeve and becomes rigidly fixed in the femur (**B**). Moreover, as it is directed into position by the sleeve, the rod is in the precise position of the press-fit stem and allows exact preparation of the distal femoral bone.

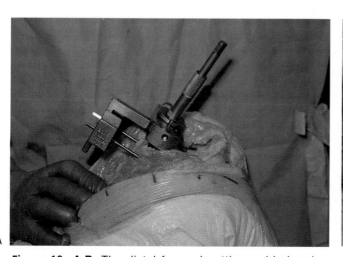
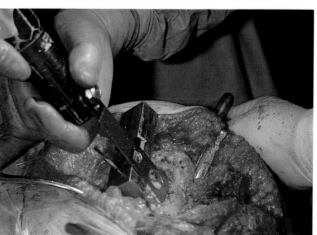

A   B

Figure 10. A,B: The distal femoral cutting guide is advanced over the I.M. rod and the distal femoral resection is performed. Based on the preoperative templating and interoperative measurements to restore the normal joint line, the choice of individual or combined distal femoral augmentation is determined and the appropriate cut is made.

Femoral rotation is determined after tibial preparation, with the caveats that internal rotation must be avoided and that slight external rotation will facilitate patellar tracking. Linking the femoral rotation to the tibial component will prevent component malrotation.

Tibial Preparation

The tibial intramedullary canal is prepared using hand reamers of increasing diameter. As on the femoral side, it is important to prepare a broad area of the diaphysis for endosteal contact rather than tip contact. It is extremely important to gently prepare this cortex by hand in order to prevent perforation. When necessary, intraoperative radiographs are made. The rod and sleeve assembly used in femoral preparation is inserted to create a rigid, fixed reference point for tibial preparation (Fig. 11). This point is identical in position and thickness to the inside

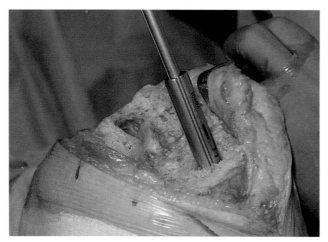

Figure 11. The tibial diaphysis is reamed in the same fashion as the femur, and the appropriate I.M. rod and sleeve are inserted.

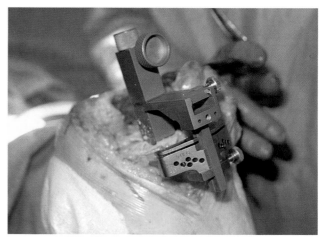

Figure 12. The intramedullary tibial guide is emplaced and tibial resection performed. The level of tibial resection is based on preoperative radiographs and the extent of bone loss on the tibial surface.

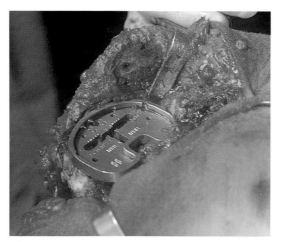

Figure 13. The appropriate size tibial base plate is fitted with an I.M. rod of appropriate outside diameter and inserted in approximate rotation as determined by the tibial tubercle. In this case a medial and posteromedial gap is present, indicating the need for a metal wedge.

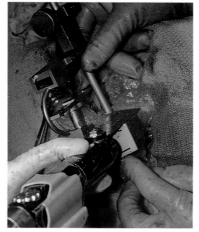

Figure 14. The angled tibial-wedge cutting guide is placed and the bony surface prepared.

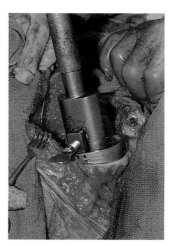

Figure 15. The trial wedge is positioned and the trial tibial component inserted to determine precision of fit.

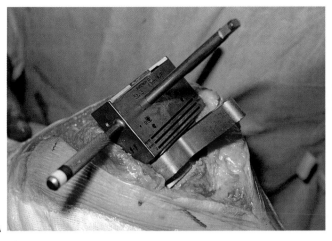
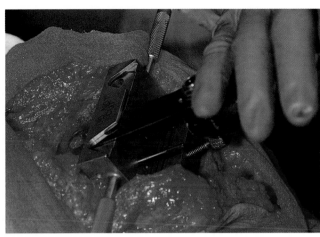

A   B

Figure 16. A,B: Final rotation of the femoral component is determined with the knee in flexion and the femoral cutting guide rotated to balance the flexion gap. The anterior and posterior cuts are made **(B)**.

diameter of the final fluted press-fit stem. The intramedullary cutting guide is affixed to the I.M. rod and tibial preparation is performed (Fig. 12). The level of resection is chosen to achieve a reasonable proximal tibial surface. Areas of bone loss are best treated with metal wedges rather than allografts. This avoids the potential risk of recrudescent infection with allografts and the uncertainty of incorporation of previously infected bone. In younger patients and those with massive bone loss in whom revision is indicated, allografts may be necessary.

Figure 13 shows a tibial base plate fitted to the appropriate size tibial stem implanted on the prepared tibial surface. A posteromedial and medial defect is noted, and restoration of bone stock by tibial wedge is chosen. The appropriate size tibial wedge cutting guide is affixed to the front of the tibial base plate and the bony cut for the wedge is made (Fig. 14). It is generally best to establish correct femoral rotation and then adjust tibial rotation to conform to the femoral component prior to making the wedge cut. Figure 15 shows the trial tibial wedge fitted into the prepared tibial bed.

Determination of Femoral Rotation

If the index femoral component was properly rotated, there are generally landmarks available to guide rotation for the femoral cuts. External rotation of the femoral component is acceptable and often preferable for three reasons. First, a slightly externally rotated femoral component will balance a tight medial flexion gap, which is common in revision situations. Second, external rotation of the femoral component tilts the trochlea slightly laterally, facing it toward a patella that may track to the lateral side. Third, external rotation of the femoral component will allow a commensurate external rotation of the tibial component, which reduces the quadriceps angle and facilitates patellar tracking. Under no circumstances should the femoral component be internally rotated.

With the trial tibial base plate and stem in place, and the femoral I.M. rod and sleeve combination fixed in the femoral intramedullary shaft, the femoral cutting block is affixed to the femoral I.M. rod (Fig. 16). A spacer block of appropriate thickness to tighten the flexion gap is emplaced and the anterior and posterior cuts are performed. A decision is implanted about posterior augmentation on the basis of the disparity between the posteromedial and posterolateral femoral bone as well as the difference between the original flexion and extension gaps. As on the tibial side, femoral augmentation following sepsis is usually performed with augmentation wedges rather than bone grafts.

Figure 17 shows the femoral housing cutting guide, which is placed over the I.M. rod and pinned, after which the rod is removed. This prepares the intramedullary femoral bone for acceptance of the cruciate housing of the femoral component, since cruciate substitution is needed to restore soft-tissue stability.

Patellar Preparation

The patellar bone is examined and the patellar thickness measured (Fig. 18). Soft tissues around the edges are trimmed to expose the peripheral bone. Resurfacing of the patella with a cemented polyethylene patellar button is preferred when possible. It is best to have a patellar bone thickness of 12 to 15 mm and the resection amount is determined by the patellar component thickness. In cases of extreme

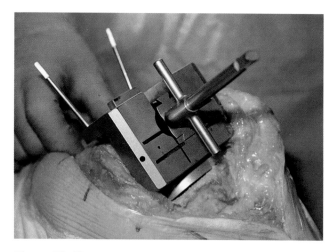

Figure 17. The chamfer guide and femoral housing guide are inserted and the bone cut for the femoral housing.

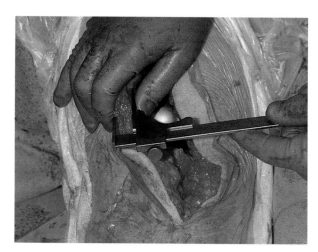

Figure 18. The remaining patellar bone is measured. If the overall thickness is greater than 12 mm and the surface is uneven, a minimal resection is made to provide a flat surface with a minimum thickness of 12 mm.

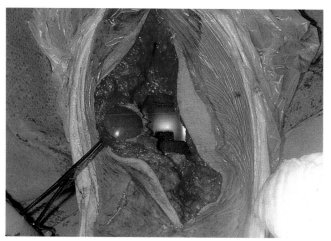

A

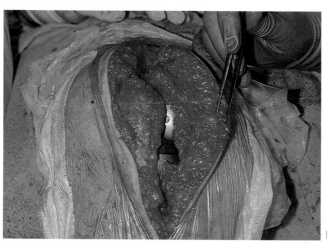

B

Figure 19. A,B: The patellar trial component is fitted **(A)**, the patella returned to the trochlea, and the knee flexed to ascertain soft-tissue balance and proper tracking **(B)**. If the patella does not remain in the groove during flexion and extension, a lateral retinacular release is performed.

bone loss a patelloplasty is performed to smooth the patellar surface in lieu of prosthetic resurfacing. The surgeon may choose to interpose a soft-tissue layer from the fat pad if available. Patelloplasty is preferable to patellectomy in cases of extremely thin patellar bone. The choice between an onlay or inset patella is surgeon specific; in some cases the patellar bone has a peripheral rim that fits an inset patella, and at times a resurfacing type patella can be inset in this peripheral bed for added stabilization.

With femoral and tibial trial inserts in place and the patellar trial insert in the patellar bed, the quadriceps mechanism is returned to the trochlea and the knee flexed (Fig. 19). If the patella does not remain in the trochlea with the medial retinaculum open, a lateral retinacular release is performed. The release is performed from inside out and is slightly posterior to the midcoronal line of the femur. Care is taken to identify and avoid, if possible, the supralateral geniculate vessels, which form the base of a triangle between the lateral femoral shaft and the vastus lateralis muscle. If a proximal turndown or TTO was necessary for exposure, patellar tracking can be tested only after the defect in the quadriceps is closed.

Assembly of the Components

Assembly of the final press-fit stem on the appropriately sized femoral component is now completed (Fig. 20). Augmentation wedges are assembled if necessary. The tibial press-fit stem on the appropriate template is assembled, and the medial wedge is secured to the undersurface of the tibial component (Fig. 21).

Cementing Components with Press-Fit Stems

Antibiotic-impregnated methacrylate (Simplex) is routinely used in delayed exchange revision for septic total knee arthroplasties. A variety of antibiotics are thermostable and available in powder form (9,11). In most cases, powdered tobramycin (600 mg per 40 g of cement) is utilized (8). The antibiotic is mixed with the partially polymerized powder prior to addition of the monomer. In cases of patient hypersensitivity or resistance of the original infecting organism to tobramycin, other antibiotics may be utilized. The most common alternative to tobramycin is cefamandole used in doses of 1 g per 40 g of cement.

In most cases the components of the new prosthesis are cemented into place separately, with the patellar component cemented at the same time as either the

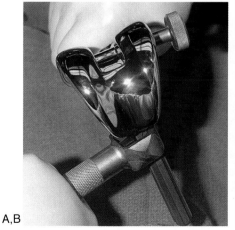
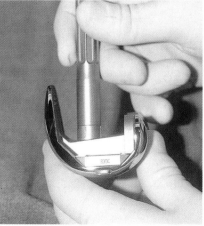

A,B

Figure 20. A,B: The appropriate press-fit stem and femoral distal/posterior combined wedge are assembled.

Figure 21. The appropriate tibial wedge and tibial press-fit stem are assembled.

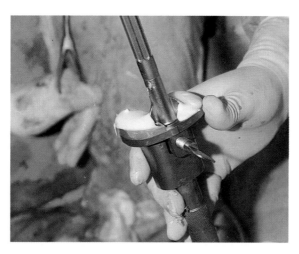

Figure 22. Antibiotic-impregnated cement is placed on the undersurface of the component but not the stem. It is also placed on the cancellous bed but not in the intramedullary area. This will allow press-fitting of the stems, with cementing at the surface of the implant.

tibial or femoral component. It is imperative to rehearse the fixation sequence using trial components in order to assure that the central eminence of the tibial plateau does not prevent insertion of the femoral component.

Prior to cementing, bony surfaces are carefully cleaned by pulsatile lavage with an antibiotic irrigant, and are thoroughly dried. The cement is applied in a doughy stage to the surface of the bone but not to the intramedullary shaft. Cement is then applied to the undersurface of each component (Fig. 22) and the component inserted. Excess cement is carefully trimmed away. The trial tibial insert of appropriate thickness and the femoral trial insert are put into place and the leg held in extension during curing of the cement. If time permits, the patellar component may be cemented at this time and a patellar clamp applied.

The femoral component is then cemented into place, using these same techniques.

Closure

The tourniquet is deflated and hemostasis achieved. The tourniquet may be reinflated for closure if necessary. The wound is thoroughly irrigated and examined for excess cement and particularly for interposed cement at the articulating interface. A two-limbed suction drain is inserted laterally and the two limbs left in the lateral gutter. The trochar is tunneled for a short distance into the subcutaneous tissue to reduce the possibility of a sinus tract developing at the drain site.

The quadriceps tendon is closed with absorbable sutures (# 0 Vicryl), with the proximal portion closed in two distinct layers with interrupted sutures. If a quadriceps turndown is performed it is closed in the same fashion (6). The knee is then flexed to test the integrity of the repair and the maximum flexion attained, and to confirm proper patellar tracking. The subcutaneous tissues are closed with absorbable sutures and the skin is closed with interrupted nylon or surgical clips. A sterile dressing and knee immobilizer are applied.

POSTOPERATIVE MANAGEMENT

The patient is maintained with a therapeutic antibiotic profile directed against the original pathogen. The antibiotics are maintained for 5 to 7 days, until negative results are returned on intraoperative cultures. If an intraoperative culture is positive, intravenous antibiotics may be continued as determined in consultation with the infectious disease specialist. Long-term suppression with oral antibiotics is not routinely utilized.

A standard postoperative physical therapy program is begun with the caveat that rehabilitation goals are usually achieved more slowly than with the index arthroplasty and even than in non-infected cases of revision.

COMPLICATIONS

Delayed exchange or revision of a total knee arthroplasty for infection is associated with a greater frequency of complication than index and even non-infected revision arthroplasties. Patients with risk factors that increase their susceptibility to infection frequently have multisystem disease, increasing their anesthetic and perioperative risks. The soft-tissue and bony abnormalities resulting from the infection and its treatment increase the patient's operative risks. The major operative risks are discussed in the following sections.

Recrudescent/Recurrent Infection

In most published series there is a small but significant incidence of recrudescent infection following exchange or revision of a total knee arthroplasty. Moreover, the risk factors increasing the susceptibility to infection also increase the patient's risk of late recurrent infection.

Following delayed exchange, the patient is covered with appropriate parenteral antibiotics until culture results are returned. If a single broth specimen of multiple intraoperative cultures is positive for an organism other than the infecting agent, it may be a contaminant. In this case the pathology is carefully reviewed to help differentiate persistent infection from contamination. If the same organism is found as was originally present and a pathology specimen is suspicious, parenteral antibiotics are continued for 3 to 4 weeks, based on discussions with the infectious disease specialist. The use of prolonged oral antibiotic suppression is controversial. In general, oral antibiotics may suppress but not eradicate an infection.

Patients who have undergone delayed exchange require careful observation over the first 2 years postoperatively, with monitoring of radiographs and acute-phase reactants, and clinical observation. If recrudescent infection is suspected, arthrocentesis and culture should be done with the patient off antibiotics. If a recrudescent (same organism) or recurrent (different organism) infection is present in the peri- or postoperative period, debridement and prosthesis removal is generally indicated. The decision to perform a second delayed exchange versus arthrodesis is made by reassessing the indications for the various options coupled with the knowledge that the patient has already failed a single delayed exchange procedure.

Infrapatellar Tendon Avulsion/Rupture

Soft-tissue injury caused by an arthroplasty infection and scarring from multiple surgical procedures increases the risk of infrapatellar tendon rupture or avulsion. Careful exposure with a proximal turndown or TTO if necessary will decrease the risk of this complication. If complete avulsion of the infrapatellar tendon occurs, with a resultant extension lag and proximal migration of the patella, surgery is necessary to restore a competent extensor mechanism. If this occurs in association with persistent infection, arthrodesis should be strongly considered. Non-surgical therapy with extension casting will not restore functional extension.

A variety of surgical techniques have been attempted for restoring the infrapatellar tendon, with little success. In my experience a technique using the gracilis and semitendinosis has restored a functional extensor mechanism following complete rupture. The infrapatellar tendon is isolated and a whipstitch using #5 Tevdek is placed through the tendon. The horizontal limb of this stitch is woven through the tendon just at the strong Sharpey's fibers at the inferior patellar pole. The stitch is secured to the tibia around a screw and washer combination in a position on the tibia that facilitates patellar tracking. Maximum lengths of the gracilis and semitendinosis tendon are harvested using a tendon stripper, with their distal attachment maintained and supplemented with a screw. The tendons are used to create a box around the infrapatellar tendon that is affixed to the medial edge, woven through the infrapatellar tendon, and affixed to the lateral edge, with the tendons then brought back to their original insertion through a drill hole in the anterior cortex of the tibia. The knee is flexed under direct visualization to determine the maximum flexion that maintains the integrity of the repair. Careful postoperative flexion with limited goals and protective weight bearing is instituted.

Skin Sloughing

Patients with infected total knees have often undergone previous surgery with multiple incisions that compromise the cutaneous blood supply on the extensor surface of the knee. Careful planning of incisions, as discussed previously, will minimize but not obviate this risk. It is often helpful to consult with a plastic surgeon preoperatively to plan incisions. Also, after making the initial incision for the revision and creating the minimal requisite flap, the tourniquet can be deflated and the viability of the flap tested by inspection. If there is a question about skin viability, the wound is closed and observed. If the wound heals with viable skin after this "sham" procedure, the definitive procedure can be performed through this incision with less concern.

If a major full-thickness skin loss occurs, it is important to establish a biologic dressing as soon as possible. In consultation with a plastic surgeon, local excision with primary closure, a gastrocnemius flap, or even a free vascularized flap may be necessary. In severe cases immediate arthrodesis may be indicated.

Patellofemoral Tracking

In most series, patellofemoral problems are the major technical problems in both primary and revision knee arthroplasty. The most important of these problems are improper patellar bone resection, component malrotation, and improper patellar soft-tissue balancing. Attention to detail in revising the patellar cut, careful testing of patellar tracking during trial reduction, and an intraoperative "skyline" radiograph if necessary will minimize these complications. Moreover, it is important to carefully close the medial capsule in two layers with interrupted sutures, and to test the integrity of this repair under direct visualization prior to closure of the skin.

If a significant mechanical problem occurs in patellofemoral tracking, it is generally necessary to correct the problem surgically in order to restore proper kinematics to the knee.

Instability

In virtually every delayed exchange procedure there is significant abnormality of the capsular tissues and ligaments. As discussed in the section on surgical technique, balancing the flexion and extension gaps and recreating the normal joint line are important in re-establishing the kinematics of the knee. In most cases the posterior cruciate ligament is either absent or nonfunctional, and a cruciate-substituting or collateral-ligament-substituting prosthesis is required. If functionally significant laxity occurs following delayed exchange revision, the patient may be placed in a cast, bivalve cast, or functional brace for several weeks in an attempt to allow postoperative scarring to stabilize the knee. Moreover, limiting postoperative flexion to 95° to 100° may be beneficial in cases of flexion instability. If significant instability persists, surgery is generally necessary to correct the etiologic factor.

ILLUSTRATIVE CASE FOR TECHNIQUE

A 71-year-old woman with osteoarthritis had undergone a right total knee arthroplasty 2 years prior to presentation. After initial rehabilitation she did reasonably well for the first postoperative year, but also noticed persistent pain, swelling for 3 to 4 weeks, and a slight bowing of her extremity. She denied having fevers, sweats, or chills, but felt her knee to be warm. Supine and standing AP radiographs (Fig. 23) revealed a marked varus deformity on standing, and a fractured tibial tray. Joint aspiration, culture, and a cell count showed a synovial white blood cell count of 34,000 mm³ and cultures positive for *S. aureus*. Because of the chronicity of the patient's symptoms, the presence of *S. aureus*, and the

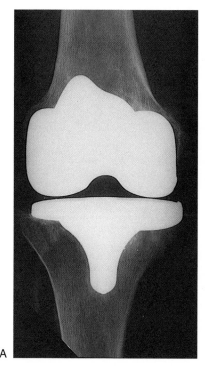
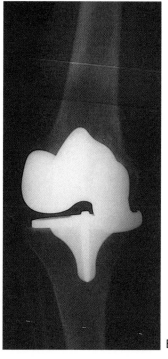

Figure 23. An AP **(A)** and standing AP **(B)** radiograph demonstrating a varus deformity and fracture of the tibial tray in a patient with an *S. aureus*-infected total knee arthroplasty.

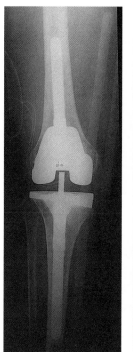
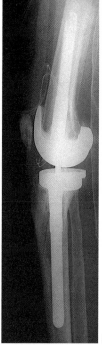

Figure 24. AP **(A)** and lateral **(B)** radiographs following delayed exchange for an infected total knee arthroplasty.

fractured tibial tray, a delayed exchange protocol was felt to be the appropriate treatment.

Figure 24 shows postoperative AP and lateral radiographs using a constrained implant with press-fit stems for revision of a failed septic total knee arthroplasty.

RECOMMENDED READING

1. Bengston, S., Knutson, K., and Lidgren, L: Treatment of infected knee arthroplasty. *Clin. Orthop.,* 245: 173–178, 1989.
2. Booth, R. E. Jr., and Lotke, P. A.: The results of spacer block technique in revision of infected total knee arthroplasty. *Clin. Orthop.,* 248: 57–60, 1989.
3. Borden, L. S., and Gearen, P. F.: Infected total knee arthroplasty. A protocol for management. *J. Arthroplasty,* 2: 27–36, 1987.
4. Poss, R., Thornhill, T. S., Ewald, F. C., Thomas, W. H., Batte, N. J., and Sledge, C. B.: Factors influencing the incidence and outcome of infection following total joint arthroplasty. *Clin. Orthop.,* 182: 117–126, 1984.
5. Schoifet, S. D., and Morrey, B. F.: Treatment of infection after total knee arthroplasty by debridement with retention of the components. *J. Bone Joint Surg.,* 72, 1383–1390, 1990.
6. Scott, R. D., and Siliski, J. M.: The use of a modified V-Y quadricepsplasty during total knee replacement to gain exposure and improve flexion in the ankylosed knee. *Orthopedics,* 8: 45–48, 1985.
7. Teeny, S. M., Dorr, L., Murata, G., and Conaty, P.: Treatment of infected total knee arthroplasty. Irrigation and debridement versus two-stage reimplantation. *J. Arthroplasty,* 5: 35–39, 1990.
8. Thornhill, T. S., and Maguire, J.: Management of infected knee arthroplasty. In: *Revision Total Knee Replacement,* edited by W. N. Scott, Grune and Stratton, New York, 1987.
9. Trippel, S. B.: Antibiotic-impregnated cement in total joint arthroplasty. *J. Bone Joint Surg.,* 68(8): 1297–1302, 1986.
10. Masini, M. A., Maguire, J. H., and Thornhill, T. S.: Infected total knee arthroplasty. In: *The Knee,* edited by W. N. Scott, Mosby, New York, 1994.
11. Walker, J. L., Gustke, K., Toney, J., and Sinnott, J.: Centrifugation of antibiotic impregnated bone cement. *Orthopedics,* 11(6): 891–893, 1988.
12. Wilson, M. G., Kelley, K., and Thornhill, T. S.: Infection as a complication of total knee-replacement arthroplasty. Risk factors and treatment in sixty-seven cases. *J. Bone Joint Surg.,* 72: 878–883, 1990.
13. Windsor, R. E., Insall, J. N., Urs, W. K., Miller, D. V., and Brause, B. D.: Two-stage reimplantation for the salvage of total knee arthroplasty complicated by infection. Further follow-up and refinement of indications. *J. Bone Joint Surg.,* 72: 272–278, 1990.
14. Windsor, R. E.: Management of total knee arthroplasty infection. *Orthop. Clin. North Am.,* 22: 531–538, 1991.

PART IV

Techniques for the Treatment of Unicompartmental Arthritis

Master Techniques in Orthopaedic Surgery,
KNEE ARTHROPLASTY, edited by P. A. Lotke,
Raven Press, Ltd., New York © 1995.

17

Unicompartmental Arthroplasty

Richard D. Scott

INDICATIONS/CONTRAINDICATIONS

Unicompartmental knee arthroplasty is an attractive alternative to proximal tibial osteotomy or tricompartmental arthroplasty in selected osteoarthritic patients with unicompartmental involvement. It should yield a higher initial success rate than osteotomy, with fewer early complications. Patients with bilateral disease can have surgery done on both knees during the same anesthesia. The time to full recovery averages 3 months.

As compared to tricompartmental arthroplasty, unicompartmental replacement has the advantage of preserving both cruciate ligaments (an absent anterior cruciate ligament is probably a contraindication to the procedure) and of preserving bone stock in the opposite compartment and patellofemoral joint. In theory, revision should be easier to accomplish after a failed unicompartmental arthroplasty than after a failed tricompartmental replacement. This was not shown in early series of revisions involving components inserted in the 1970s. Large condylar fins or lugs, excessive bone resection, and excessive cement penetration required augmentation methods in many cases. More conservative techniques used in the 1980s have resulted in easier revisions.

Factors weighed in deciding between osteotomy and arthroplasty include age, weight, occupation, avocation, range of motion, deformity, and subluxation. Osteotomy is favored in younger, heavier, active patients with a functional range of motion, while unicompartmental replacement is more appropriate in older, lighter, sedentary patients with some restrictions of motion. Patients with severe deformity and subluxation are best treated by tricompartmental replacement in order to properly align and balance the knee.

R. D. Scott, M.D.: Department of Orthopedic Surgery, Harvard Medical School, Boston, MA 02120.

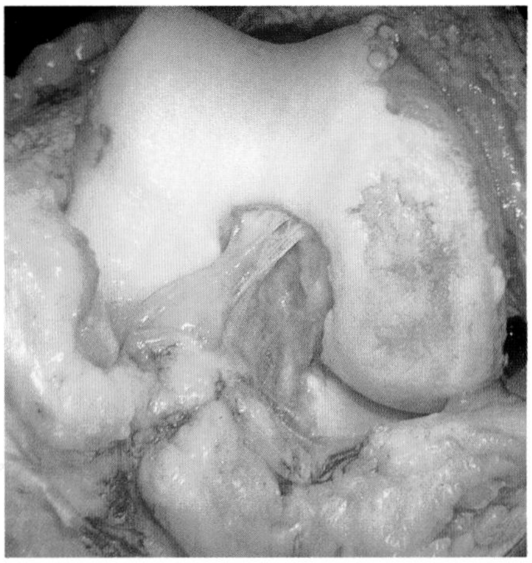

Figure 1. An intraoperative view of an ideal candidate for unicompartmental replacement.

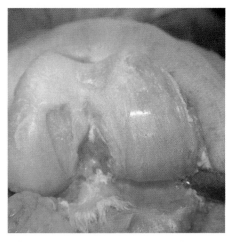

Figure 2. Secondary erosion of the medial aspect of the lateral femoral condyle due to subluxation. The anterior cruciate ligament is absent. There is eburnated bone on the trochlear groove.

Once the decision is made to perform an arthroplasty rather than an osteotomy, the choice between an unicompartmental versus a tricompartmental procedure is made intraoperatively. All three compartments are carefully inspected. The compartment with primary involvement will exhibit eburnated bone. The opposite compartment should have a full cartilaginous surface without focal chondromalacia and certainly without exposed subchondral bone (Fig. 1). As deformity progresses in the varus knee, early subluxation occurs and a secondary lesion may appear on the medial aspect of the lateral femoral condyle. This usually consists of a focal erosion and an associated osteophyte. If the lesion is small it can be debrided and unicompartmental arthroplasty performed. A large lesion implies significant lateral tibial subluxation, and a deficient anterior cruciate ligament is usually observed (Fig. 2).

The patellofemoral compartment can exhibit more involvement than the opposite compartment and still be acceptable for arthroplasty. However, most surgeons consider eburnated patellar bone a contraindication to unicompartmental arthroplasty.

Another intraoperative contraindication involves the status of the synovium. Long-term follow-up shows a higher incidence of failure due to progression of disease to the opposite compartment in patients with inflammatory osteoarthritis, gout, or pseudogout, making unicompartmental replacement less appropriate in these patients.

Poor flexion is not a contraindication to unicompartmental arthroplasty, but poor passive extension is if not correctable to −15° or better by the procedure.

A lax medial collateral ligament is a contraindication in the valgus knee with lateral compartment involvement. If this ligament has developed more than 2 mm of laxity, it can stretch even after adequate passive correction of the deformity, causing late failure of the arthroplasty.

A final intraoperative contraindication to the unicompartmental technique involves an assessment of the technique for restoring alignment and stability without overcorrection and with proper congruency between the articulating surfaces of the prosthetic components. The unicompartmental procedure should be abandoned intraoperatively if it fails to meet the standards outlined in the remainder of this chapter.

PREOPERATIVE PLANNING

The patient has presented with an angular deformity in varus or valgus, and with eburnated bone in one compartment as confirmed by physical examination and radiograph (Fig. 3). Non-surgical treatment has failed and the patient feels that the pain and disability associated with the deformity are severe enough to warrant surgery. Because of the factors outlined previously, arthroplasty is preferred over osteotomy. The patient is scheduled for unicompartmental surgery versus total knee replacement, depending on the findings at surgery.

Two units of autologous blood are donated to avoid a possible homologous transfusion. The patient is instructed to complete any anticipated dental or urologic procedures prior to the knee arthroplasty, and is instructed in the use of the prophylactic antibiotic therapy that will be implemented postoperatively.

Coumadin is prescribed to begin on the night before surgery. Random surgical prescreening tests are scheduled, including standard anteroposterior (AP), lateral, and "skyline" radiographs of the affected knee and a standing 3-foot AP radiograph of both knees from hips to ankles, with the knees in neutral rotation. This view is invaluable in the planning and execution of the surgery. If it shows lateral subluxation of the tibia on the femur, unicompartmental arthroplasty will probably not stabilize the knee (Fig. 4). A mechanical axis deviation of more than 15 degrees probably contraindicates a unicompartmental arthroplasty. The procedure is first planned on the radiographs. A varus knee with medial compartment involvement will be used as an example.

A proposed line of tibial resection is drawn 10 mm distal to the lateral compartment joint line at an angle of 90° to the longitudinal axis of the tibia (Fig. 5). This line approximates the normal tibial resection for a routine bicompartmental knee

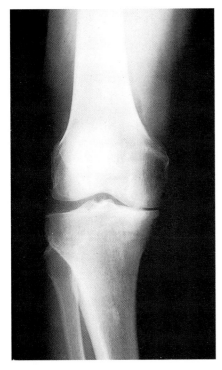

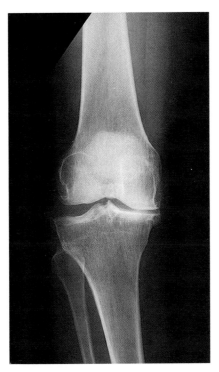

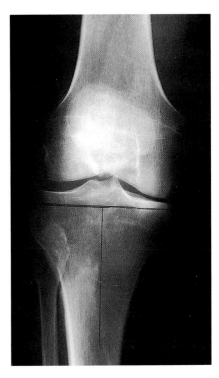

Figure 3. Presenting radiograph of a patient with a varus deformity and medial compartment osteoarthritis.

Figure 4. A preoperative standing radiograph showing early lateral subluxation of the tibia on the femur.

Figure 5. A proposed line of tibial resection for bicompartmental replacement, indicating an appropriate medial resection for unicompartmental arthroplasty.

replacement, which accommodates 10 mm of tibial component thickness. For the varus knee this line is extended medially to the medial cortex. It usually suggests a minimal medial tibial resection of 0 to 2 mm of bone as measured at the periphery. During surgery, it is helpful to refer back to this planned resection as the procedure is executed.

SURGERY

Technique

The patient is put in the supine position on the operating table, with spinal or epidural preferred over general anesthesia. A pulsatile compression stocking can be placed on the opposite leg to decrease the chance of phlebothrombosis in this limb. The initial dose of prophylactic intravenous antibiotic agents is given and a bladder catheter is inserted. A thigh tourniquet is applied and a blanket roll or sandbag can be anchored to the operating table at the level of the midcalf to support the flexed knee during the procedure.

The entire leg is prepped, from toes to tourniquet, and a full leg stockinette is applied. This is cut open from the midthigh to the ankle to expose the external landmarks, and a clear sterile adhesive is applied to seal off the area.

The surgical exposure can be made through an anteromedial approach for either the medial or lateral compartment, a submedialis approach for a varus knee, or a lateral approach for a valgus knee. For a medial compartment replacement, care is taken to protect the coronary ligament lateral to the midline, along with the anterior horn of the lateral meniscus. Similarly, for a lateral compartment replacement, the medial coronary ligament and anterior meniscal horn are preserved.

After eversion of the patella, the knee is flexed and the joint thoroughly inspected to confirm that unicompartmental replacement is appropriate. An intact ligamentum mucosum usually indicates that unicompartmental disease will be encountered (see Fig. 1). The anterior cruciate ligament should be intact. The opposite compartment should appear grossly normal, or nearly so, without any significant areas of chondromalacia. As noted previously, there may be signs in a varus knee of early lateral subluxation of the tibia on the femur, represented by cartilage erosion on the medial aspect of the lateral femoral condyle. This is often accompanied by an intercondylar osteophyte. If the erosion is small (less than 2 or 3 mm wide) it can be debrided along with the osteophyte, and unicompartmental replacement can be performed (Fig. 6). If the erosion is large and deep it represents significant lateral subluxation, and unicompartmental arthroplasty is contraindicated (see Fig. 2).

Some chondromalacia of the patellar surface is acceptable as long as there are no large areas of eburnated bone exposed on both the patellar and trochlear sides of this compartment. In a varus knee there is often some minor wear on the periphery of the medial facet where the latter articulated in flexion with eburnated bone on the distal medial femoral condyle (Fig. 7). Like the intercondylar erosion, this is often accompanied by a peripheral osteophyte and can be debrided.

The synovium should be evaluated for evidence of inflammatory disease indicating a generalized arthritic condition rather than a focal mechanical problem and mitigating against unicompartmental replacement.

Finally, the procedure should be abandoned in favor of bicompartmental total knee replacement if acceptable alignment, stability, or prosthetic congruency cannot be established with trial components. The author estimates that for any of the reasons stated above, unicompartmental replacement is aborted in 50% of patients thought to be possible candidates prior to arthrotomy.

After exposure and inspection, moist wound towels are sewn to the capsule to cover the soft tissues and protect them against drying out. An additional moist

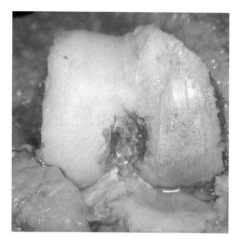

Figure 6. An intraoperative view of a small secondary lesion on the medial aspect of the lateral femoral condyle that can easily be debrided.

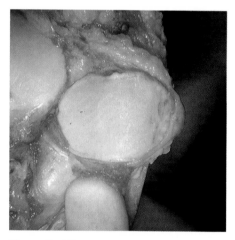

Figure 7. Minor wear of the medial facet of the patella, acceptable for unicompartmental arthroplasty.

towel is placed over the opposite compartment and patella to protect the cartilage from desiccating and to prevent any debris generated by the bone preparation from entering the normal compartment. Any intercondylar erosions or osteophytes are debrided with osteotomes or rongeurs. Peripheral osteophytes are removed from the femur and tibia to relieve their effect of tenting up the medial collateral ligament and medial capsule. This maneuver defines the local anatomy and should produce as much of a medial release as is necessary to correct a varus deformity.

Preparation of the Femur

Most unicompartmental prostheses are designed so as to require the removal of little or no bone from the distal femur, in order to support the femoral component of the prosthesis on hard subchondral bone and resist subsidence or loosening. Those that require no removal of distal bone require increased tibial resection to accommodate the appropriate thickness of the tibial component. A reasonable compromise might call for removing 4 mm of distal bone, leaving 4 to 6 mm intact for the normal distal resection in a bicompartmental knee, should revision later be necessary. Furthermore, if 4 mm of distal condyle are removed and replaced with 6 mm of metallic prosthesis (assuming 2 mm of cartilage loss) the femoral joint line is properly restored.

Sizing of the femoral component is keyed by the distance between the "tide mark" (the junction of eburnated distal condylar bone and intact trochlear cartilage) and the posterior femoral condyle (Fig. 8). The femoral component should restore the AP dimension of the knee, with the leading edge of the femoral runner extending anteriorly enough to assure good metal-to-plastic contact in full extension.

An intramedullary alignment guide is the most accurate means of determining the proper distal femoral condylar resection. A hole is made into the femoral medullary canal several millimeters anterior to the origin of the posterior cruciate ligament (Fig. 9). The guide rod is advanced slowly through the hole to the diaphyseal isthmus. The appropriate angle of distal resection is chosen, usually 5° for varus knees and 7° for valgus knees (Fig. 10). The principle in selecting the angle of resection is to err toward slight undercorrection of the deformity to allow load-sharing by the prosthetic components and avoid overcorrection that might prevent secondary wear in the unresurfaced opposite compartment. A distal femoral cut-

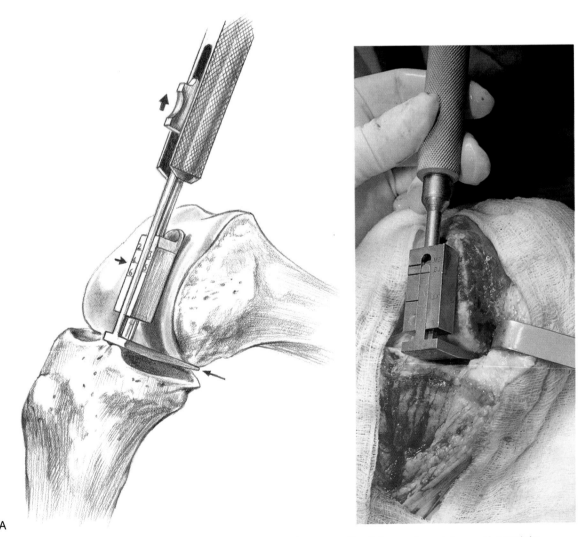

A   B

Figure 8. A,B: Sizing the femur between the tide mark and femoral condyle.

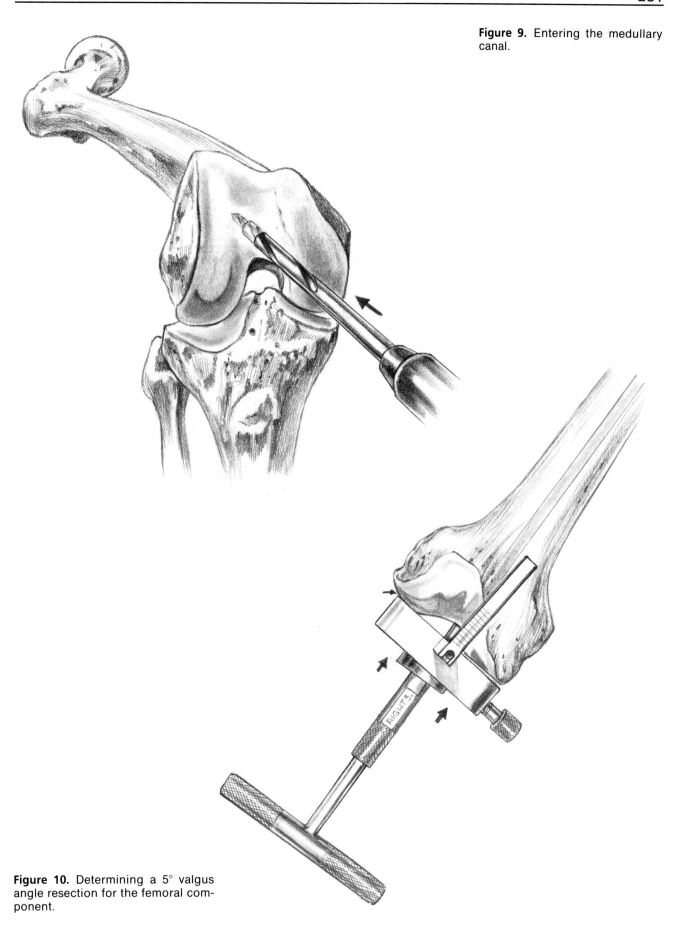

Figure 9. Entering the medullary canal.

Figure 10. Determining a 5° valgus angle resection for the femoral component.

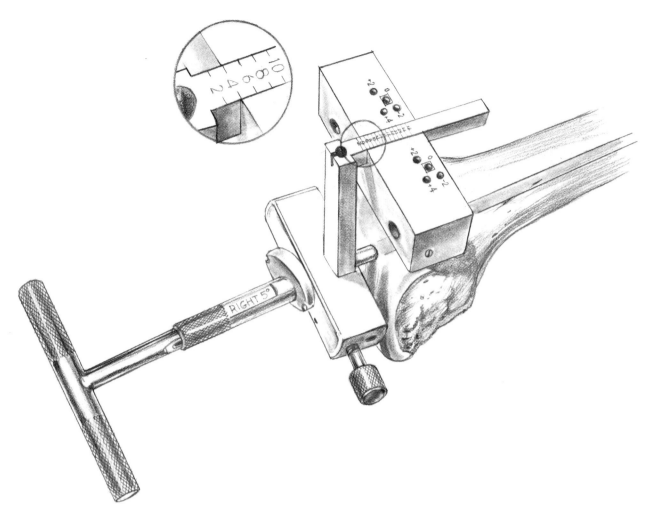

Figure 11. Bone resection is set for 4 mm, to be replaced with a 6-mm-thick femoral component. Assuming that 2 mm of normal distal femoral cartilage has been eroded, the femoral joint line is properly restored.

ting block is assembled to the alignment device and set for 4 mm of bone resection in neutral flexion extension (Fig. 11). The block is pinned to the femur and the resection performed with an oscillating saw.

Preparation of the Tibia

Next, the level and angle of the tibial resection are determined and linked to the femoral resection. To assure a conservative tibial resection, an estimated line of resection is drawn on a preoperative AP radiograph. This line is 8 to 10 mm distal to the intact lateral joint line and perpendicular to the long axis of the tibia (see Fig. 5); the line represents a proposed routine resection for bicompartmental replacement, and can be used to determine a conservative medial resection that will permit easy conversion to bicompartmental arthroplasty intraoperatively or at a later date. The extent of peripheral resection of the medial plateau is recorded. This usually measures between 0 to 2 or 3 mm from the periphery of the involved medial plateau (Fig. 12). With the knee flexed at 90°, a tibial resection guide can now be placed at this level, set for 0° to 3° of posterior slope, and adjusted into slight varus or valgus until it is perpendicular to the rotational alignment chosen

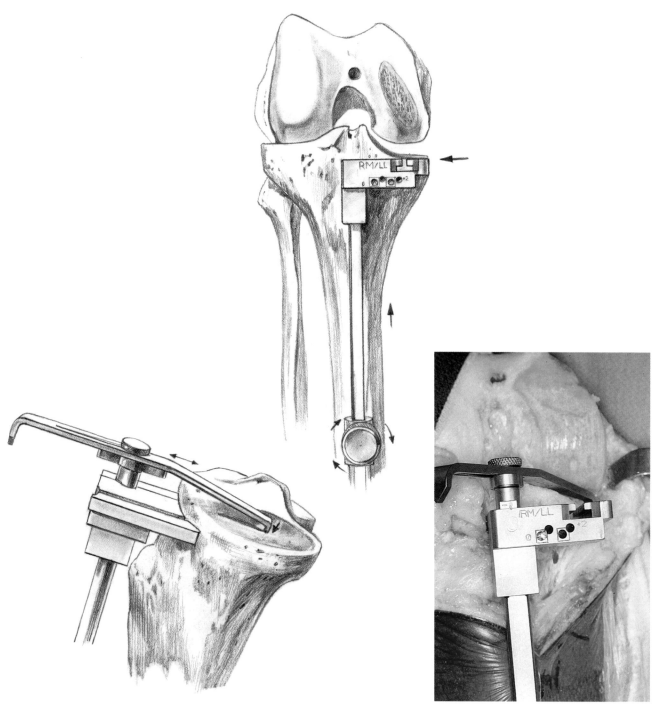

Figure 12. A,B: The medial tibial resection is determined by preoperative planning.

for the femoral component (Fig. 13). The guide is pinned and the tibial resection is performed with an oscillating saw. A reliable medial-lateral reference point for the tibial cut is halfway up the slope of the medial tibial spine and in line with the chondro-osseous wear pattern of the plateau (Fig. 14). Final tibial rotation may be adjusted after trial reduction with the femoral trial implant.

Assessment of Extension and Flexion Gaps

With the leg in extension and a slight valgus stress applied to the knee, the extension gap can now be measured (Fig. 15). It should be at least 14 mm to accommodate a 6-mm femoral component and 8-mm tibial component. If the gap is less than 14 mm it should be increased to this minimal size by more distal femoral or proximal tibial resection at the surgeon's discretion.

The final balancing step is the creation of a similar or slightly larger flexion gap. In unicompartmental arthroplasty, excessive tightness in flexion must be avoided, while slight laxity in flexion is tolerated because of the intact cruciate ligaments and opposite compartment. Therefore, before the final AP positioning and sizing of the femoral component is established, the knee is placed in 90° of flexion to determine if the flexion gap is appropriate, A spacer block 6 mm thinner than the measured extension spacer block is inserted between the prepared tibial plateau

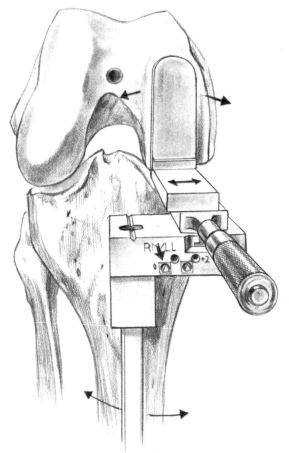

A

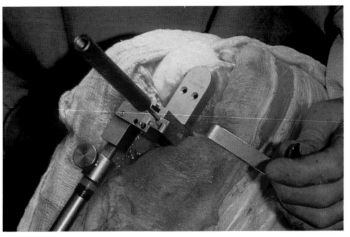

B

Figure 13. A,B: The varus/valgus alignment of the tibial resection can be linked to the proper rotatory alignment of the femoral component to assure good congruency in flexion.

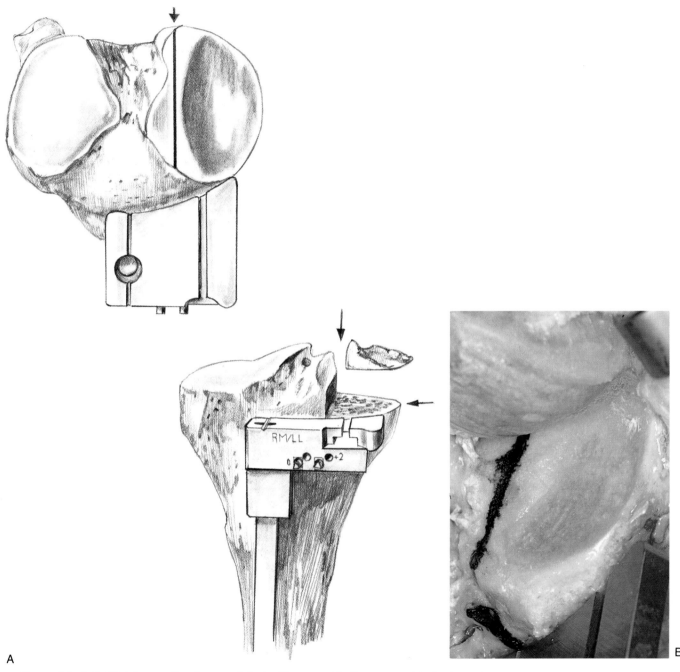

Figure 14. A,B: Tibial resection is completed with an oscillating saw, with the lateral extent of the resection halfway up the tibial spine and in line with the chondro-osseus wear pattern.

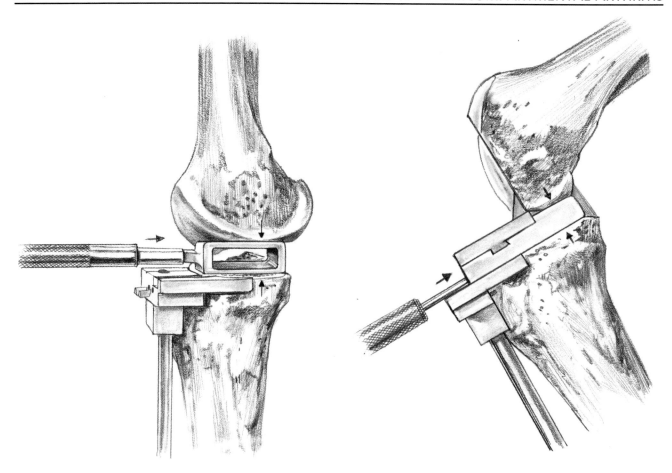

Figure 15. Assessing the extension gap with the leg in extension.

Figure 16. Assessing the flexion gap with the knee in 90° of flexion.

and unresected posterior femoral condyle (Fig. 16). The ease with which it passes through this space reflects the final ligament tension in flexion if the sizing and posterior condylar resection proceed anatomically. If the gap is too small in flexion, it is easily enlarged by skiving off the appropriate amount of posterior condylar bone or retained cartilage with an oscillating saw. This will move the leading edge of the femoral component anteriorly by the same distance as the amount of posterior condyle that is removed, and in rare cases may require downsizing of the previously chosen femoral component.

Completing Femoral Preparation

Once the gaps are balanced, the femoral preparation is completed, using the appropriate cutting jigs to resect the posterior condyle and prepare any chamfered surfaces and lug holes (Fig. 17). After final femoral preparations, spacer blocks of the same size should span and stabilize the flexion and extension gaps.

Sizing the Tibial Component and Trial Insertion

The tibial plateau is sized for maximum AP and medial-lateral capping of the resected bone. A trial insert of the appropriate size and thickness is placed on the plateau, and a trial femoral component is inserted onto the distal femur. The

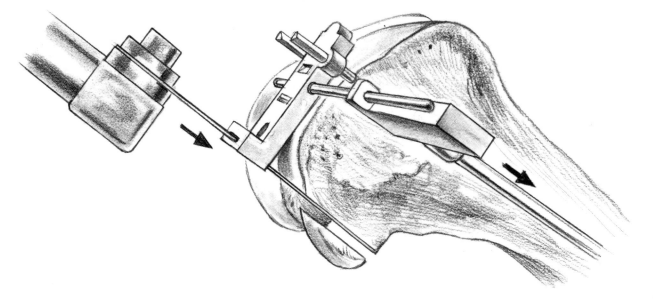

A

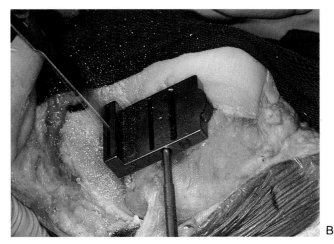

B

Figure 17. A,B: Completing femoral resection.

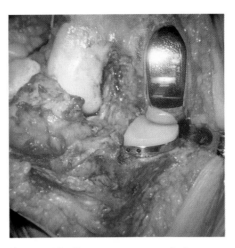

Figure 18. Congruency must be assessed in extension rather than flexion because the everted quadriceps will artificially externally rotate and laterally subluxate the tibia on the femur.

stability and congruency of the components are assessed as the knee is brought through a full range of motion with the patella returned to the trochlear groove. There must be good medial-lateral and rotational congruency with the knee in full extension (Fig. 18). The conservatively cut tibial spine resection is modified as necessary to achieve this. If overcorrection or tibial/femoral subluxation is suspected and cannot be corrected by thinner components or slight modification of the resections, an intraoperative radiograph may be useful to confirm these possibilities. The unicompartmental procedure should be abandoned for bicompartmental arthroplasty if the surgeon is not fully satisfied with the alignment, balance, and congruency it provides.

Cementing Components

The implantable components of the prosthesis are brought onto the operating field. The bone surfaces of the femur and tibia are cleansed with pulsatile lavage. Methylmethacrylate is mixed; usually one half of a pack is sufficient. The tibial component is cemented first. Care is taken to avoid an excessive posterior application of cement, leading to a possible posterior extrusion of cement that will be difficult to see and retrieve. If the flexion space will not easily admit the posterior lug of the component, a small "ramp" leading to the posterior lug hole can be created on the tibial plateau. This should be assessed prior to the application of cement.

The tibial component of the prosthesis should be inserted onto the bed of cement so that it first makes contact posteriorly with the anterior edge of the component at a point several millimeters above the prepared tibial plateau. As seating occurs, this causes cement to extrude anteriorly, where it can be seen and cleared. The tibial component, whether solid or modular, can be held in position as the cement polymerizes, or the surgeon can proceed to simultaneous cementing of the femoral component. To accomplish this, additional cement is applied to the prepared femoral site. None is placed on the posterior condylar bone, but rather into the cement recess of the prosthesis, so as to minimize the chance of posterior extrusion of cement. The femoral component is positioned and seated with an impactor. Excess cement is cleared from the margins and the knee is extended to increase and maintain pressurization during polymerization. To avoid possible disturbance of

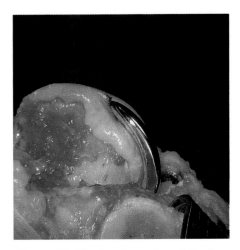

Figure 19. The leading edge of the femoral component must be recessed to avoid patellar impingement.

the prosthesis–cement and bone–cement interfaces, the knee should not be flexed again until the methacrylate has cured. After this the knee can be ranged and any further extruded cement excised. As the knee is flexed and extended, the articulating margins of the components should be observed for possible impingement on bone or cement. An especially vulnerable area is the edge of the tibial component that runs along the tibial spine, which can impinge on retained intercondylar cement or osteophytes.

Patellar tracking is also assessed. The patella should not impinge on the leading edge of the femoral component at the junction between the trochlear cartilage and the prosthesis (Fig. 19). Any impinging peripheral medial osteophytes should also be excised.

The tourniquet is deflated and a second dose of prophylactic antibiotics administered. Bleeding is controlled with electrocautery. Suction drains are placed at the surgeon's discretion. The capsule is closed anatomically with interrupted sutures. Flexion against gravity is measured and recorded to determine the potential range of the patient's postoperative motion. After skin closure, a dressing and a pulsatile stocking are applied and the knee is placed on a continuous passive motion (CPM) machine in the recovery room. If a continuous epidural anesthetic is functioning, the machine is usually set for 90° of flexion. In the case of a spinal or general anesthetic the range is decreased to 30°.

POSTOPERATIVE REHABILITATION

If tolerated, the CPM machine is allowed to run continuously throughout the night following surgery, in conjunction with bilateral pulsatile stockings. Prophylactic intravenous antibiotics are given at appropriate intervals. Oral intake begins, supplemented by intravenous fluids. The bladder remains catheterized. A second dose of warfarin sodium (Coumadin) (usually 5 mg) is given in the evening. Suction knee drainage is monitored. If bilateral prostheses have been implanted under the same anesthesia, the CPM machine is used on one knee and an immobilizer on the other. These are alternated every 12 hours.

The drains are pulled on the first day after surgery. The CPM machine is now used at intervals lasting several hours in the morning and several hours in the afternoon. Between these intervals the patient begins quadriceps exercises and wears a knee immobilizer in extension at night. Intravenous antibiotics continue. The dose of Coumadin now depends on the results of a daily prothrombin time, with a goal of elevating the test result to between 14 and 16 seconds. If possible, the epidural analgesia begun at the time of surgery is continued, or patient-controlled analgesia or intramuscular medications are given for pain relief.

The dressing is changed on the second day after surgery and the epidural analgesia is discontinued. Supplementary pain relief can be provided with pills or by injection. The patient leaves bed for a chair, and may be able to use a commode. The bladder catheter is removed. Intravenous antibiotics are discontinued, but oral antibiotics are begun to cover bladder organisms until the patient is voiding normally. Active assisted exercises begin. The CPM machine continues to be used during the day, increasing the angle of flexion by 10° to 20° per day as tolerated until 90° of flexion is achieved. Daily anticoagulation continues with Coumadin.

On the third day the patient begins ambulation with a walker and graduates to partial weight-bearing with two crutches. The patient is taught how to perform activities of daily living (ADL) and to negotiate stairs. Baseline radiographs, including a recumbent AP, lateral, and "skyline" view, are obtained. A baseline venous ultrasound examination can be used to screen for deep vein thrombosis. If the examination is positive, the appropriate treatment is initiated. If it is negative, Coumadin prophylaxis may continue at the surgeon's discretion for 6 weeks.

Discharge plans are made for continued physical therapy at home, a skilled nursing facility, or a rehabilitation hospital, depending on the patient's individual needs.

The initial postoperative visit occurs approximately 6 weeks after surgery. At this time the patient graduates from crutches to a cane outdoors and no support when walking around the house. Permission is now given to drive a car if the right leg was involved (earlier for the left leg). The patient can also begin to ascend stairs with the help of a handrail, using the treated leg, and may return to work at a job that can be performed while using a cane.

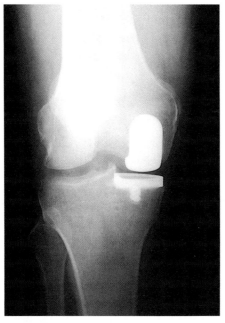

Figure 20. Follow-up radiograph of a unicompartmental arthroplasty with no signs of loosening.

At this time also, preoperative instructions about the use of prophylactic antibiotics during dental and certain medical procedures are reviewed with the patient in the form of a letter.

An office visit is optional at 12 weeks, and is usually omitted in favor of a phone call or postcard from the patient with a progress report and any new questions. Return to full activity is permitted if the patient is ready. Athletic activities such as golf or doubles tennis can be started. The patient is reminded that lifting objects weighing more than 20 lb (especially from a bent-knee position) should be avoided. Impact forces to the knee, such as those in jumping or jogging, should also be avoided. Single-racquet sports are to be avoided. Downhill skiing is discouraged, but is not as dangerous as with a bicompartmental replacement because both cruciate ligaments are intact.

Annual visits are recommended at postoperative years 1, 2, 3, 5, 7, 10, 12, 15, 17, and 20. At each of these visits, a knee rating is obtained with the Knee Society Scoring system, and a radiographic evaluation including AP lateral, and "skyline" views are also obtained to assess the bone–cement interface (Fig. 20).

COMPLICATIONS

Early Complications

Complications that occur within the first year after surgery are rare. These include inadequate pain relief in approximately 1% or 2% of patients. Deep vein thrombosis may be discovered by venous ultrasound examination in 1% to 5% of patients, while clinically apparent pulmonary embolism occurs in less than 0.5% of cases. The early infection rate in a large series of patients should range from 0.1% to 0.3%. Pes anserinus bursitis is probably the most frequent clinically apparent complication, being noted in 10% of patients in one early series of unicompartmental arthroplasties. In recent series it has not been reported with as high a frequency. Patients with such bursitis present with medial pain just below the joint line, as well as significant local tenderness and possible swelling. The pain is often of a burning nature and occurs at rest as well as with weight bearing. It usually resolves with time, antiinflammatory medication, or a local injection of steroid.

Late Complications

Late complications that lead to secondary surgery after unicompartmental arthroplasty occur at the rate of approximately 1% per year of follow-up for the first 10 years after arthroplasty. In the second decade, with earlier prosthetic designs and implantation techniques, late complications have been more frequent. The problems most commonly requiring repeat surgery include loosening or subsidence of one or both components, secondary degeneration of the opposite compartment, wear of the polyethylene articulating surface, or metastatic infection to the joint. The relative incidence of these complications (other than infection) will vary with patient selection, surgical technique, and the prosthetic components that are utilized. For example, loosening and subsidence are more frequent in heavy, active patients whose deformities have been undercorrected and who have an undersized prosthesis. Secondary degeneration of the opposite compartment is more apt to occur in a heavy, active patient with overcorrection and a previously undiagnosed inflammatory condition such as chondrocalcinosis or a rheumatoid variant. Polyethylene wear is most often seen in metal-backed components with a polyethylene thickness of less than 6 mm and poorly congruent articulating surfaces.

ILLUSTRATIVE CASE FOR TECHNIQUE

A 55-year-old woman presented with progressive pain and disability secondary to arthritis in the medial compartment of the right knee. She was employed in a sedentary clerical occupation. She was active athletically in her youth, enjoying tennis and skiing. Ten years before her presentation she had sustained a torn medial meniscus and undergone an arthroscopic meniscectomy. She did well for approximately 8 years but now notes an increasing varus deformity and medial pain on weight-bearing. She occasionally requires a cane to walk outdoors. She limits the distance of her walking to less than three blocks, and ascends and descends stairs one step at a time, leading with her left leg up and right leg down. She needs arm support to rise from a chair. She takes acetaminophen for pain relief. Antiinflammatory medications have not helped, and the patient received three intraarticular injections of steroid. The first injection helped for 3 months, the second for 2 weeks, and the third was of no benefit.

Examination showed a female patient 5 feet 5 inches tall, weighing 135 lb. She walked with an antalgic gait on the right and had a standing anatomic varus alignment of 5°. The deformity was passively correctable to neutral. There was a mild effusion. The knee flexed to 115°, with −5° of active and passive extension. There was painful bony crepitus in the medial compartment with varus stress.

Radiographs including standing AP, lateral, and "skyline" views confirmed the varus deformity and showed complete loss of the joint space in the medial compartment, with good preservation of the lateral and patellofemoral joint spaces. There was no lateral subluxation of the tibia on the femur (Fig. 21). At arthrotomy, the patient was an excellent candidate for unicompartmental arthroplasty (Fig. 22).

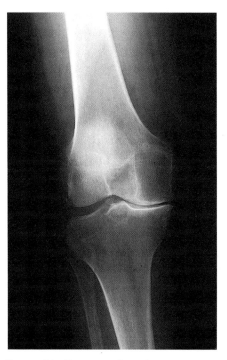

Figure 21. Preoperative view indicates varus malalignment.

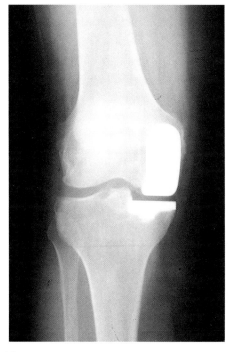

Figure 22. Postoperative view after unicompartmental arthroplasty. The patient is pain free and has returned to normal activities.

RECOMMENDED READING

1. Barnes, C. L., and Scott, R. D.: Unicompartmental arthroplasty. pp. 309–314. In: *Instructional Course Lectures,* Vol. 42, edited by J. Heckman. American Academy of Orthopaedic Surgeons, Chicago, 1993.
2. Blunn, G. W., Joshi, A. B., Lilley, P. A., et al.: Polyethylene wear in unicondylar knee prostheses. *Acta. Orthop. Scand. J.,* 63(3): 247–255, 1992.
3. Capra, S. W. Jr., and Fehring, T. K.: Unicondylar arthroplasty: a survivorship analysis. *J. Arthroplasty,* 7(3): 247–251, 1992.
4. Kozinn, S. C., and Scott, R.: Unicondylar knee arthroplasty. *J. Bone Joint Surg.,* 71A: 145–150, 1989.
5. Marmor, L.: Unicompartmental knee arthroplasty: ten- to 13-year follow-up study. *Clin. Orthop.,* 226: 14–20, 1988.
6. Padgett, D. E., Stern, S. H., and Insall, J. N.: Revision total knee arthroplasty for failed unicompartmental replacement. *J. Bone Joint Surg.,* 73A: 186–190, 1991.
7. Scott, R. D., Cobb, A. G., McQueary, F. G., et al.: Unicompartmental knee arthroplasty: eight- to twelve-year follow up with survivorship analysis. *Clin. Orthop.,* 271: 96–100, 1991.
8. Scott, R. D., and Santore, R. F.: Unicondylar unicompartmental replacement for osteoarthritis of the knee. *J. Bone Joint Surg.,* 63A: 233–238, 1981.

Master Techniques in Orthopaedic Surgery,
KNEE ARTHROPLASTY, edited by P. A. Lotke,
Raven Press, Ltd., New York © 1995.

18

High Tibial Osteotomy

Russell E. Windsor

INDICATIONS/CONTRAINDICATIONS

Osteotomy for the correction of limb deformities is among the oldest of surgical operations. Volkmann published the first known report on osteotomy performed on the tibia. Corrective osteotomy in osteoarthritis has been done to relieve pain from varus malalignment due to arthritis.

There are two theories for why high tibial osteotomy relieves pain after correction of the mechanical axis of the knee. The first concept hypothesizes that osteotomy redistributes the load passing across the knee joint, with associated modification of the blood circulation. A reduced intraosseous venous pressure that the osteotomy provides relieves the pain built up by the abnormal forces across the medial side of the knee. The second theory is purely mechanical, holding that pain relief is obtained by simply restoring the normal alignment of the knee.

High tibial osteotomy is indicated in persons under 60 years of age with osteoarthritis and varus deformity of less than 15°. The ideal candidate is one who wishes to maintain a very active lifestyle and does not desire the limitations imposed by knee replacement. A prosthetic knee in an excessively active individual will either wear prematurely or loosen. Thus, the concept of "young" must be individualized from one patient to another.

High tibial osteotomy is contraindicated in conditions that affect the entire joint, such as rheumatoid arthritis and other metabolic arthritides. Valgus deformity is not predictably corrected by high tibial osteotomy, since the articular surface becomes tilted into excessive varus, causing pain, joint line obliquity, and early failure. It is also not indicated for varus deformities of more than 15° in which there is usually joint subluxation and collateral ligament instability. The operation should also not be done on knees with limited motion. Additionally, flexion con-

---

R. E. Windsor, M.D.: Department of Orthopaedic Surgery, Cornell University Medical College, New York, NY 10021.

tracture exceeding 10° and overall motion of less than 90° contraindicates the procedure. Radiographic patellofemoral osteoarthritis by itself does not contraindicate osteotomy, since the procedure restores somewhat normal patellofemoral mechanics. Older patients with a more limited lifestyle would generally be better candidates for total knee replacement now that the long-term results of the proce-

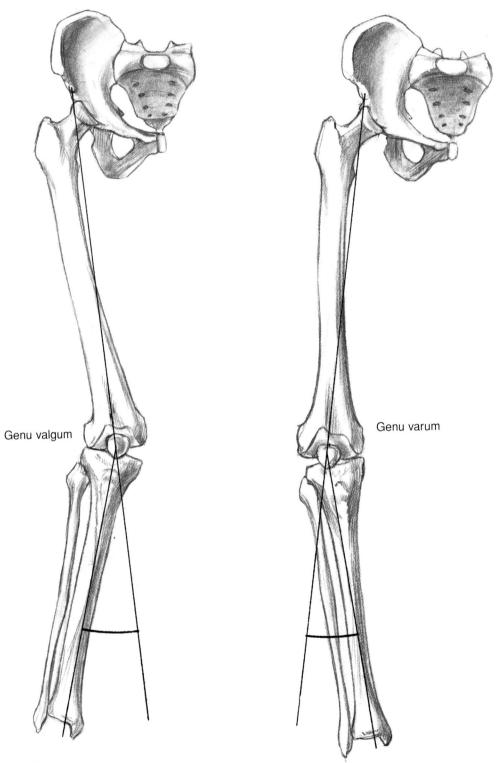

Genu valgum

Genu varum

Figure 1. Varus and valgus mechanical axes of the knee. High tibial osteotomy is indicated for varus deformity. (Redrawn from ref. 5.)

dure have shown durability and predictable pain relief. However, each patient should be treated individually, since there may be an occasional older patient having a "physiologic" age of 60 years who wishes to continue very aggressive activities and sports. This latter patient would be best served with osteotomy.

PREOPERATIVE PLANNING

A standing full-length anteroposterior (AP) radiograph of the knee should be obtained to plan the osteotomy. The mechanical axis and femorotibial axis should be evaluated.

The mechanical axis is determined using standing radiographs that include the hip, knee, and ankle (Fig. 1). The normal mechanical axis passes through the knee and the middle of the ankle joint distally. It extends proximally straight through the center of the femoral head. High tibial osteotomy is indicated for correction of varus deformities of less than 15°.

The femorotibial angle is demonstrated in weight-bearing radiographs. Radiographs of supine or unstressed subjects will not demonstrate loss of substance or ligament laxity. The normal angle is 175°, or 5° of valgus.

The alignment of the knee is assessed preoperatively (Fig. 2). After the amount of varus deformity is known, the wedge of bone to be resected should be determined. The recommended amount of correction should be enough to bring the knee to a valgus alignment of 8° to 12°. The wedge of bone is triangular, with its base located at the lateral cortex. For small individuals, 1 mm of bone represents 1° of correction. For taller individuals, 10 mm of bone removal generally provides 8° of correction. There are currently available numerous guides that may be utilized intraoperatively to assess the appropriately angled wedge (Fig. 3).

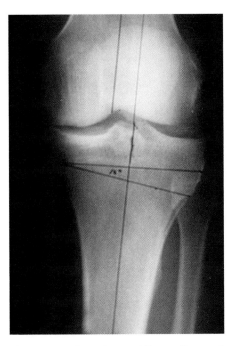

Figure 2. Standing AP radiograph showing varus alignment, with lines drawn along the center of the intramedullary shafts of the femur and tibia. The wedge needed for proper correction during osteotomy is outlined. The base of the wedge is located along the lateral tibial cortex.

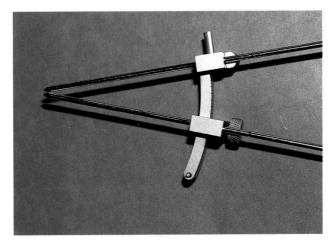

Figure 3. Osteotomy guide used to determine the appropriate angle of the wedge. For this guide the Steinmann pins should meet at the medial tibial cortex. Each Steinmann pin has a notch in which the guide should be positioned so that a reproducible angle may be created.

SURGERY

Patient Positioning

The patient is placed in the supine position. A tourniquet is applied on the proximal thigh and tested before sterile preparation and draping of the limb. The leg is draped free with see-through plastic drapes so that alignment can be assessed using the landmarks of the ankle malleoli and the anterior superior iliac spine of the pelvis.

Choice of Incision

I prefer to use an anterior midline longitudinal incision for exposure. This incision is quite extensile and may be readily utilized if there is a need for a later total knee replacement. However, some surgeons utilize a transverse horizontal incision (Fig. 4), which provides more limited exposure and can be used with smaller fixation devices. An alternative incision is the lateral longitudinal incision (Fig. 5). This provides extensile exposure for the osteotomy but may complicate the choice of incision if total knee replacement later becomes necessary.

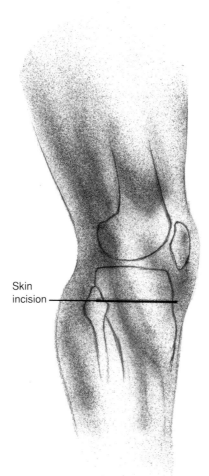

Skin incision

Figure 4. Horizontal transverse incision. This incision permits only small fixation devices. It is the incision generally used when cast fixation is chosen to keep the tibial bone fragments aligned.

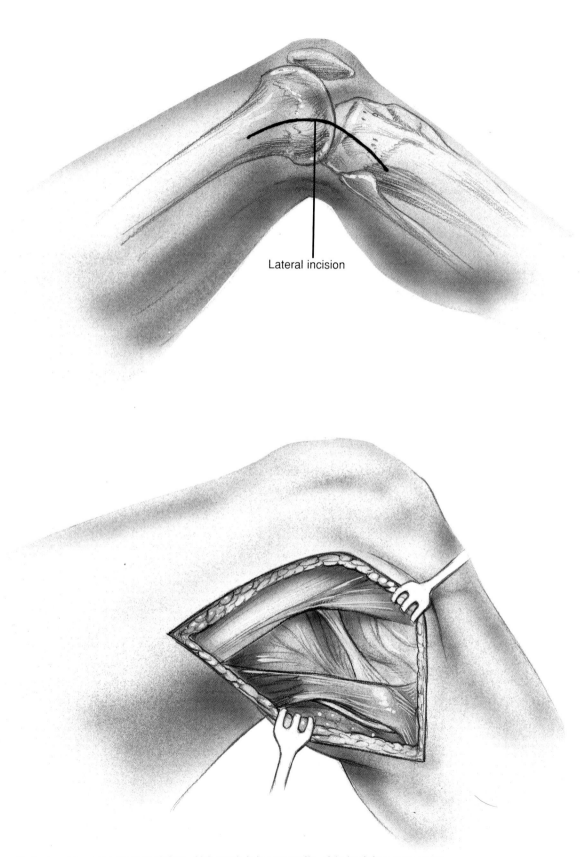

Figure 5. Lateral longitudinal incision. Although it is extensile, this incision may pose difficulties in terms of choosing an incision if future total knee replacement becomes necessary.

Options for Anesthesia

Epidural anesthesia is my anesthesia of choice whenever possible. Patient-controlled analgesia or continuous epidural anesthesia in the postoperative period is not recommended, since it may interfere with proper assessment of the neurovascular function of the leg.

Procedure

After the patient is placed in the supine position and the leg is prepped and draped in a sterile manner, a midline longitudinal incision is made from the level of the patella to just distal to the tibial tubercle (Fig. 6). An incision is made on the lateral tibial flare through the periosteum and extended distally about 4 cm distal to the tibial tubercle. This incision is extended proximally along the lateral margin of the patellar ligament. Another incision is made at the level of Gerdy's tubercle and follows the lateral proximal flare of the tibia posteriorly to the tibiofibular joint. The musculature of the anterior compartment is stripped off the tibia subperiosteally to expose the posterior tibial cortex. A periosteal elevator is used to strip the posterior periosteum as best as possible, in order to allow placement of a Bennett retractor to protect the posterior anatomic structures during the osteotomy itself.

The proximal fibula should be mobilized to allow the bone to migrate proximally when later coaptation of the osteotomy is required. My preference is to disrupt the tibiofibular joint with a blunt, wide periosteal elevator, taking care to completely disrupt the joint. Otherwise, easy closure of the osteotomy will not be possible and the osteotomy may spring open. Other surgeons resect the fibular head or do a cuff resection of the fibular shaft more distally. However, these latter two techniques put the peroneal nerve in great jeopardy of being injured.

An instrument guide is placed around the proximal tibia, with its most proximal end at the level of the joint line. It guides the placement of the first proximally

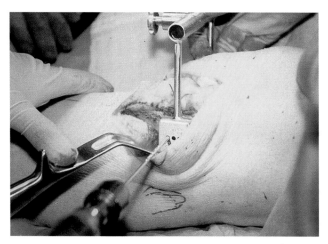

Figure 6. The midline longitudinal incision is extensile and permits fixation with any type of device. A positioning guide is placed to accurately position a nonthreaded Steinmann pin 2 cm distal to the joint line. This distance is sufficient to allow placement of a blade plate while leaving a safe amount of proximal tibia for protection against fracture after the osteotomy.

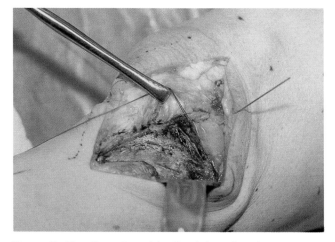

Figure 7. Needles placed in the joint give the surgeon a reference point for the location of the tibial articular surface.

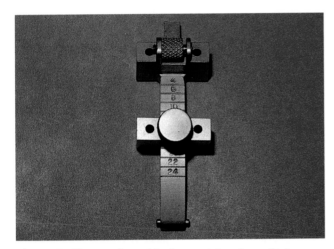

Figure 8. The angle guide is used to place Steinmann pins in the correct alignment for the subsequent placement of the cutting blocks.

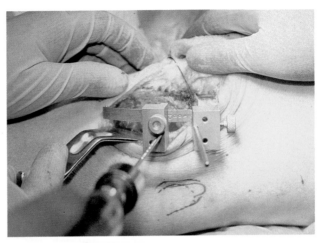

Figure 9. A distal Steinmann pin is placed after the angle guide is positioned parallel to the long axis of the anterior tibia.

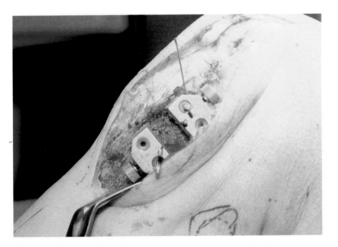

Figure 10. Cutting blocks are placed over the Steinmann pins after the angle guide is removed.

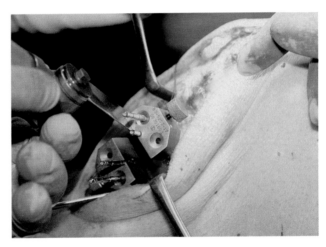

Figure 11. The osteotomy is started with an oscillating saw.

placed Steinmann pin at a level 2 cm away from the joint line. This distance is needed to provide a safe amount of bone stock for placement of a buttress plate. It is helpful to place straight needles into the medial and lateral joint lines to assess the location of the tibial articular surface (Fig. 7).

An angle guide is placed over the first Steinmann pin (Fig. 8). Once this guide is in place, care should be taken to align it along the anterior shaft of the tibia before it is fixed into position by a second, distally placed Steinmann pin. The angle of correction that was determined preoperatively should be set before the pin is drilled into the bone. The Steinmann pins should pass medially just to the level of the medial tibial cortex (Fig. 9). After the location of the pins is found to be satisfactory, the angle guide is removed and the cutting blocks are affixed (Fig. 10). An oscillating saw is used to begin the osteotomy and cuts are made through the lateral cortex proximally and distally (Fig. 11). A half-inch straight osteotome is used to complete the osteotomy. I consider this method to be safer, since osteotomes do not create local heat necrosis of the bone surfaces, which could predispose to delayed healing of the osteotomy (Fig. 12). A second half-inch straight osteotome is placed to complete the distal aspect of the osteotomy (Fig. 13). After both osteotomes are inserted the surgeon can get a good idea of the overall angle of the wedge that will be resected. While using the osteotomes, care should be given to directing them away from the tibial articular surface, so that inadvertent perforation into the joint will be prevented (Fig. 14). The osteotomes should extend

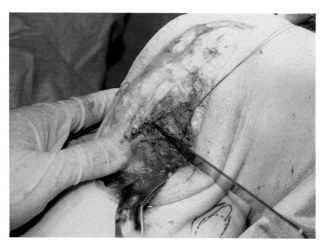

Figure 12. An osteotome is placed into the proximal cut to complete the osteotomy and avoid heat necrosis caused by the oscillating saw.

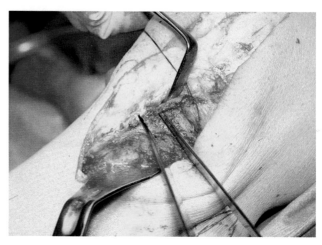

Figure 13. Another half-inch osteotome is placed into the distal cut made by the oscillating saw. The two osteotomes give the surgeon a good visual estimate of the wedge that will be taken.

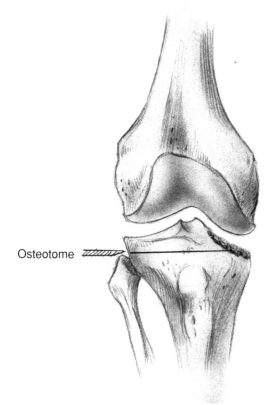

Osteotome

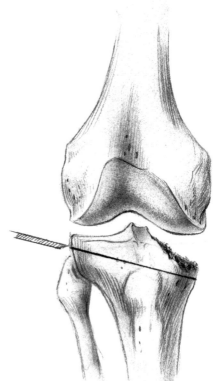

Incline is distal and medial

Figure 14. Intaarticular perforation with the osteotome should be avoided. This serious complication can be avoided by angling the proximal osteotomy slightly distally. Starting the osteotomy 2 cm distal to the tibial articular surface also protects against this complication. (Redrawn from ref. 5.)

almost to the medial tibial cortex, so that a periosteal sleeve remains intact as a hinge (Fig. 15). On the other hand, if too much bone remains medially, vigorous closure of the osteotomy may result in an intra-articular fracture (Fig. 16). Excessive force should not be applied to close the osteotomy. In this situation the osteotomy should be extended more medially and the tibiofibular joint should be re-examined to make sure it is fully released.

The bone wedge is removed whole or piecemeal (Fig. 17). I inspect the osteotomy site before closing it, and make sure that there is no residual bone left in the

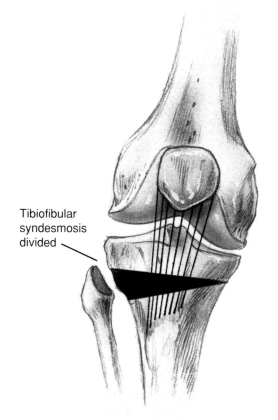

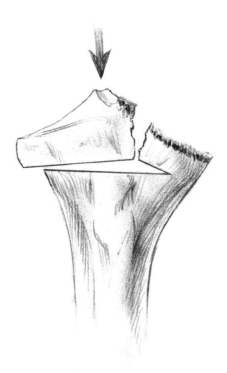

Figure 15. The osteotomy should just reach the medial tibial cortex, so that the latter may act as a hinge when the osteotomy is closed. (Redrawn from ref. 5.)

Figure 16. Failure to make the osteotomy end at the medial cortex may leave a bridge of bone that may cause an intraarticular fracture if excessive force is used to close the osteotomy. (Redrawn from ref. 5.)

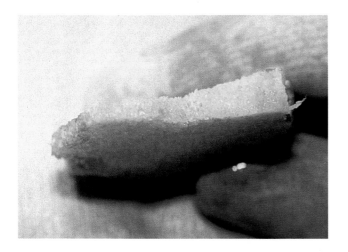

Figure 17. The bone wedge may be removed whole or piecemeal.

space (Fig. 18). Further thrusts with the osteotomes may be necessary at this stage to adequately mobilize the two tibial fragments.

Miniature buttress plates are used to fix the osteotomy fragments according to accepted fracture management techniques (Fig. 19). These plates are small and come with different sized proximal offsets. Once the osteotomy is closed, the plate is applied and screwed into place (Fig. 20). Other methods of fixation have been described. A blade plate may be utilized, but a larger exposure is required to fit it along the lateral tibial cortex (Fig. 21). Surgical staples have also been used, but provide tenuous fixation strength at best (Fig. 22). A cylinder cast with three-point fixation at the thigh, knee, and ankle may also be used without the need for internal fixation (Fig. 23). This latter method provides the ability to slightly modify the alignment of the leg in the postoperative period. However, the prolonged immobilization that is sometimes necessary may cause muscle atrophy and stiffness.

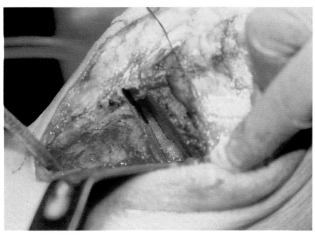

Figure 18. View of the osteotomy space after removal of the bone wedge. Note the presence of bone at the medial tibial cortex. Other bone fragments may be removed from this space by rongeurs prior to closing it.

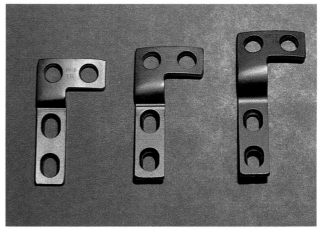

Figure 19. Miniature buttress plates with different sized proximal offsets may be used to fix the bone fragments.

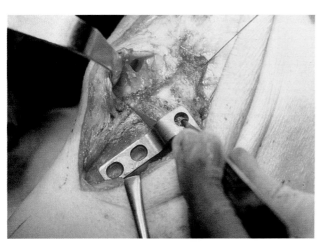

Figure 20. The plates are applied to bone according to accepted fracture fixation techniques. Care should be taken to make sure the bone fragments are properly apposed before securing the plate with screws.

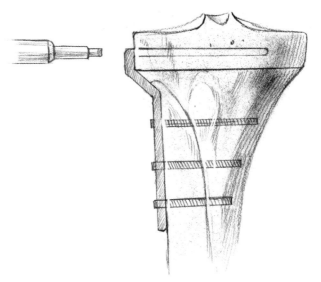

Figure 21. Blade plates may also be utilized to fix the osteotomy fragments, but greater exposure may be needed. (Redrawn from ref. 5.)

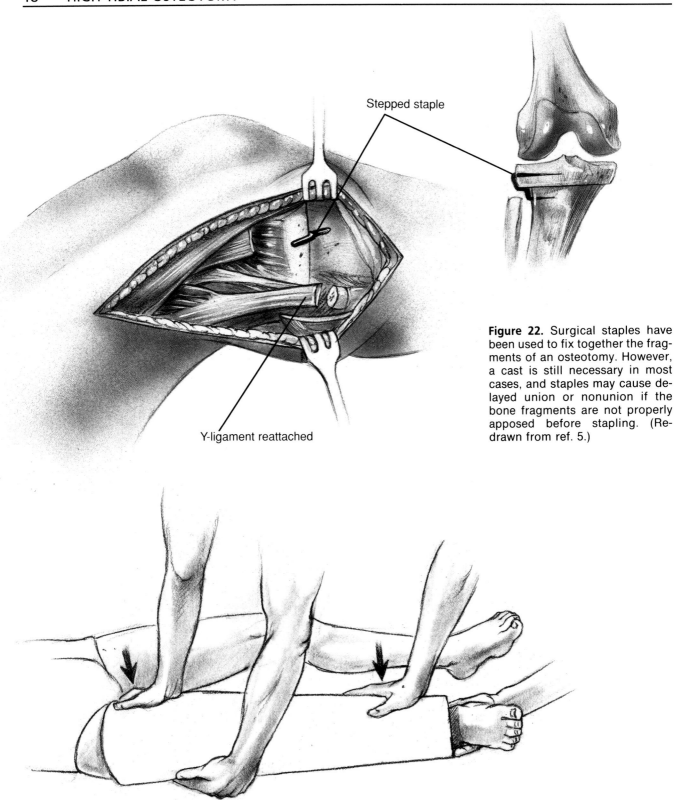

Stepped staple

Y-ligament reattached

Figure 22. Surgical staples have been used to fix together the fragments of an osteotomy. However, a cast is still necessary in most cases, and staples may cause delayed union or nonunion if the bone fragments are not properly apposed before stapling. (Redrawn from ref. 5.)

Figure 23. The cylinder cast technique makes use of three-point fixation of the limb to secure the alignment. The points of fixation are the medial tibia just above the medial malleolus, the lateral side of the knee, and the proximal medial thigh. (Redrawn from ref. 5.)

The deep fascia is closed loosely with interrupted absorbable sutures after a drain is placed. The subcutaneous tissue is closed with interrupted absorbable sutures, and stainless steel staples are used to close the skin. Betadine-soaked gauze and sterile dressings are applied to the wound, and the leg is wrapped with elastic bandages uniformly placed around it.

POSTOPERATIVE MANAGEMENT

The patient's dressing is kept in place for 2 days. The drain is removed after 1 day and the knee is placed in a continuous passive motion (CPM) apparatus. The limb is checked every 2 hours during the first day to assess its neurovascular status. The hospitalization usually lasts 5 to 7 days, until the patient can handle crutches comfortably.

The patient should expect to remain on partial weight bearing for 1 month, followed by progression to full weight bearing over the next month. Unassisted walking will probably not occur for 2 to 3 months. The ultimate result should not be expected for 1 year. Aggressive activity generally commences after 6 months.

Clinical Results

Good to excellent relief of arthritic pain can be expected in 80% to 85% of cases of high tibial osteotomy (1). Success hinges greatly on proper patient selection and technique. A few long-term follow-up studies have been done on high tibial osteotomy. Coventry found that after 10 years, 61.8% of patients rated themselves as having less pain than before osteotomy (2). Coventry further followed his osteotomies beyond 10 years and found that the satisfactory results were maintained if the patient was not overweight and the correction obtained was at least 8° of valgus (3). Insall followed 95 knees for a mean of 8.5 years. At follow-up, 63% were in the excellent or good categories and 37% were fair or poor. Subsequently, 24 knees were revised to total knee arthroplasties (4). The general consensus in the literature is that a minimum correction of at least 8° to 12° of valgus is necessary to achieve long-standing successful rates. However, results do deteriorate with time, with an associated progression of osteoarthritis and pain (5).

COMPLICATIONS

Insall collected the data from all published reports on osteotomy and evaluated the complications in a total of 804 high tibial osteotomies.

Peroneal Nerve Palsy. Among the 804 high tibial osteotomies, in his investigation, Insall found that 56 peroneal nerve palsies had been observed, 37 of them associated with transfixation pins. Because of this high incidence of palsy with the use of transfixation pins, these pins are generally not recommended for use in fixing the osteotomy fragments. Of the three different methods of mobilizing the fibula, disruption of the tibiofibular joint is the safest with regard to injuring the peroneal nerve. Resection of the fibular head or removal of a segment of fibular shaft distal to the tibiofibular joint is associated with a higher incidence of peroneal nerve injury. It is generally treated by observation, and in most cases peroneal nerve function will return to normal after 6 months.

Infection. Sixty infections were reported in the 804 osteotomies examined by Insall. Fifty-five were superficial and 5 were deep. Thirty-seven occurred with the use of transfixation pins, constituting another reason why this method of fixation is contraindicated.

Arterial Injury. High tibial osteotomy poses the risk of injury to the anterior tibial or peroneal arteries. There have been no reported injuries to the popliteal nerve, but every effort must be made to protect these structures during the procedure .

Nonunion/Delayed Union. This complication is usually associated with improper internal fixation of the tibial bone fragments. Staples may keep the fragments apart if they are not appropriately placed after being compressed manually.

Intraarticular Fracture. This complication occurs when the osteotome perforates the tibial articular surface. The surgeon should direct the osteotome away from the articular surface and take into account the 3° medial tilt of the proximal tibial surface. Fracture can also occur if excessive force is exerted during closure of the osteotomy. The proximal tibia can fracture if too much bone is left medially.

ILLUSTRATIVE CASE FOR TECHNIQUE

A 48-year-old man with osteoarthritis of the knee and a 5-degree varus deformity developed increasing pain over a 3-year period (Fig. 24). His physical examination showed good ligamentous stability with an ROM from full extension to 130 degrees. There was no extension lag or flexion contracture. The patient underwent high tibial osteotomy using the cast method (Fig. 25). The osteotomy healed after 8 weeks and the patient is still free of pain after 9 years.

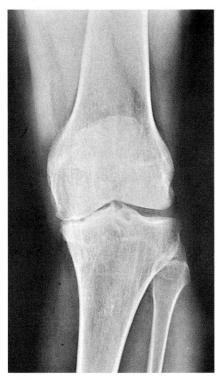

Figure 24. Preoperative standing AP radiograph showing medial osteoarthritis with varus malalignment.

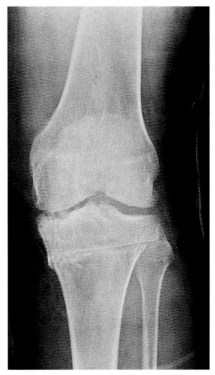

Figure 25. Postoperative AP radiograph with the knee fixed in a cylinder cast, showing the line of osteotomy. Healing occurred in 2 months.

Acknowledgment.   Figures 1, 4, 5, 14, 15, 16, 21, 22 and 23 were redrawn from Insall, J. N.: *Surgery of the Knee,* 2nd ed., New York: Churchill Livingstone, 1993; Chapter 22: 643–649, with permission of the publisher.

RECOMMENDED READING

1. Aichroth, P. M., Cannon, D. W., and Patel, D. V.: *Knee Surgery. Current Practice.* Raven, New York, 1993.
2. Coventry, M. B.: Upper tibial osteotomy for osteoarthritis. *J. Bone Joint Surg.,* 67A: 1136, 1985.
3. Coventry, M. B., Ilstrup, D. M., and Wallrichs, S. L.: Proximal tibial osteotomy. A critical long-term study of eighty-seven cases. *J. Bone Joint Surg.,* 75A: 196, 1993.
4. Insall, J. N., Joseph, D. M., and Msika, C.: High tibial osteotomy for varus gonarthrosis: A long-term follow-up study. *J. Bone Joint Surg.,* 66A: 1040, 1984.
5. Insall, J. N.: Osteotomy. p. 635. In: *Surgery of the Knee,* 2nd ed. edited by J. N. Insall, R. E. Windsor, W. N. Scott, M. A. Kelly, and P. Aglietti. Churchill Livingstone, New York, 1993.

Master Techniques in Orthopaedic Surgery,
Knee Arthroplasty, edited by P. A. Lotke,
Raven Press, Ltd., New York © 1995.

19

Distal Femoral Varus
Osteotomy for Genu Valgum

Bernard F. Morrey

INDICATIONS/CONTRAINDICATIONS

Distal femoral osteotomy as a realignment procedure is most commonly performed for lateral gonarthrosis (6,7). The male-to-female ratio of the procedure is approximately 1 to 10. Distal femoral osteotomy is the treatment of choice to realign a valgus deformity with a tibiofemoral angle of more than 15 degrees. The procedure is also indicated if the joint alignment is in 10 or more degrees of valgus tilt (6). Osteotomy in general is preferred in individuals under the age of 60 years and those with modest activity levels. Total knee arthroplasty is employed in those over the age of 65. Individuals between 60 and 65 years of age are considered in a "gray zone," with such individual features as weight, activity, and expectations, dictating the final choice of procedure.

A valgus angulation of less than 10 degrees away from anatomic alignment is in my experience best corrected with a varus-producing proximal tibial osteotomy (1). If the joint has less than 5 degrees of valgus tilt, and if less than 10 degrees of anatomic valgus alignment is to be corrected, then osteotomy at the distal femur should be avoided, and proximal tibial osteotomy is preferred. This prevents a varus orientation of the joint-line surface. Older individuals (over 65 years) are most reliably treated with joint-replacement arthroplasty. Osteotomy should not be seriously considered if moderate osteoporosis is present.

PREOPERATIVE PLANNING

A full-length radiograph including the hip and ankle is important in planning for an adequate correction. The relationship between the anatomic axis, or femoral

B. F. Morrey, M.D.: Department of Orthopedic Surgery, Mayo Clinic and Mayo Foundation, and Mayo Medical School, Rochester, MN 55905.

tibial axis, and the mechanical axis, consisting of the line connecting the center of the hip and center of the ankle joint, must be appreciated (Fig. 1). The desired corrected anatomic angle is typically recommended to be about 0 degrees (2,3,5). This results in a mechanical axis that is in approximately 5 degrees of varus (6). A varus anatomic (tibiofemoral) axis is to be avoided. The preoperative planning should also involve cutouts to estimate the proper size of the wedge and the angular orientation of the joint upon completion of the osteotomy (Fig. 2) (4). The determination of the alignment guides and the internal fixation are also considered during the preoperative planning phase. I feel that the easiest method of determining the desired angular correction is to calculate the angle (alpha) formed by the mechanical axis from the hip to the knee (HK) and the mechanical axis from the ankle to the knee (AK) (Fig. 3).

SURGERY

The patient is placed supine on a routine operating table. A fluoroscopic C-arm is available to obtain films during the procedure. The leg is draped free.

Technique

A medial incision is made from just distal to the medial joint line across the adductor tubercle and approximately 10 cm proximal along the line of the posterior

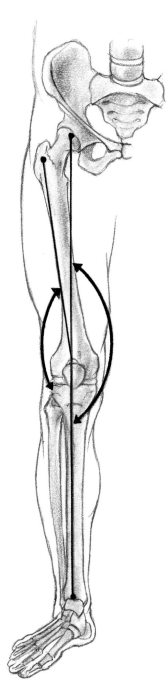

Figure 1. The mechanical aspect represents alignment from the center of the hip through the center of the knee and the center of the ankle.

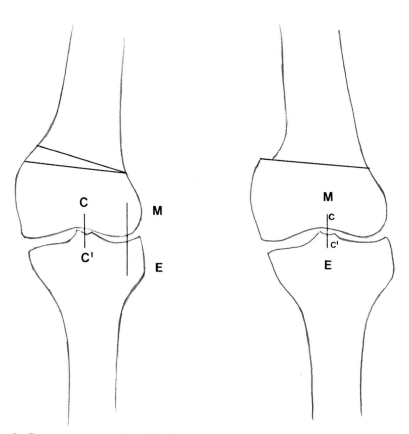

Figure 2. Proper preoperative planning requires cutouts of the abnormal and corrected alignments. An accurate estimation of the location and size of the wedge can be reliably made.

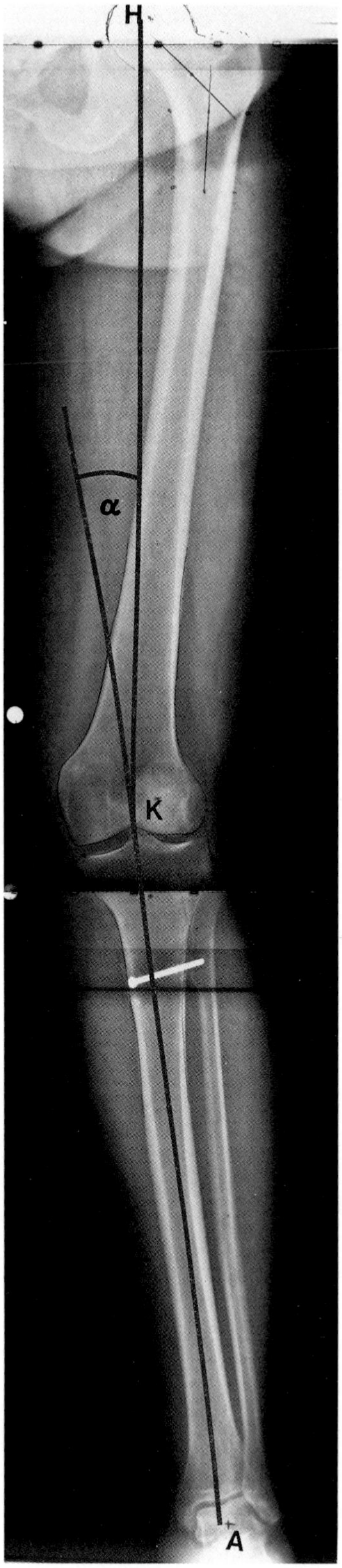

Figure 3. The desired angle of correction is most easily determined from the angle (alpha) formed by the proximal and distal mechanical axis created by the line from the center of the hip through the center of the knee and the distal mechanical axis from the center of the ankle through the center of the knee. This requires a hip-to-ankle roentgenogram.

aspect of the vastus medialis (Fig. 4). The posterior aspect of the vastus medialis is identified (Fig. 5) and is elevated from the intermuscular septum, thus exposing the medial aspect of the femur (Fig. 6). The dissection is carried distally to identify and cauterize the epiphyseal vessels, which are at the level of the adductor tubercle. Because the fixation passes through the region of the adductor tubercle, the dissection is carried only several centimeters distal to this landmark.

Planning the Osteotomy

Using the fluoroscope, a guide pin is placed from the adductor tubercle across the distal femur (Fig. 7). I prefer a 100-degree plate, and 10 degrees of varus distal

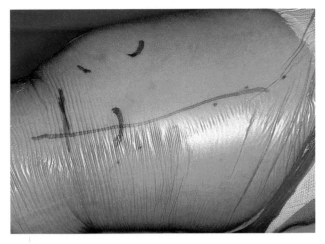

Figure 4. The skin incision is medial at the margin of the vastus medialis proximally and progresses distally over the abductor tubercle, ending approximately 2 cm distal to the joint line.

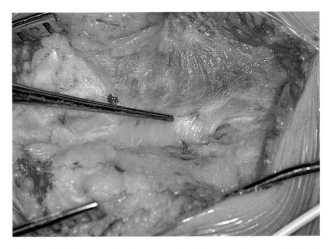

Figure 5. The posterior agent of the vastus medialis is identified and elevated.

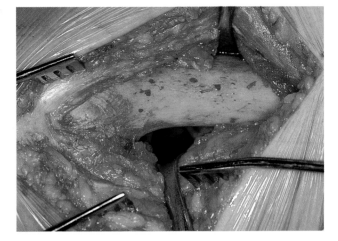

Figure 6. By elevating the vastus medialis, the distal medial aspect of the femoral shaft is identified.

alignment must therefore be obtained with the guide pin referable to the bone. The osteotome is driven across the distal femur in line with the distal pin (Fig. 8). This is done while the femur is intact in order to avoid displacing the distal fragment after the wedge has been taken. A second guide pin is placed across the femur at the distal level of the intended osteotomy. The position is verified with a spot film (Fig. 9).

The Osteotomy

The osteotome is removed and the distal femur is transected at the level of the proximal guide pin, which represents the distal cut of the wedge and measures

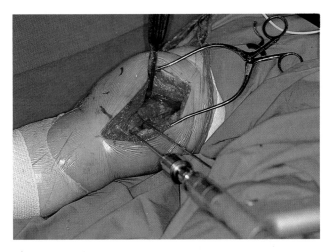

Figure 7. A fluoroscope is used to accurately place the pin just distal to the abductor tubercle and in the 10-degree varus alignment referable to the joint surface of the femoral condyles. This accommodates the 100-degree plate, which I prefer.

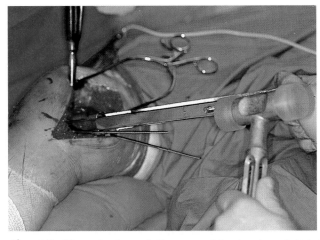

Figure 8. The osteotome follows a guide pin placed distal to the adductor tuberosity. The position is verified with a fluoroscopic spot film.

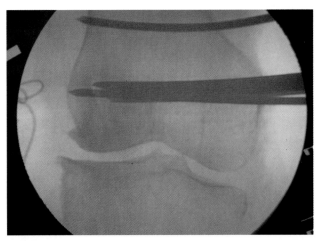

Figure 9. The proximal aspect of the osteotomy is identified with a second guide pin and the position is verified by fluoroscopy.

about 2 to 2.5 cm above the position of the osteotome (Fig. 10). Care is taken not to violate the opposite cortex with the osteotomy cut, so as to maintain stability when the plate is driven across the distal femur. The appropriate width of wedge is marked on the femur, based on preoperative planning. Angular guides are used to confirm the precise width and angular correction to be obtained (Fig. 11). A second pin may be inserted at the position of the proximal cut and the amount of correction verified. The proximal portion of the osteotomy is then completed, assuring that the wedge has an apex at the lateral cortex. The width of the wedge is reassessed and the wedge is removed (Fig. 12). The appropriateness of the wedge may be further evaluated with special instruments designed for this purpose (Fig. 13).

Fixation

The 100° AO osteotomy plate is then driven across the distal femur (Fig. 14), and its position is verified by radiography (Fig. 15). The opposite cortex is cracked with a 7-mm osteotome and the osteotomy is closed. If the above steps are properly executed, the plate will rest flush against the femur (Fig. 16). Position and closure

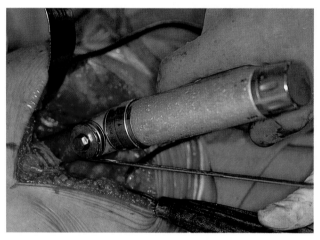

Figure 10. The osteotome is removed and the oscillating saw follows the guide pins in order to perform the osteotomy in an accurate fashion.

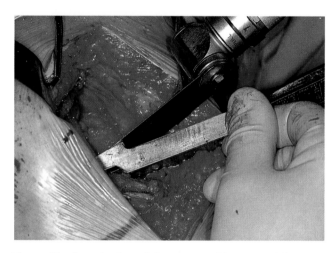

Figure 11. Angular templates are used to accurately measure the width of the desired wedge.

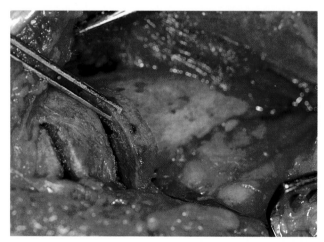

Figure 12. After the second cortical cut is made, the width of the cortex is measured and an appropriate measurement is confirmed.

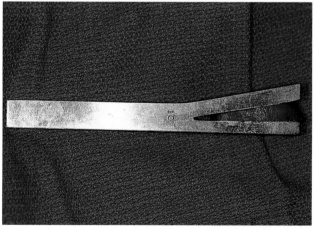

Figure 13. The wedge when removed is evaluated with an instrument to verify that it matches the wedge that was desired in the preoperative planning.

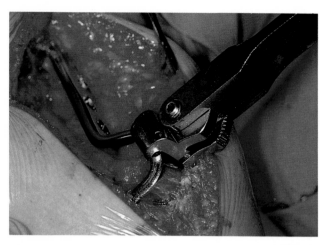

Figure 14. The 100-degree AO plate is driven across the distal femur.

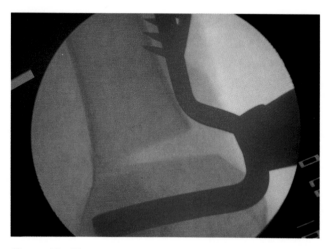

Figure 15. The position of the plate is verified radiographically before the osteotomy is closed.

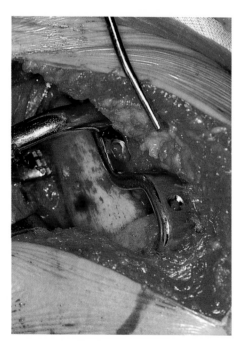

Figure 16. If the preoperative planning has been correct and the wedge accurately removed, the plate rests flush against the cortex of the femur.

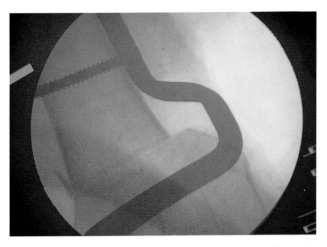

Figure 17. The apposition of the osteotomy surfaces is confirmed by fluoroscopy.

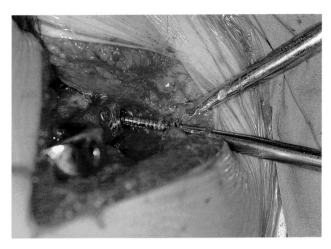

Figure 18. AO screws are placed routinely. The first is used in a compression mode.

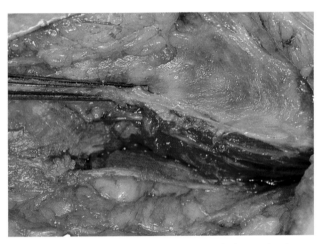

Figure 19. The vastus medialis obliquus is brought down over the plate, and closure is routine.

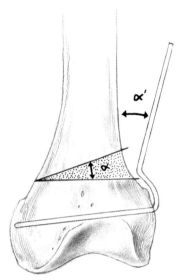

Figure 20. The angular correction from the distal femur corresponds to the angle formed by the shaft of the femur and the distal condylar plate.

appositioning are verified by fluoroscopy (Fig. 17). Routine insertion of AO cortical screws is then done to secure the plate (Fig. 18). The first screw is placed closest to the osteotomy and in the dynamic compression mode. To effect closure, the vastus medialis obliquus is sewn to the intermuscular septum (Fig. 19). The remainder of the closure is routine.

Technical Note

The fluoroscopy is most valuable with regard to the accurate execution of this procedure. This both determines the proper orientation and facilitates the localization of three major aspects of the technique: (i) that of the plate across the femur;

(ii) the distal cut; and (iii) the proximal cut. The side plate of the AO device should make the same angle on the femoral shaft as the wedge to be removed (Fig. 20). This allows close coaptation of the osteotomized surfaces as the plate is brought flush against the femur. Care should be taken to provide counterpressure to the distal femur when the plate is being inserted, in order to avoid translation of the distal fragment from overzealous impaction of the device.

POSTOPERATIVE MANAGEMENT

The patient is placed in a pressure dressing and started on physical therapy the day after surgery. Protected weight bearing with crutches or a walker is required until early healing is achieved. This will last for 3 to 4 months, after which the patient may use a cane. During the early phases of rehabilitation, gentle range-of-motion activities are encouraged. The patient should regain his or her preoperative range of motion within 3 weeks of surgery.

RESULTS

There are very few reports in the literature of the results of distal femoral osteotomy. In two previous studies reported in the last 5 years, a satisfactory result of approximately 85% to 90% was reported (3,5). The Mayo Clinic experience has recently been described by Edgerton and Morrey (2). If the complications due to inadequate fixation with the use of a staple are ignored in the Mayo series, satisfactory results were observed in approximately 90% of cases, which even with longer follow-up is comparable to that in the other reports. Edgerton correlated the results with the preoperative knee score, and noted a statistically significant correlation, with better results among those patients with higher preoperative scores. This clearly indicates that those with more severe arthrosis should be considered candidates for total knee arthroplasty rather than osteotomy. Another important factor shown by the Mayo study was that if a satisfactory result is present 2 to 3 years after surgery, there is a smaller tendency for deterioration with time, as is seen with proximal tibial osteotomies (8).

COMPLICATIONS

A major complication of distal femoral osteotomy is nonunion, which continues to occur in approximately 5% of cases even with contemporary surgical techniques. Consolidation may be slow and can take up to 6 months. After this period, union is considered to be delayed, and this is particularly worrisome in older individuals. The infection rate is approximately 1% to 2%, which is higher than would be expected for joint-replacement arthroplasty. Neural injury is uncommon in procedures that approach the medial aspect of the distal femur.

ILLUSTRATIVE CASE FOR TECHNIQUE

This 58-year-old woman has a significant valgus deformity and lateral joint-line pain (Fig. 21). The radiograph demonstrates moderate lateral gonarthrosis, with 13

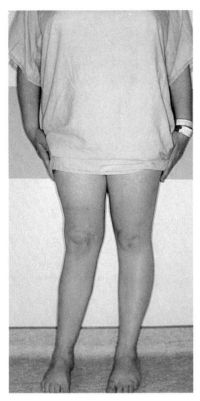

Figure 21. Moderate valgus alignment in a 58-year-old woman with marked pain and valgus thrust during gait.

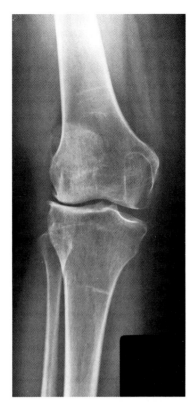

Figure 22. Radiograph demonstrating the lateral arthritic changes in the patient in Figure 21.

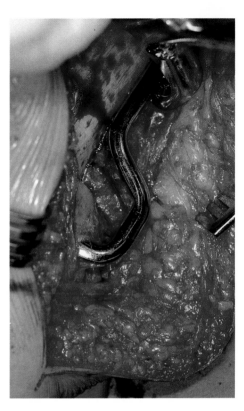

Figure 23. A varus-producing distal femoral osteotomy was done in the manner described above.

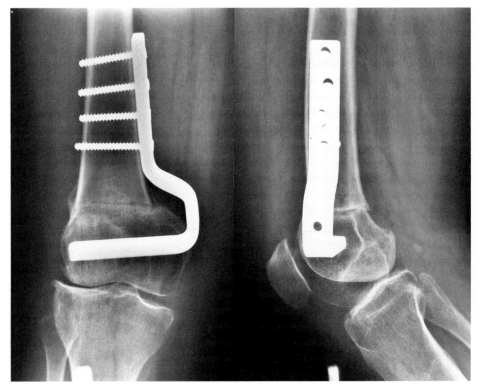

Figure 24. At 4 months the osteotomy is healed.

degrees of valgus in the anatomic axis (Fig. 22). A varus-producing distal femoral osteotomy, using the technique described above, was done (Fig. 23). The osteotomy healed in 4 months (Fig. 24) and the patient was ambulating without a cane at 5 months after surgery. Her arc of motion is currently 0 to 110 degrees and her leg alignment is straight. She has no pain and is satisfied with the procedure 1 year after surgery.

RECOMMENDED READING

1. Coventry, M. B.: Proximal tibial varus osteotomy for osteoarthritis of the lateral compartment of the knee. *J. Bone Joint Surg.*, 69A: 32, 1987.
2. Edgerton, B. C., Mariani, E. M., and Morrey, B. F.: Distal femoral varus osteotomy for painful genu valgum: A 5–11 year follow-up. *Clin. Orthop.*, 288: 263–269, 1993.
3. Healy, W. L., Anglen, J. O., Wasilewski, S. A., and Krackow, K. A.: Distal femoral varus osteotomy. *J. Bone Joint Surg.*, 70A: 102, 1988.
4. Maquet, P.: The treatment of choice in osteoarthritis of the knee. *Clin. Orthop.*, 192: 108, 1985.
5. McDermott, A. G., Finklestein, J. A., Farine, I., Boynton, E. L., MacIntosh, D. L., and Gross, A.: Distal femoral varus osteotomy for valgus deformity of the knee. *J. Bone Joint Surg.*, 70A: 110, 1988.
6. Morrey, B. F., and Edgerton, B. C.: Distal femoral osteotomy for lateral gonarthrosis. AAOS Instructional Course Lectures, Vol. 41, pp. 77–85, 1982.
7. Soundry, M., and Insall, J. N.: Supracondylar femoral osteotomy for valgus knee deformities. *Orthop. Trans.*, 9: 25, 1985.
8. Stuart, M. J., Kelly, M., and Morrey, B. F.: Late recurrence of varus deformity after proximal tibial osteotomy. *CORR*, 260: 61–66, 1990.

PART V

Techniques for Other Reconstruction

Master Techniques in Orthopaedic Surgery,
KNEE ARTHROPLASTY, edited by P. A. Lotke,
Raven Press, Ltd., New York © 1995.

20

Patellectomy

John B. Meding and Merrill A. Ritter

INDICATIONS/CONTRAINDICATIONS

Prior to deciding to perform a patellectomy, the surgeon must carefully consider the significant role of the patella in knee function. The patella aids knee extension throughout its entire range of motion by lengthening the lever arm of the quadriceps mechanism; providing an articular surface with a low coefficient of friction and a wider distribution of compressive forces; protecting the femur from trauma; protecting the quadriceps from attritional wear; and improving cosmesis (1,8).

Because the patella is important to the function of the knee, there are many conditions in which a patellectomy will be the treatment of choice. These conditions include irreducible comminuted and displaced fractures; isolated patellar femoral arthrosis (frequently used after patellar fracture); pain associated with severe chondromalacia patellae; refraction to conservative treatment; chondral defects (with arthroscopic or imaging documentation); and tumors (rare).

In general, patellectomy is indicated after total knee replacement and in certain cases of patellar fracture. It is also indicated in cases of failed attempts at open reduction and internal fixation procedures, loosening of a patellar component, and failure of a patellar component.

PREOPERATIVE PLANNING

Individual evaluation prior to patellectomy will be directed toward a patient's specific pathology. In all cases, however, preoperative consideration must be given to the biomechanical alterations in knee function.

J. B. Meding, M.D.: Kendrick Memorial Hospital, and Sports Medicine & Joint Reconstructive Surgery, P.C., Center for Hip and Knee Surgery, Mooresville, IN 46158.

M. A. Ritter, M.D.: Department of Orthopaedic Surgery, Indiana University Medical Center, Kendrick Memorial Hospital, and, Sports Medicine & Joint Reconstructive Surgery, P.C., Center for Hip and Knee Surgery, Mooresville, IN 46158.

Prior to patellectomy the patient should be evaluated for extensor and flexor imbalance, extensor maltracking, and range of motion. Kaufer (7) has shown experimentally that as much as 30% more quadriceps force may be required for full knee extension following patellectomy. Watkins and associates (13) reported that peak quadriceps torque may be reduced as much as 50% after patellectomy. The increased force requirements are of noteworthy concern in this older patient population. Stair climbing may be particularly difficult, especially if both cruciate ligaments have been sacrificed, thus preventing normal femoral roll back and shortening of the extensor moment arm (12). An intact posterior cruciate ligament thus appears desirable preoperatively. Along with guidance about deficient extensor power and difficulty in using stairs, patients should also be counseled about a decreased stance phase in flexion, compromised function of both the quadriceps and the hamstrings, an increased incidence of knee instability, and a poor cosmetic appearance of the knee (8).

SURGERY

The draping procedure should be performed so that there is wide access to the entire lower extremity. We use a 30-second alcohol prep and then completely surround the knee with Ioban drape (9).

As many surgical procedures on the knee as possible should be performed through an anterior longitudinal incision (Fig. 1), so that future surgery will not be hampered by bouts of necrosis between two incisions. The entire extensor retinaculum is then exposed. Since damage to the extensor mechanism may vary, especially with patellectomy for fractures, we shall describe four different techniques the surgeon should consider in patellectomy.

Longitudinal Repair (Boyd-Hawkins)

A longitudinal incision is made in the midline of the quadriceps and the patellar tendons that are connected along the anterior aspect of the patella. The patella is then osteotomized in the longitudinal plane (Fig. 2A). The two patellar fragments are then everted and the patella is shelled out of the extensor mechanism (Fig. 2B). Inspection of the interior of the knee can be accomplished at this time. Repair is by imbrication of the two flaps on the medial and lateral sides so as to tighten up some of the slack (Fig. 2C).

Transverse Repair

The expansion of the quadriceps tendon and extensor retinaculum of the patella is incised transversely and the patella shelled from the remaining periosteum and extensor tendons. Repair is then accomplished by imbricating the two surfaces (Fig. 3). This can then be reinforced with part of the vastus medialis (Fig. 4). Most important is the repair of the extensor retinaculum medially and laterally.

Some attempts have been made to make a V incision into the quadriceps tendon after closure of the transverse repair (Fig. 5A), thus bringing a flap of the quadriceps tendon down to reinforce the repair and give more bulk in this area. The V incision is then closed into a Y incision (Fig. 5B) (10).

Text continues on page 331.

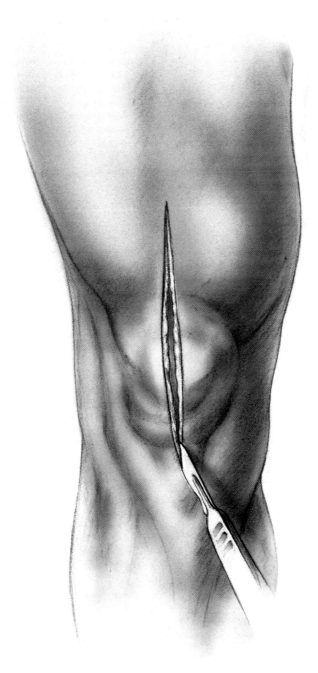

Figure 1. To prevent necrosis between two incisions, as many operative procedures to the knee as possible should be performed through an anterior longitudinal incision.

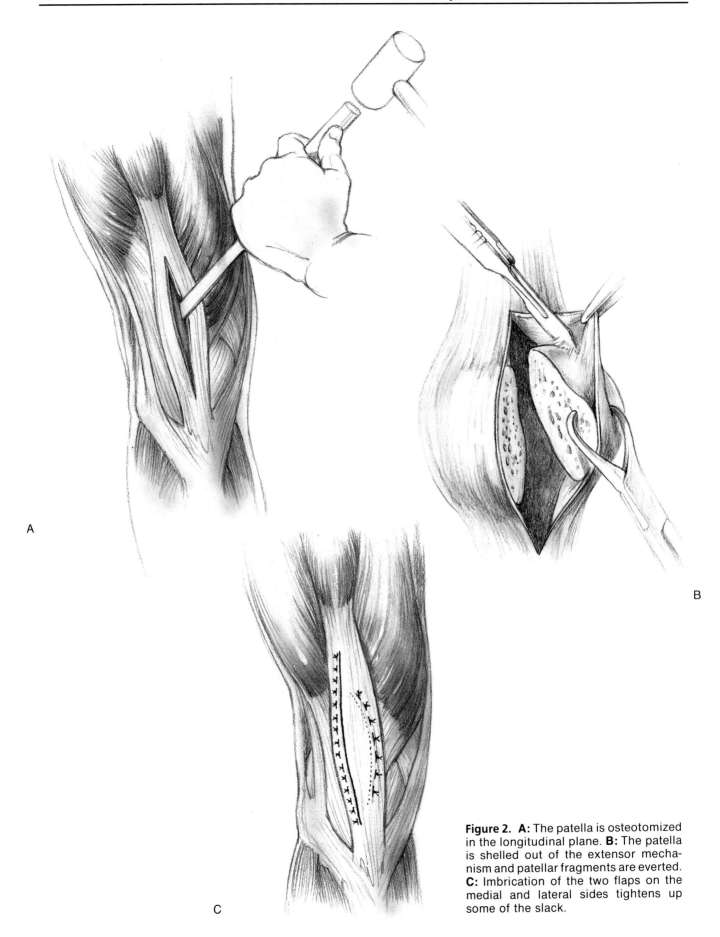

A

B

C

Figure 2. A: The patella is osteotomized in the longitudinal plane. **B:** The patella is shelled out of the extensor mechanism and patellar fragments are everted. **C:** Imbrication of the two flaps on the medial and lateral sides tightens up some of the slack.

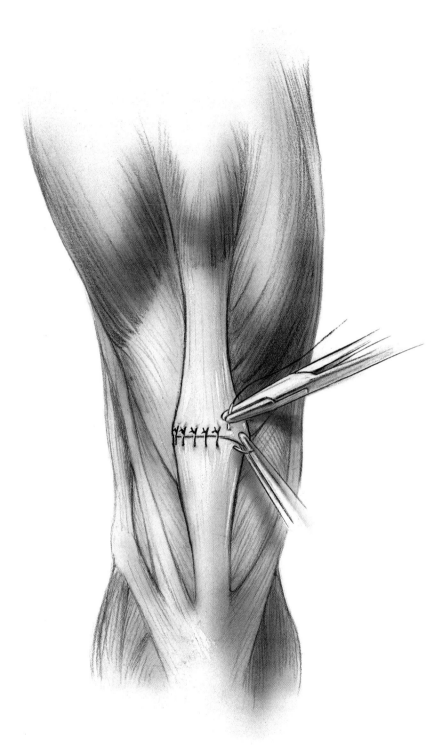

Figure 3. The transverse repair is accomplished by imbricating the two surfaces.

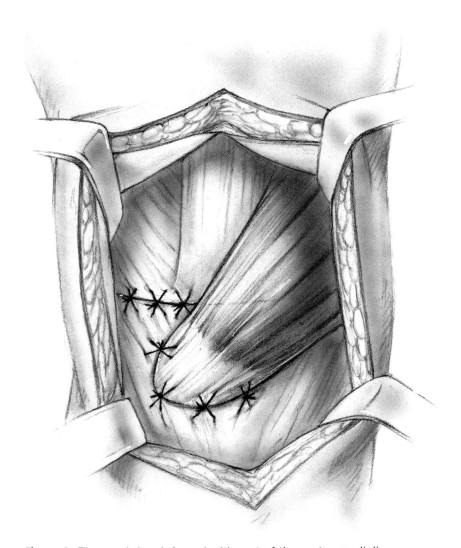

Figure 4. The repair is reinforced with part of the vastus medialis.

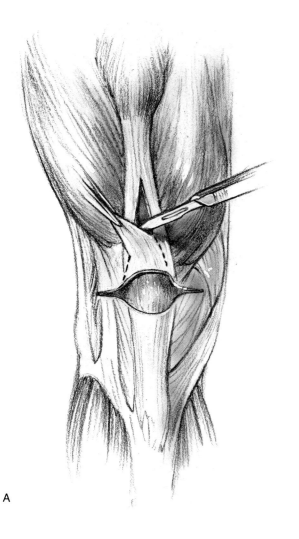

A

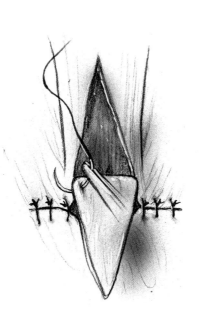

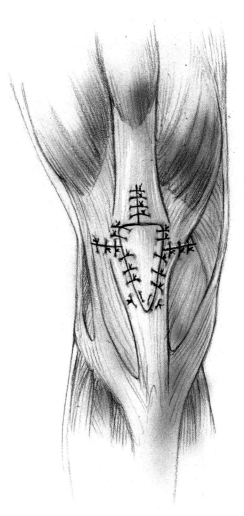

Figure 5. A: A flap of the quadriceps tendon is brought down to reinforce the repair and give more bulk to this area. **B:** The V incision is closed into a Y incision.

B

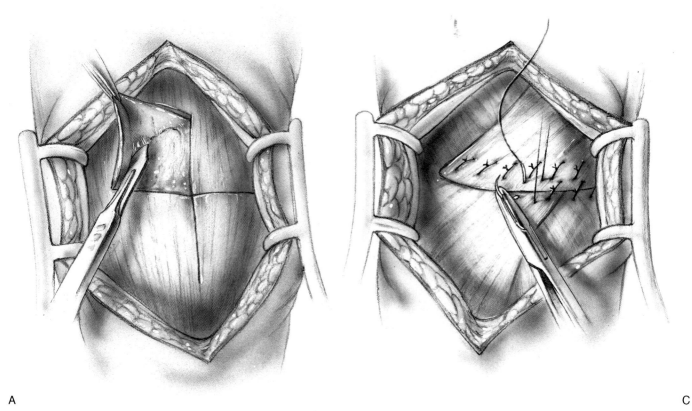

A

C

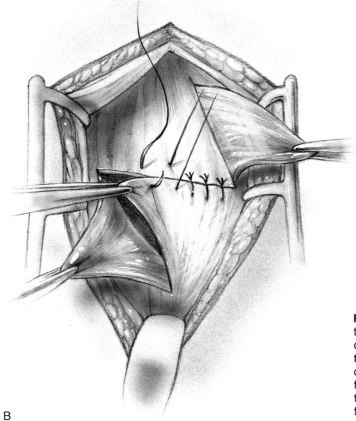

B

Figure 6. A: All four flaps are raised subperiosteally from the patella, and the extensor retinaculum is cut in a cruciate fashion. **B:** The central apex flaps are brought to the extreme edges of the lateral and medial portions of the incision and sutured closed. **C:** In order to reinforce the repair and add some bulk to the central portion of the patella, the superior medial and inferior lateral flaps are crossed.

Cruciate or Z Plasty

The extensor retinaculum over the patella is cut in a cruciate fashion and all four flaps are raised subperiosteally from the patella (Fig. 6A). Removal of the patella is then accomplished without difficulty. The interior of the joint can be visualized easily. The fat pad is left if at all possible. The central apex of the inferior medial and the superior lateral flaps are then brought to the extreme edges of the lateral and medial portions of the incision, respectively, and sutured closed (Fig. 6B). Next, the superior medial and inferior lateral flaps are crossed in the same fashion and closed, reinforcing the repair and adding some bulk to the central portion of the area of the patella (Fig. 6C).

Tube

A medial parapatellar retinacular incision is made. The patella is inverted and shelled from the quadriceps tendon. A lateral release is performed and the medial borders of the quadriceps, patellar extension, and patellar tendon are wrapped underneath to attach to the lateral aspect of the lateral release, and are secured with sutures. This then forms a tube. Next, the vastus medialis is closed to the area that was directly anterior to it, and has now rotated to the medial side (Fig. 7).

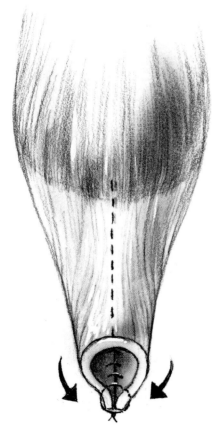

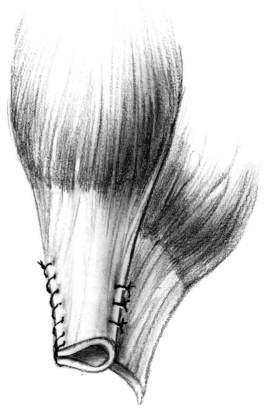

A   B

Figure 7. A,B: A tube is fabricated utilizing a lateral release and wrapping the medial borders of the quadriceps, patellar extension, and patellar tendon underneath and securing them with sutures. The vastus medialis has now rotated to the medial side and is closed to the area that was originally directly anterior to it.

We do not always release the tourniquet following knee surgery. However, in this particular situation the tourniquet should be dropped so that the circumferential pressure around the quadriceps muscle can be removed. The knee is put through a range of motion and the anastomosis observed. This helps to provide reassurance about the quality of postoperative care.

A compression dressing should be applied with a posterior splint that brings the knee out into full extension. If a knee immobilizer is used and full extension cannot be maintained, a posterior splint should be utilized. Full extension is a must.

POSTOPERATIVE CARE

Postoperative management should consist of a rigid splint applied posteriorly to help control the extension of the knee. Ambulation is begun on the first day after surgery. Weight bearing is allowed as tolerated, with external support. For the next 6 weeks, range-of-motion exercises are encouraged with the use of continuous passive motion or controlled physical therapy. Strengthening is discouraged except for straight leg raising and quad setting.

At the end of 6 weeks and for up to 12 weeks, range of motion exercise is assisted and strengthening is moderately resisted. After 12 weeks a strengthening program should be the predominant component of the rehabilitation program so that the extensor lag can be reduced to zero.

COMPLICATIONS

Many of the complications reported after patellectomy are a direct result of the biomechanical changes created by the procedure. Effects on the extensor mechanism, altered patterns of knee loading and gait during both walking and stair climbing, and cosmetic changes are all unavoidable following patellectomy and have been discussed (8).

Extensor lag and decreased quadriceps excursion may be minimized by observing the anastomosis and adjusting quadriceps tension during surgery. Other reported complications following patellectomy include prolonged postoperative pain, boutonniere deformity, heterotopic ossification, necrosis of the patellar tendon, disruption of the extensor mechanism by infection, inadequate repair, overly vigorous rehabilitation (3%), and subluxation or dislocation of the remaining extensor mechanism (3,12). Of these remaining complications the surgeon has the greatest control over the adequacy of the repair and progression of the patient during rehabilitation.

Reports in the literature of the results of total knee replacement after patellectomy have included mixed results (12). At the Center for Hip and Knee Surgery, most results were rated as good or excellent at 2 years. The posterior cruciate ligament was retained in all cases, and all tibial components were cemented. Pain results were excellent in all patients. At final follow up (average, 5.8 years) there were only 2 fair and 2 poor results among 22 patients. Instability was not clinically evident, and only one patient was noted to have a 5-degree flexion contracture. In this review, stair climbing was somewhat compromised by patellectomy. Therefore, patients should be instructed that only about 30% will be able to walk stairs normally (reciprocally and without support).

ILLUSTRATIVE CASE FOR TECHNIQUE

A 49-year-old woman had had knee problems dating back to a diagnosis of chondromalacia of the patella during her young adulthood. She had had a patellar debridement 15 years before her current presentation, at which time she was told that she had a significant chondromalacic defect in her articular surface. In the preceding 5 years she has had three arthroscopic procedures with additional debridement of the retropatellar surface. Each time she was told that there were denuded areas of articular cartilage and subchondral bone articulating against areas of subchondral bone on the femoral side of the knee. She elected to have a patellectomy because of progressive disability and pain (Fig. 8).

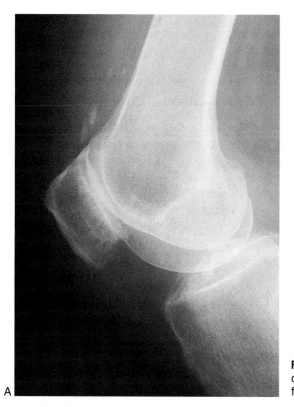

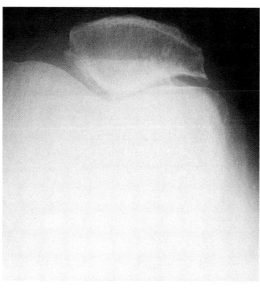

Figure 8. A,B: Lateral roentgenogram and merchant view demonstrating significant patellofemoral arthrosis.

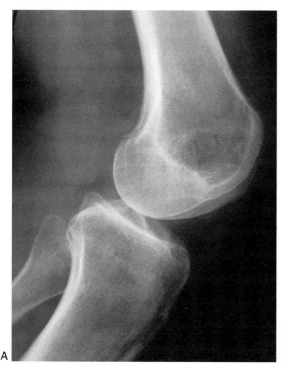

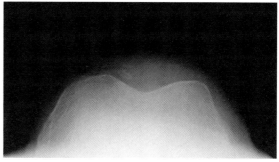

Figure 9. A,B: Postoperative patellectomy roentgenograms. The patient had no pain but complained of weakness when walking down stairs.

Postoperatively she gradually began increasing range-of-motion and muscle-strengthening exercises. Her wound healed well, the patellar tendon maintained its track in the intercondylar groove, and she gradually increased her activities. One year after surgery she was comfortable, had no pain, and was pleased that she had undergone the surgery. Her chief complaint at this time was a sense of weakness when coming down stairs, but other than this she has resumed a normal lifestyle and is happy with the relief of her pain (Fig. 9).

RECOMMENDED READING

1. Brick, G. W., and Scott, R. D.: The patellofemoral component of total knee arthroplasty. *Clin. Orthop.*, 231: 163, 1988.
2. Boyd, H. B., and Hawkins, B. L.: Patellectomy. A simplified technique. *Surg. Gynecol. Obstet.*, 86: 357, 1948.
3. DeMaio, M., and Drez, D. J.: Patellectomy. *(Submitted for publication.)*
4. Dennis, D. A.: Patellofemoral complications in total knee arthroplasty. *Am. J. Knee Surg.*, 5: 156, 1992.
5. Ficat, R. P., and Hungerford, D. S.: *Disorders of the P-F Joint*. Williams and Wilkins, Baltimore, 1977.
6. Grace, J. N., and Rand, J. A.: *Extensor Mechanism in Joint Replacement Arthroplasty*, edited by B. F. Morrey. pp. 1039–1049. Churchill Livingstone, New York, 1991.
7. Kaufer, H.: Mechanical function of the patella. *J. Bone Joint Surg.*, 53A: 1551, 1971.
8. Kelly, M. A., and Insall, J. N.: Patellectomy. *Orthop. Clin. North Am.* 17: 289, 1986.
9. Ritter, M. A., and Campbell, E. D.: Retrospective evaluation of an Iodophor-incorporated antimicrobial plastic adhesive wound drape. *Clin. Orthop.*, 228: 307, 1988.
10. Shorbe, H. B., and Dobson, C. H.: Patellectomy: Repair of the extensor mechanism. *J. Bone Joint Surg.*, 40A: 1281, 1958.
11. Stevres, P. A., Gradisar, I. A., Hoyt, W. A., and Chu, M.: Patellectomy: a clinical study and biomechanical evaluation. *Clin. Orthop.*, 144: 84, 1979.
12. Szalapski, E. W., Siliski, J., King, T. V., and Ritter, M. A.: Total knee replacement in the patellectomized knee. *(Submitted for publication.)*
13. Watkins, M. P., Harris, B. A., Wender, S., Zarins, B., and Rowe, C. R.: Effect of patellectomy on the function of the quadriceps and hamstrings. *J. Bone Joint Surg.*, 65A: 390, 1983.

Master Techniques in Orthopaedic Surgery,
KNEE ARTHROPLASTY, edited by P. A. Lotke,
Raven Press, Ltd., New York © 1995.

21

Arthrodesis for the Failed Total Knee Arthroplasty

James A. Rand

INDICATIONS/CONTRAINDICATIONS

Arthrodesis is a traditional salvage technique for the knee severely damaged by arthritis, infection, or ligamentous instability. The most frequent indication for arthrodesis is failure of a total knee arthroplasty, usually from sepsis or mechanical failure, in the young individual. Arthrodesis should be considered in those individuals who have a failed arthroplasty and still put a high demand on the knee. Arthrodesis should also be considered for those individuals with infections caused by highly virulent microorganisms, especially when the host is immunocompromised, since recurrent infection with reimplantation might present a life-threatening risk to the patient.

Relative contraindications to arthrodesis would include ipsilateral ankle or hip disease, severe segmental bone loss, contralateral leg amputation, or bilateral knee disease. Although Charnley (3) has reported satisfactory results with bilateral knee arthrodeses, this presents a significant functional handicap and should generally be avoided.

PREOPERATIVE PLANNING

The patient presenting with failure of a total knee arthroplasty for which arthrodesis is being considered must be carefully evaluated (14). The etiology of the failure is of paramount importance. Aseptic and septic failure represent different problems in management, and will necessitate different techniques for salvage by

J. A. Rand, M.D.: Division of Orthopedic Surgery, Mayo Clinic Scottsdale, Scottsdale, AZ 85259.

arthrodesis. Septic failure may demonstrate increasing radiolucency at the bone–cement interface, with periosteal new bone formation or significant attritional bone change (Fig. 1). Differential technetium-99m or indium-111 bone scanning can be performed with an 84% accuracy rate (11). Aspiration of the knee can be useful when a positive culture is obtained, but a negative aspiration does not exclude infection. Sometimes, multiple aspirations will be necessary to recover the organism. With three aspirations of a knee, 90% of infections will be detected. Synovial fluid should also be evaluated for its glucose concentration and cell count. An increased cell count or depressed glucose concentration would be suggestive of infection. Other etiologies for failure of an arthroplasty must be carefully evaluated. The patient with chronic pain due to reflex sympathetic dystrophy or chronic pain syndrome may present requesting arthrodesis. Unfortunately, if the underlying problem (such as reflex sympathetic dystrophy) is not corrected, the patient's pain will persist. These patients are not good candidates for arthrodesis and should not be considered for it. Care must also be taken to be sure that the patient's pain is not referred from the low back or hip, since pathology in this area would clearly not be corrected by addressing the knee. Finally, it is important to counsel the patient about the functional disability that will follow arthrodesis. Occasionally, a trial of immobilization in a cylinder cast will help the patient to understand this functional deficit.

Once arthrodesis has been selected as the means of salvage for a failed total knee replacement, the technique must be selected. The basic options are external fixation or internal fixation using an intramedullary nail or plates. External fixation would be planned for the patient who has septic failure with acute infection, since it allows wound management, does minimal damage to the bone vascularity, and allows compression across the bone surfaces. External fixation certainly facilitates wound management, since it leaves the wound exposed and leaves no retained long-term foreign body. Conversely, external fixation has the disadvantages of providing less than rigid fixation and potential problems with the pin tracts. Internal fixation provides much more rigid fixation than external fixation but is generally not recommended in the case of acute sepsis about the knee. Internal fixation for arthrodesis would be selected for those patients who have non-septic failure of a knee arthroplasty, or those who have had septic failure and in whom the sepsis is quiescent after failed initial attempts at arthrodesis or resection arthroplasty. The knee must be carefully evaluated to be sure there is no evidence

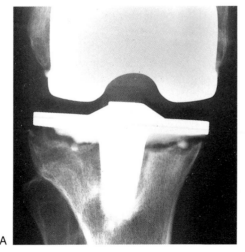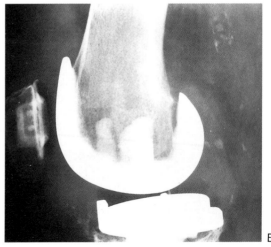

A   B

Figure 1. AP **(A)** and lateral **(B)** radiographs of an infected kinematic condylar prosthesis. There is a circumferential radiolucent line about the tibial compartment, with bone resorption in the tibial plateau. (Reprinted with permission from Rand, J. A.: Knee arthrodesis. Instructional Course Lectures 36: 330, 1986.)

of residual acute infection, which may spread into the medullary canals with rod fixation or create recurrent infection with plate fixation.

Other important considerations in preoperative planning for arthrodesis are the amount of tibiofemoral valgus angulation in which to place the knee, and the degree of flexion. If external fixation is going to be utilized, a position of approximately 3° to 5° of tibiofemoral valgus is selected, since this provides the most physiologic loading across the limb. A position of 0° of tibiofemoral valgus would be selected with intramedullary nail fixation. For plate fixation an angulation of between 3° and 5° of valgus would be selected. The degree of flexion of the knee will depend upon the degree of shortening anticipated. Generally, the shortening following arthrodesis is approximately 3 cm (13). With increasing shortening of the limb, a position closer to full extension should be selected for arthrodesis, and in no cases should knee flexion be greater than 20°. The objective should be to allow the limb to clear the floor without the need for a circumduction gait.

Preoperative radiographs should include a full-length, standing, anteroposterior radiograph of the lower extremity, and anteroposterior and lateral radiographs of the knee with radiographic markers that can be utilized to template bone size (Fig. 2). These radiographs become critical in the case of internal fixation with an intramedullary nail, but are less critical if a plate or external fixation is being utilized. Radiographs can be very valuable in assessing the extent of bone loss

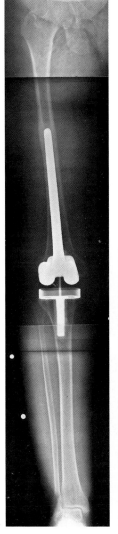
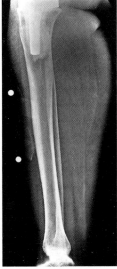

A,B

Figure 2. Full length AP **(A)** and lateral **(B)** radiographs of a failed total knee arthroplasty with radiographic markers for magnification, which assist in sizing the intramedullary canal.

preoperatively, with the anticipated amount of bone loss usually greater than that visualized in the preoperative radiographs.

SURGERY

Arthrodesis with External Fixation

Exposure for removal of the total knee arthroplasty must be considered. The exposure should utilize a preexisting incision used for total knee arthroplasty, since this reduces the risk of wound-healing complications following arthrodesis. In general, an anteromedial approach has proven quite effective in exposing the knee for the removal of implants. Exposure of the knee should include excising all scar tissue in the suprapatellar pouch and medial and lateral gutters in order to allow eversion of the patella and flexion of the knee to 90°. An additional short incision across the rectus tendon proximal to the patella will facilitate exposure of the stiff knee. All of the hypertrophic synovium and scar must be excised from the joint to expose healthy vascularized tissue. If vascularized tissue is not exposed, the chance of union is diminished. Implant removal needs to be planned to avoid any loss of bone. Bone preservation is essential to minimize the extent of shortening of the limb. To remove the implant, flexible osteotomes or a high-speed cutting instrument should be used. It is best to dissect prosthetic cement or the prosthesis–bone interface in order to remove the implant with as little bone loss as possible (Fig. 3). Next, the cement is carefully removed from the remaining bone. In the case of infection, all foreign material and granulation tissue must be removed to prevent a late recurrence of infection around any retained foreign material (Fig. 4). Once a thorough debridement is performed, the bone ends will be ready for preparation (Fig. 5).

The tibia is cut using the extramedullary cutting instruments used for total knee arthroplasty, removing 1 to 2 mm of bone to expose healthy vascular cancellous bone (Fig. 6). Once the tibia has been cut, the limb can be aligned in the desired degree of tibiofemoral valgus and flexion, and the distal femur cut in a reciprocal manner, removing 1 to 2 mm of bone (Fig. 7). The objective should be to expose healthy, vascular cancellous bone that can be apposed in a stable configuration

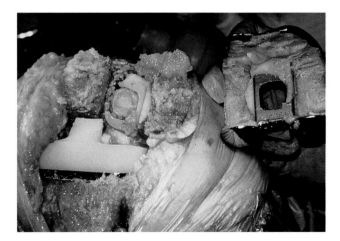

Figure 3. Removal of femoral component with minimal loss of bone.

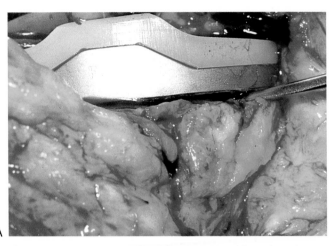
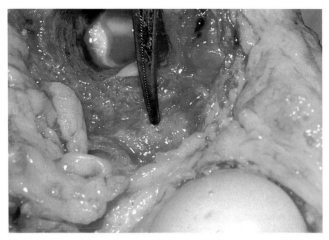

A   B

Figure 4. A: Intraoperative photograph of interface beneath the tibial component of the knee shown in Figure 1. **B:** All of the infected granulation tissue must be removed. **(A,** from ref. 9.)

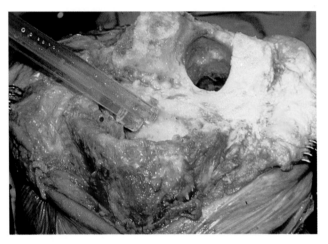
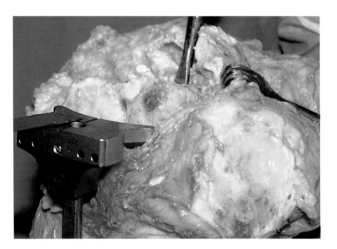

Figure 5. Appearance of bone following debridement.

Figure 6. Extramedullary cutting guide for total knee arthroplasty is used to resect 1 to 2 mm of bone from the proximal tibia.

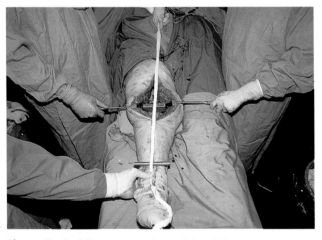
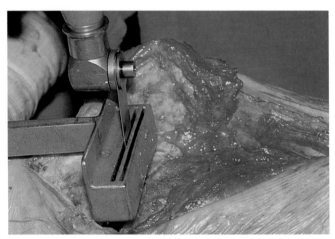

A   B

Figure 7. A: After preparation of the tibia, overall limb alignment is selected. **B:** One to 2 mm of distal femur are resected.

in the desired degree of valgus and flexion, based on the preoperative plan (Fig. 8). Once the tibia and femur have been prepared, the bone ends can be approximated and the external fixator applied. I prefer to use biplanar external fixation since this helps control anteroposterior bending forces (Fig. 9) (6). I most often use the Ace–Fischer apparatus, which employs three transfixing pins in the proximal and distal fragments and two anterior half pins in the proximal and distal fragments for fixation, combined with a semicircular ring (13). The pins on the femoral side are placed from a medial to lateral direction (Fig. 10) to avoid the

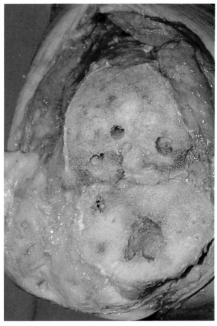

Figure 8. Effective arthrodesis depends on the presence of healthy, vascular cancellous bone that can be apposed in a stable configuration.

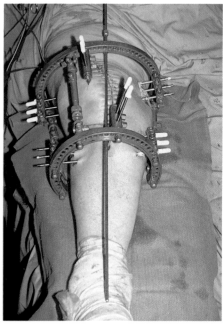

Figure 9. Biplanar external fixation using the Ace–Fischer apparatus for arthrodesis.

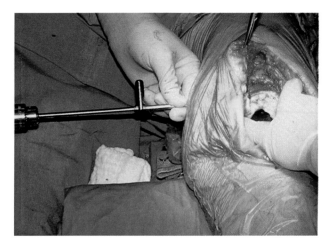

Figure 10. The femoral pins are placed from the medial to the lateral side to avoid the neurovascular structures in this left knee. A cannula protects the soft tissues during drilling and pin placement.

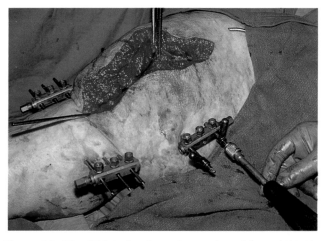

Figure 11. The tibial pins have been placed from lateral to medial to avoid the neurovascular structures in this right knee.

neurovascular structures, and on the tibia from a lateral to medial direction (Fig. 11). The frame is assembled (Fig. 12) and the anterior half pins are placed in the bone. In order to improve fixation, the anterior half pins should be placed proximal to the proximal ring and distal to the distal ring, so as to put the greatest distance between the pins and the arthrodesis site (Fig. 13). Once the apparatus has been applied, radiographs in the anteroposterior and lateral planes should be obtained to be sure that the threaded portion of the pins lies within bone, and that the arthrodesis site is well apposed in the proper orientation (Fig. 14).

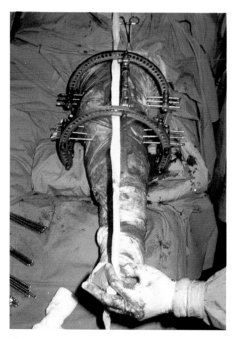

Figure 12. Assembled external fixation frame with transfixing pins. Femoral alignment is correct.

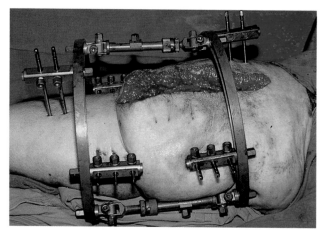

Figure 13. Anterior half pins are placed proximal and distal to the ring.

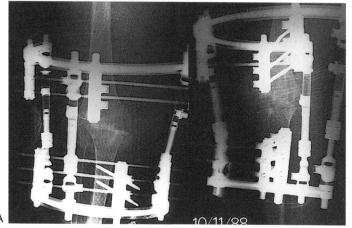

Figure 14. AP **(A)** and lateral **(B)** radiographs showing properly applied external fixation.

Arthrodesis with Intramedullary Nail Fixation

Intramedullary nail fixation is a demanding procedure that is of long duration, involves high blood loss, and has a 50% complication rate (5). In order to perform intramedullary nailing, a careful preoperative plan is essential for ensuring the proper nail size. The diameter of the intramedullary nail is determined by the size of the intramedullary canal of the tibia. The anterior bow of the femur will stabilize the rod by three-point fixation. The length of the intramedullary nail should extend from the tip of the greater trochanter to the distal tibial metaphysis (Fig. 15). Judgment by the surgeon about the amount of bone loss that will occur and subsequent limb shortening at the time of removal of the arthroplasty will determine the final rod length. For this reason it may be wise to have more than one size of nail available, and to rely on intraoperative measurement to be sure that the nail is not going to be too long or too short. If the nail is too long it will protrude at the hip and cause irritation about the gluteal muscles. If the nail is too short and ends in the isthmus of the tibia, stress fractures may occur at the tip of the nail (4).

Wide preparation and draping are necessary for intramedullary nail fixation for arthrodesis, and an image intensifier and image table are necessary. The patient should be placed in the supine position with a roll under the hip to elevate and expose the greater trochanter. A sterile tourniquet can be placed on the thigh and then removed at the time of nail insertion in an effort to minimize blood loss during

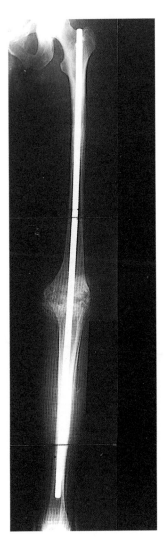

Figure 15. AP radiograph of intramedullary nail used for arthrodesis. The nail extends from the greater trochanter to the distal tibial metaphysis.

removal of the arthroplasty and preparation of the knee. Exposure of the knee, removal of the implants, and preparation of the bony bed are similar to that in external fixation for arthrodesis. However, a position of 0° of valgus angulation and usually minimal flexion will be required in order to pass the nail and maintain bone apposition at the arthrodesis site.

The intramedullary canal of the tibia should first be reamed with flexible reamers to determine its size (Fig. 16). A rod of the same type and diameter as ultimately used for arthrodesis should be trial-fit into the medullary canal of the tibia to be sure that it will fit securely but not impact in the canal (Fig. 17). The femur is then reamed in an antegrade direction from the hip (Fig. 18), as well as in a retrograde direction from the knee to the point of the same diameter as that of the tibia. The intramedullary nail is introduced from the hip, and with the knee reduced is driven across the knee into the tibia to the distal tibial metaphysis (Fig. 19). Attention must be given to ensuring that correct rotational alignment is maintained during insertion of the nail, and that the knee does not distract with insertion of the nail as it engages the tibia. The image intensifier is very helpful in making these determinations and observing the progress of the intramedullary nail during its insertion.

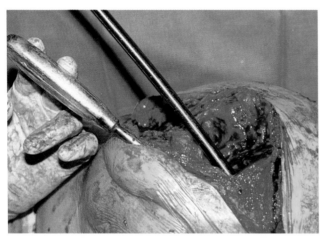

Figure 16. Reaming of the tibial intramedullary canal is performed to determine its diameter.

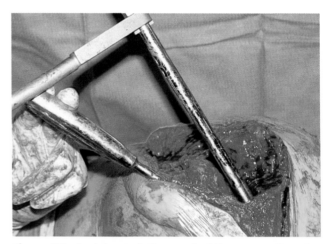

Figure 17. An intramedullary rod of the same diameter and type as will ultimately be used for arthrodesis should be trial fitted in the tibia.

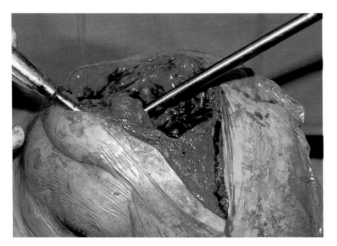

Figure 18. Antegrade reaming of the femur is performed to the same diameter as was utilized for the tibia.

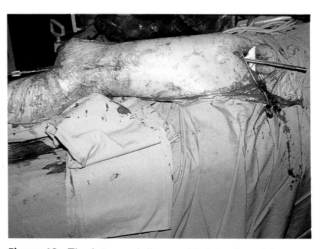

Figure 19. The intramedullary rod is introduced from the hip and driven across the knee while visualizing its passage with an image intensifier.

Plate Fixation

Plate fixation for arthrodesis can be done either with a single plate or two contoured plates (8). Plates are generally placed anterolaterally and anteromedially, to provide two-plane fixation to the arthrodesis site (Fig. 20), or as a single anterolateral plate (Fig. 21). The exposure and preparation of the bone ends for plate fixation are similar to those for external fixation. A 4.5-mm dynamic compression plate is selected in order to engage six bicortical screws proximal and distal to the arthrodesis site. It is important to determine whether there will be adequate soft-tissue coverage prior to applying a second plate, since limb shortening often makes soft-tissue coverage over the anterior aspect of the knee difficult. Consequently, there may be inadequate soft tissue to cover two plates and achieve adequate wound closure.

Bone Grafting

Bone grafting is useful to achieve knee arthrodesis and improve the rate of union. Bone grafting is recommended if there is less than 50% bone apposition at the time of arthrodesis. Grafting should not be performed at the time of the initial arthrodesis in the presence of acute infection, but serial debridements should be performed. Once the infection has resolved, bone grafting is done with ground, cancellous allograft bone to create particles approximately 5 mm in diameter, mixed with autogenous iliac cancellous bone (Fig. 22). Cortical bone should be avoided, especially in the presence of prior infection. Since the intramedullary canals of the tibia and femur have been compromised by the prior implants and

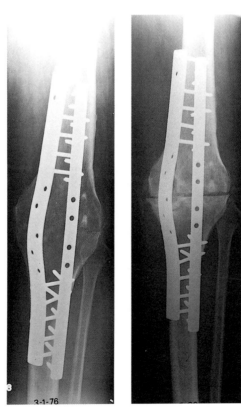

Figure 20. Dual plate fixation for arthrodesis. (From ref. 10.)

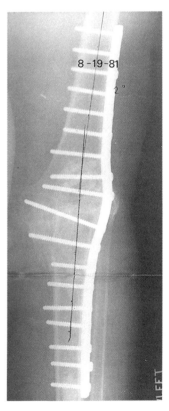

Figure 21. Single-plate fixation for arthrodesis.

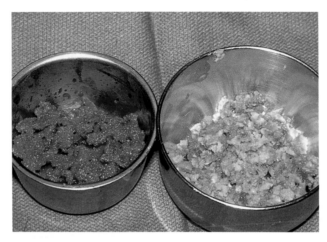

Figure 22. Iliac-crest autograft and cancellous allograft bone for bone grafting.

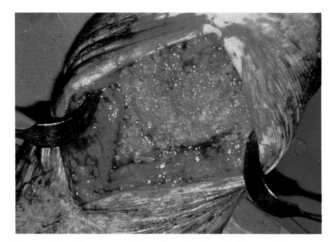

Figure 23. Bone graft is placed about the periphery of the arthrodesis site to allow revascularization from the surrounding soft tissues.

cement, it is best to place the bone graft peripherally about the arthrodesis site, in order to allow revascularization from the surrounding soft tissues (Fig. 23). If bone grafting is contemplated it is essential to place the posterior graft before compressing the arthrodesis with the external fixator, inserting the intramedullary nail, or rigidly fixing the arthrodesis with plates. With plate fixation, the room in which to engraft additional bone is often limited. The best source for an iliac crest graft is the posterior ilium, from which bone is harvested with the patient lying prone, prior to beginning the arthrodesis procedure.

Wound Coverage

Wound closure after arthrodesis may be difficult. As the limb shortens with removal of the implant, there is a tendency for the soft tissues to bulge medially and laterally about the arthrodesis site, making closure of the wound difficult. Patellectomy may assist in achieving soft-tissue coverage. The patella is another potential source of a bone graft. Removing the patella avoids another potential source of nonunion, which may occasionally involve the patella and be a source

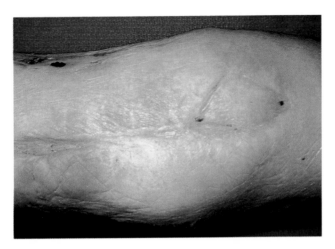

Figure 24. Appearance at 4 months after a gastrocnemius muscle flap for coverage of a knee arthrodesis.

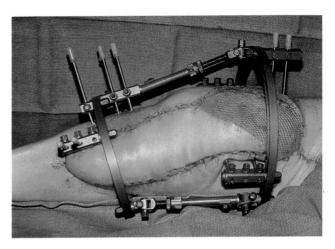

Figure 25. Appearance of free flap for soft-tissue coverage following arthrodesis.

of pain after an otherwise successful arthrodesis. If the patella is retained, it can be used as a vascularized graft across the arthrodesis site. In this situation it should be rigidly fixed on both sides of the arthrodesis site, avoiding excess tension across the soft tissues. In the event of difficulty in achieving a direct soft-tissue closure of the wound, the use of medial, lateral, or combined medial and lateral gastrocnemius flaps is recommended (Fig. 24). These can be followed by appropriate skin grafting at 4 or 5 days once the muscle flap has been determined to be viable. Only in extremely unusual cases with deficient anterior soft tissues would free-flap coverage be necessary about the knee (Fig. 25).

POSTOPERATIVE MANAGEMENT

Following arthrodesis, the patient is managed in a bulky Robert Jones dressing for 3 to 5 days until wound healing is assured. If external fixation is being utilized, the bulky dressing is removed and routine care of the pin sites begun. It is important to tighten the external fixator after 2 to 3 days and apply some additional compression, since the fixators often tend to loosen slightly. External fixation is maintained for 8 to 10 weeks or until the arthrodesis is solid. With appropriate pin-site care, we have maintained external fixation in some patients for as long as 6 months. After the external fixator is removed under intravenous sedation, a cylinder cast should be applied and maintained for an additional 4 to 6 weeks. Additional bracing may be required until the arthrodesis is solid. In some instances it has taken as long as one year for solid union to occur following arthrodesis with external fixation (12).

With internal fixation with an intramedullary nail for arthrodesis, a long leg cast with a pelvic band is applied to provide additional rotational control. The cast is worn for a period of 6 weeks. The patient is allowed progressive weight bearing as tolerated within the cast. Ancillary bracing is usually unnecessary after cast removal.

Postoperative management after plate fixation consists of utilization of a long leg or cylinder cast for 6 to 8 weeks to provide additional support to the arthrodesis site. Ancillary bracing is usually not required following cast removal.

The time to union following arthrodesis depends upon several factors including the technique of arthrodesis used, the size of the bone deficiency, the vascularity, and the healing capabilities of the patient. The time to union has varied from as little as 2 months following a failed resurfacing prosthesis (2) to as long as 22 months following a hinged arthroplasty (16). Patience and persistence will usually result in success, although the latter may require additional attempts at arthrodesis. The overall rate of success of arthrodesis has been in the 50% to 60% range following failure of hinged prostheses, while the prognosis in cases involving the resurfacing prosthesis has been better, with arthrodesis having an 80% to 90% success rate (2). The patient with a successful arthrodesis is generally free of pain and able to walk unlimited distances, but is often dissatisfied with the lack of motion in the knee. It must be remembered that energy expenditure is increased by as much as 20% after arthrodesis (7), and that this may result in a functional limitation for the elderly patient with limited cardiopulmonary reserve.

COMPLICATIONS

The most frequent complication following attempted arthrodesis is failure of union (Fig. 26) (12). Other potential complications include recurrent sepsis, pintract infection, fracture, and neurovascular injury. Many of these problems can be avoided by attention to surgical technique.

The incidence of nonunion as a complication of arthrodesis varies from 30% to 50%, and is greater among patients with extensive bone deficiency. Prevention of nonunion is best achieved by obtaining proper bone apposition and using rigid fixation combined with prolonged immobilization. Bone grafting is indicated for the patient with bone deficiency. Once nonunion is established to exist, a decision about its treatment is made on the basis of the patient's functional disability. Some arthrodeses without union will be reasonably stable because of fibrous union, will cause minimal pain, and will be adequately controlled by bracing. Nothing further

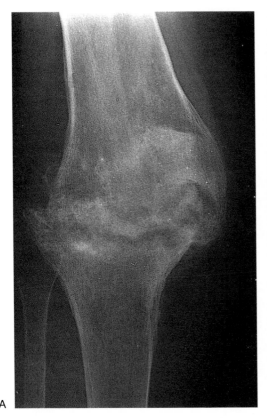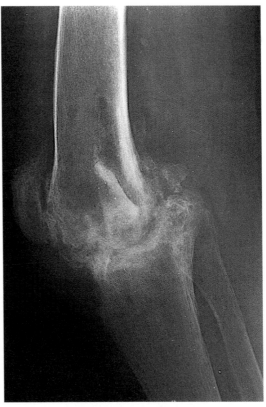

A   B

Figure 26. AP **(A)** and lateral **(B)** radiographs of nonunion following attempted arthrodesis.

need be considered for these patients. However, in many cases, patients with nonunion will have persistent pain and instability, and repeated attempts at arthrodesis are indicated (12). Prior to a repeat surgical procedure it is important to determine whether infection has been eradicated, since persistent sepsis is one reason for nonunion (2). If infection is present, repeat debridement and antimicrobial therapy are necessary to eliminate it. Management of the aseptic nonunion is a more frequent problem. Although a variety of techniques can be considered for this, including electrical stimulation (1), repeat external fixation, or internal fixation, internal fixation is the technique of choice. Either plate fixation or the use of a long intramedullary rod is the most predictable way to achieve union in the presence of a failed arthrodesis. The principles of repeat surgery for nonunion are the same as they are for the initial arthrodesis.

Pin-tract infections are inherent to the technique of external fixation. They can be prevented by careful attention to soft-tissue releases to prevent tethering of the skin on the pin and minimizing motion of the soft tissues over the pin. Predrilling of the pin holes before placing the pins in the bone will prevent thermal necrosis and ring sequestra. Also, a threaded pin provides better purchase within the bone, with less pin motion and less potential for pin-tract infection. Neurovascular injury during pin insertion relates to errors in surgical technique. By carefully incising the skin alone, and using a blunt obturator through the soft tissues to bone and then drilling only through the bone, the risk of potential neurovascular injury will be minimized. Proper technique for placement of the pins from the medial side on the femur and from the lateral side on the tibia will allow the pins to avoid the neurovascular structures.

Pin-site fractures (Fig. 27) or a fracture of the ipsilateral limb after arthrodesis are problems that may occur in up to 10% to 15% of patients (15). These fractures

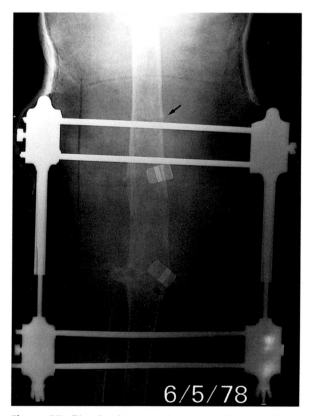

Figure 27. Pin-site fracture *(arrow)* at the proximal pin of a Charnley compression clamp used for knee arthrodesis.

most commonly occur through a pin site that acts as a stress riser. The local stress-concentrating effect of the pin site, plus the long lever arm of the arthrodesed limb, focuses tremendous stresses at these areas and leads to this complication. The complication is again best avoided by a period of immobilization after the removal of external fixation, to be sure that all pin tracts have a chance to heal and fill with bone. Any area of nonhealing due to residual pin-tract infection should be debrided. If the defect is large, bone grafting should be performed. If a fracture does occur, its treatment is similar to that of any other fracture, with the choices being intramedullary nail or plate fixation or cast immobilization.

ILLUSTRATIVE CASE FOR TECHNIQUE

A 73-year-old woman is noted to have sudden onset of pain, swelling, fevers, and chills one year after a total knee replacement. *Staphylococcus aureus* is cultured from the knee and the patient is treated with an arthroscopic debridement that fails. Six months later she has persistent synovitis and pain despite suppressive antibiotics. Radiographs show progressive loosening, bone lysis, and radiolucencies about the prosthetic components (Fig. 28). Because of the amount of bone loss and extensive involvement of bone by infection, an arthrodesis is elected. After adequate debridement, a compression arthrodesis (Fig. 29) is completed and eventually goes on to heal.

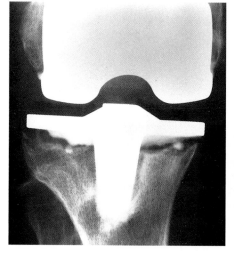
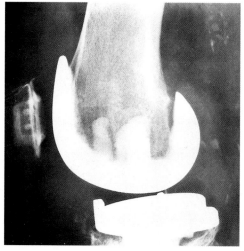
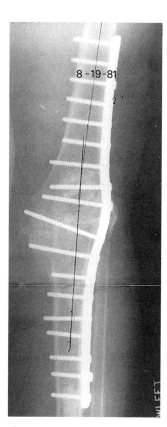

Figure 28. Preoperative AP **(left)** and lateral **(right)** views show loosening and radiolucencies about the prosthetic component.

Figure 29. A single-plate compression arthrodesis was performed and the patient's knee healed well.

RECOMMENDED READING

1. Bigliani, L. U., Rosenwasser, M. P., Caulo, N., Schink, M., and Bassett, C. A. L.: The use of pulsing electromagnetic fields to achieve arthrodesis of the knee following failed total knee arthroplasty. *J. Bone Joint Surg.,* 65A: 480–485, 1983.

2. Brodersen, M. P., Fitzgerald, R. H., Peterson, L. F. A., Coventry, M. B., and Bryan, R. S.: Arthrodesis of the knee following failed total knee arthroplasty. *J. Bone Joint Surg.,* 61A: 181–185, 1979.

3. Charnley, J.: Arthrodesis of the knee. *Clin. Orthop.,* 18: 37–42, 1960.

4. Donley, B. G., Matthews, L. S., and Kaufer, H.: Arthrodesis of the knee with an intramedullary nail. *J. Bone Joint Surg.,* 73A: 907–913, 1991.

5. Ellingsen, D., and Rand, J. A.: Intramedullary arthrodesis after failed total knee arthroplasty. *J. Bone Joint Surg.,* 76A: 870–877, 1994.

6. Knutson, K., Bodelind, B., and Lidgren, L.: Stability of external fixators used for knee arthrodesis after failed knee arthroplasty. *Clin. Orthop.,* 186: 90–95, 1984.

7. Mazetti, R. F.: Effect of immobilization of the knee: An energy expenditure during walking. *J. Bone Joint Surg.,* 42: 533, 1960 (abstr.).

8. Nichols, S. J., Landon, G. C., and Tullos, H. S.: Arthrodesis with dual plates after failed total knee arthroplasty. *J. Bone Joint Surg.,* 73A: 1020–1024, 1991.

9. Rand, J. A.: Knee arthrodesis. Instructional Course Lectures 36: 330, 1986.

10. Rand, J. A.: Sepsis in total knee arthroplasty. In: *Total Knee Arthroplasty,* edited by J. A. Rand, p. 36. Raven Press, New York, 1993.

11. Rand, J. A., and Brown, M. K.: The value of indium-111 leukocyte scanning in the evaluation of the painful or infected total knee arthroplasty. *Clin. Orthop.,* 259:179–182, 1990.

12. Rand, J. A., and Bryan, R. S.: The outcome of failed knee arthrodesis following total knee arthroplasty. *Clin. Orthop.,* 205:86–92, 1986.

13. Rand, J. A., Bryan, R. S., and Chao, E. Y. S.: Failed total knee arthroplasty treated by arthrodesis of the knee using the Ace–Fischer apparatus. *J. Bone Joint Surg.,* 69A: 39–45, 1987.

14. Rand, J. A., Bryan, R. S., Morrey, B. F., and Westholm, F.: Management of infected total knee arthroplasty. *Clin. Orthop.,* 205: 75–85, 1986.

15. Stolz, M. R., and Ganz, R.: Fracture after arthrodesis of the hip and knee. *Clin. Orthop.,* 115: 177–181, 1976.

16. Vahvanen, V.: Arthrodesis in failed knee replacement in eight rheumatoid patients. *Ann. Chir. Gynecol.,* 68: 57–62, 1979.

Master Techniques in Orthopaedic Surgery,
KNEE ARTHROPLASTY, edited by P. A. Lotke,
Raven Press, Ltd., New York © 1995.

22

Arthroscopic Synovectomy

Alexander A. Sapega

INDICATIONS/CONTRAINDICATIONS

Partial arthroscopic synovectomy combined with articular debridement and joint lavage is useful as a palliative treatment for degenerative joint disease in a significant percentage of cases. The synovectomy portion of such surgery represents the less demanding elements of a total, four-compartment synovectomy, given that direct access to the posteromedial and posterolateral compartments is rarely required.

Complete, four-compartment synovectomy of the knee is generally indicated in primary synovial diseases such as rheumatoid arthritis, other rheumatic diseases that induce chronic proliferative synovitis, pigmented villonodular synovitis, synovial chondromatosis, and occasionally secondary synovial disorders such as hemophilic arthropathy. The symptoms of chronic knee swelling and recurrent effusion should be present for at least 6 months, and unresponsive to medical treatment, before such surgery is considered.

The objective of synovectomy is to rid the joint of intrinsically pathologic or pathologically inflamed synovial tissue that is causing chronic knee swelling, effusion, and pain. Synovectomy alone cannot be expected to eliminate the pain associated with destructive articular changes. In most cases a simple debulking of most of the synovium in the affected joint is indicated, whereas in other circumstances, such as diffuse pigmented villonodular synovitis, as complete a synovectomy as possible is desired.

The frequency and severity of postoperative problems associated with traditional open synovectomy have led many surgeons to favor arthroscopic synovectomy whenever this is technically feasible. Open synovectomy is the less demanding of the two surgical techniques, and can generally be accomplished with

---

A. A. Sapega, M.D.: Department of Orthopaedic Surgery, University of Pennsylvania Sports Medicine Center, Philadelphia, PA 19104.

significantly less operating-room time. My usual preference for arthroscopic syno-vectomy is based on my desire to minimize postoperative morbidity and maintain knee joint function at the highest possible level. In younger patients who have the diffuse form of pigmented villonodular synovitis, cosmesis is also often a consideration.

In cases in which the menisci can be sacrificed, open synovectomy can provide at least as complete a resection of the synovial joint lining as will an arthroscopic procedure, assuming that direct open access to the posteromedial and posterolat-eral compartments is also undertaken. When the menisci cannot be sacrificed, or when only an anterior open surgical approach is contemplated, then arthroscopic synovectomy is likely to result in a more complete synovial resection than tradi-tional open techniques.

Arthroscopic synovectomy of the knee is a difficult and tedious procedure that requires expert skill with both the arthroscope and the motorized synovectomy instrumentation. The procedure requires entry into the most difficult access zones within the complicated synovial spaces of the knee. Complete arthroscopic syno-vectomy should not be attempted by any surgeon who does not have great profi-ciency in surgical arthroscopy of the knee.

PREOPERATIVE PLANNING

Patients being considered for arthroscopic synovectomy should be screened to make sure they do not have any known or latent coagulopathies. Weight-bearing preoperative radiographs are useful to assess whether any destructive articular changes are present, and their degree. They will also provide a crude assessment of bone stock, which is useful if the patient's joint motion is limited by contracture, possibly requiring joint manipulation.

Magnetic resonance imaging (MRI) of the knee can be useful in some synovial diseases, particularly diffuse pigmented villonodular synovitis (PVNS). Special, hemosiderin-weighted pulse sequences can generate pictures that clearly show hemosiderin-laden synovium in the various joint compartments. It is my routine practice to obtain such MRI scans of every preoperative patient with PVNS. In a limited series of cases I have found that chronic, diffuse PVNS often demonstrates extraarticular extension, either into popliteal cysts or in and about the fibular head and proximal tibiofibular joint, via the popliteus hiatus or direct synovial connections. Preoperative evidence of extraarticular involvement should lead to a surgical plan that includes the open excision of extraarticular tissue masses following the arthroscopic portion of the procedure. Hemosiderin-weighted MRI scanning is most useful before the *initial* attempt at resection of PVNS. The scar tissue left after prior surgical treatment decreases the clarity and specificity of subsequent MRI scans, but they are still worth obtaining when planning repeat synovectomy surgery for recurrent PVNS disease. Arthrography does not have any specific advantage over a combination of plain radiographs and an MRI scan, and the latter is preferred.

A properly performed, complete arthroscopic synovectomy does not result in more than 200 to 300 cc of blood loss, and preoperative blood-cross matching or autologous blood donation is therefore not deemed necessary unless the patient is either anemic or extremely apprehensive about the remote possibility of blood transfusion.

High-quality arthroscopic equipment is just as essential to successful synovec-tomy as the skill required to use it. Because arthroscopic visualization is often made difficult enough by thick, proliferative synovial tissue, no further hindrance is needed from second-rate or improperly functioning arthroscopes and video equipment. The motorized shaver should be a high-speed unit that accommodates many different, disposable blades. The blades of choice are generally 3.5 mm, 4.5

mm, and 5.5 mm full-radius or "synovial-resector" type blades without serrated cutting edges. The use of aggressive, serrated-edge cutting blades should be limited to fat-pad resection, since using these blades for other portions of the synovectomy can easily result in capsular resection as well. A standard synovectomy blade is designed to allow complete resection of the synovial lining, down to the recognizably white capsular fibrous tissue, but leaving the latter intact. In some areas in which the capsule is exceptionally thin, such as the suprapatellar pouch, partial resection of the capsular lining is unavoidable, but is not specifically harmful. However, excision of capsule in the posterior compartment or in the medial/lateral gutters is potentially harmful, and should be avoided. The less aggressive blades are also useful in performing a synovectomy about the cruciate ligaments without damaging them.

Because of the magnification and superior visualization provided by an arthroscope, arthroscopic synovectomy in the intercondylar notch is generally more complete than that accomplished by any open technique. Occasionally, a curved or angled blade may be necessary, particularly in difficult access zones. One should make sure that a variety of blades are available prior to the procedure, and that a motorized backup resector and control unit are available in case the primary system malfunctions during the course of the surgery.

A tourniquet is almost universally used for at least some portion of each case. Since arthroscopic synovectomies can be quite long and tedious, I prefer to begin without a tourniquet, carrying on as long as possible in this way until visualization is compromised, at which point the limb is exsanguinated and the tourniquet inflated. General anesthesia has the advantage of allowing controlled hypotension in the patient, which minimizes bleeding and the need for high-pressure saline infusion to maintain visualization. Epidural anesthesia is perfectly satisfactory, but it is useful to consult with the anesthesiologist at the beginning of the case with regard to blood-pressure control. Pharmacologic pressure modulation can be most helpful in minimizing total tourniquet time. Epidural blockade is the anesthesia of choice when it is anticipated that a concomitant manipulation or capsular release is going to be needed for the treatment of preexisting contracture. These patients are in much more pain postoperatively and are at a great risk of losing joint motion, even if continuous passive motion is used. Therefore, continuous postoperative epidural analgesia for 24 to 48 hours is extremely helpful.

During surgery, I prefer that the joint is distended with saline via gravity inflow from a height of approximately 5 feet above the patient. Avoiding the use of a high-pressure saline infusion pump minimizes extracapsular saline extravasation. When severe, the latter condition can make surgical access all the more difficult (particularly when working in the posterior compartments) and can even induce a transient calf- or thigh-compartment syndrome. Because even gravity inflow can result in saline extravasation near skin portals, however, I prefer to leave the posteromedial and posterolateral compartments until the latter part of the arthroscopic procedure. If they are done first, and major posterior saline extravasation subsequently occurs and pressurizes the calf or thigh, one may be tempted to stop the arthroscopic procedure and continue via an open arthrotomy. The only disadvantage of working in the posterior compartments last is that it entails dealing with these potentially difficult areas at a time when one may already be somewhat fatigued from the first portion of the case. Preoperatively, each surgeon should weigh these advantages and disadvantages according to his or her own personal judgement in planning the optimal sequence for a synovial resection.

In my experience, the morbidity of a complete, four-compartment synovectomy can be rendered almost trivial if the procedure is done arthroscopically in an inpatient surgical setting and with postoperative continuous passive motion. A 24- to 36-hour admission should be planned and arrangements made for the patient to have a continuous-passive-motion machine brought home for use over the next 7 to 14 days.

Postoperative, self-administered, faradic electrical muscle stimulation of the quadriceps is most useful for minimizing postsurgical quadriceps inhibition. A small rental unit can be obtained preoperatively and programmed. Placement of a sterile electrode over the rectus and vastus medialis can be done in the operating room prior to application of the elastic compression dressing. Stimulation should be continued until the patient is capable of stationary bicycle exercise, which is usually at 1 to 2 weeks after arthroscopy.

SURGERY

Routine patient positioning and draping are employed in arthroscopic synovectomy. A leg holder or flip-up stress post should be available and utilized when necessary, particularly when attempting to debride parameniscal synovial tissue underneath the menisci. A rapid diagnostic arthroscopy and synovial biopsy are first performed. Tourniquet hemostasis is not initially employed, and is withheld as long as possible.

Technique

It is strongly recommended that synovial biopsies be taken from multiple sites about the knee. In the case of diffuse, pigmented villonodular synovitis, the most diagnostic histologic findings (foam cells and giant cells) may not be present in all pathologic synovial tissue. On occasion, a semidiffuse, "multinodular" form of the disease may be encountered. In such cases I have found that biopsy of the largest and best developed nodules is more diagnostic than biopsy of even very proliferative non-nodular tissue. Complete synovectomy is obviously not the treatment of choice for the single-nodular form of the disease, and comments on the treatment of this particular pathologic entity are therefore beyond the scope of this chapter.

One can either begin the formal synovectomy in the anterior compartment and intercondylar notch or in the suprapatellar pouch, according to preference. My preference is to start in the anterior compartment, using a high medial "utility" portal for the arthroscope. The first surgical portal employed is an anterolateral portal, made at the level of the joint line and just lateral to the lateral border of the infrapatellar tendon (Fig. 1). Through this approach, most of the fat pad can be resected and synovectomy can be performed in the anterolateral compartment. A complete synovectomy of the lateral gutter is then done, gradually bringing the knee out toward full extension as one works toward the suprapatellar pouch. The knee is then brought back into flexion, and with applied varus stress the parameniscal synovium above and below the lateral meniscus can be excised. By using a curved resector blade one can even reach to some degree down into the meniscotibial recess to resect pathologic tissue. Care should be taken not to damage the popliteus tendon. Meniscectomy is only performed when these structures are damaged or no longer functioning because of severe degenerative breakdown.

A portion of the cruciate ligament synovectomy can now be performed, and is completed by switching the scope to the lateral portal and introducing the motorized tissue resector through the anteromedial utility portal. Care must be taken not to remove ligamentous tissue. The anterior two-thirds of the synovial sheaths of the cruciate ligaments can be almost completely stripped away using this approach. At this time, any synovium or fat pad left about the internal entrance of the medial portal (where the arthroscope was first inserted) can be directly visualized and resected.

For medial compartment synovectomy, the arthroscope can either be maintained in the lateral portal or switched to the anteromedial utility portal. A medial

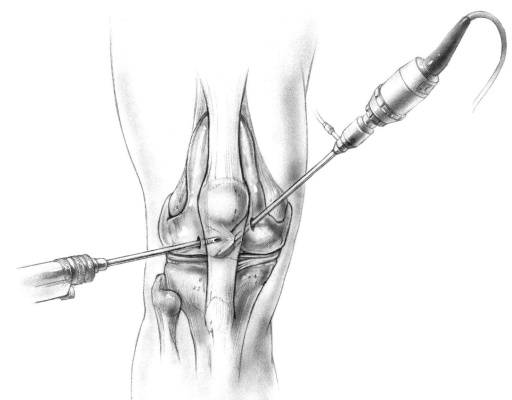

Figure 1. Starting portals used for anterior compartment synovectomy and work in intercondylar notch.

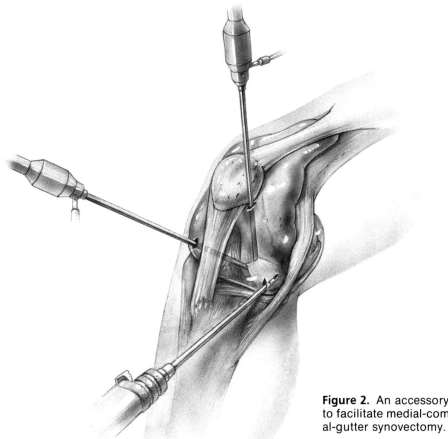

Figure 2. An accessory medial surgical portal is utilized to facilitate medial-compartment debridement and medial-gutter synovectomy.

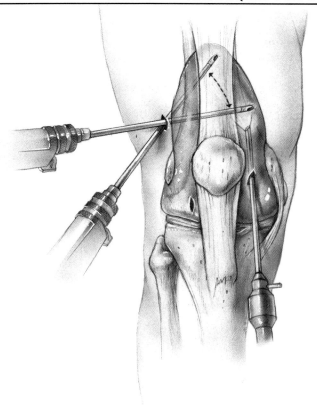

Figure 3. Technique for synovectomy in the suprapatellar pouch.

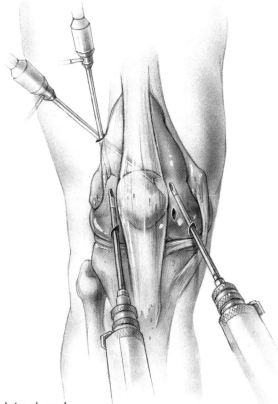

Figure 4. Technique for removal of medial, lateral, and proximal peripatellar synovium.

surgical portal for the resector is made at the level of the joint line, just above the medial meniscus and 5 to 10 mm anterior to the medial collateral ligament (Fig. 2). Valgus stress is then applied and the medial parameniscal synovium is removed in a manner similar to that described for the lateral compartment. The posteromedial portion of the synovial sheath of the posterior cruciate ligament can often be debrided at this time if the knee is not too tight. Medial gutter synovectomy is then performed, working from distally to proximally and gradually bringing the knee toward full extension as one approaches the suprapatellar pouch with the resector.

Pouch synovectomy is begun simply by advancing the motorized resector proximally with the knee in full extension. A complete and careful resection must be done of all synovial lining tissue. In most cases the suprapatellar pouch is enlarged and contains an extensive amount of synovial tissue. Therefore, use of the 5.5-mm synovial resector blade is recommended at this stage to quicken the pace of the procedure. This blade can be introduced through a lateral suprapatellar portal for easy, quick access to the remainder of the pouch cavity (Fig. 3).

Several "blind zones" immediately adjacent to the patella make the resection of all peripatellar synovium somewhat difficult. In order to see this tissue, one must first switch the arthroscope out of the utility portal (if it is being used) and to a portal that is further away from the patella. The medial and lateral surgical portals usually suffice for this purpose, keeping the resector in the lateral suprapatellar portal for the time being. All peripatellar synovial tissue that can be seen is removed and the scope is then switched up to the lateral suprapatellar portal. All remaining peripatellar synovium is resected, as shown in Figure 4. The secret to seeing the tissue in the blind spots just adjacent to the patellar margin is to move the arthroscope as far away from the patella as possible and to inspect the circumferential margin from multiple directions.

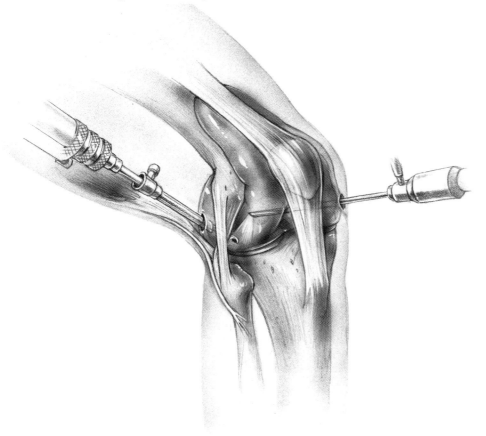

Figure 5. First stage of synovectomy in the posterolateral compartment.

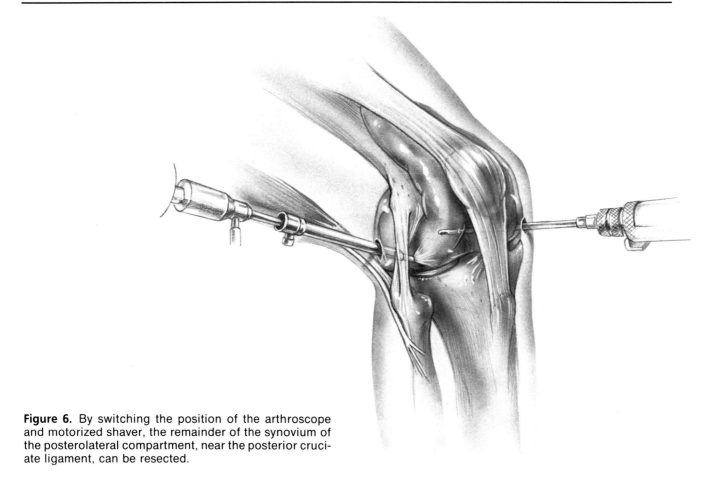

Figure 6. By switching the position of the arthroscope and motorized shaver, the remainder of the synovium of the posterolateral compartment, near the posterior cruciate ligament, can be resected.

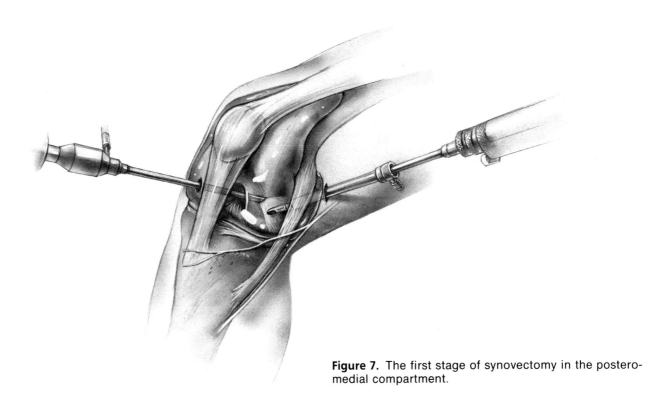

Figure 7. The first stage of synovectomy in the postero-medial compartment.

Once synovectomy has been completed in the anterior compartment, intercondylar notch, medial/lateral gutters, medial/lateral tibiofemoral compartments, and suprapatellar pouch, it is begun in the posterior compartment. I generally prefer to engage the posterolateral compartment first, since there tends to be less extravasation of saline following posterolateral portal entry than after posteromedial portal entry. I save posteromedial surgical access for the end of the procedure.

As shown in Figure 5, a 70-degree arthroscope is inserted across the intercondylar notch and into the posterolateral compartment, via the anteromedial utility portal. With the knee in 50 to 70 degrees of flexion, the lateral collateral ligament and biceps tendon are palpated externally and marked with a skin pencil as landmarks. Staying anterior to the biceps tendon and posterior to the lateral collateral ligament, entry into the posterolateral compartment is made under direct interior visualization with the 70-degree arthroscope. The 4.5-mm motorized shaver blade is introduced and all visible synovium in the posterolateral compartment is removed. It is important to note that the 70-degree arthroscope may have a small blind zone that hides some tissue near the posterior outlet of the intercondylar notch. It is easiest to check this by switching to a 30-degree arthroscope passed into the posterolateral surgical portal so as to look back to where the 70-degree scope had been. If residual synovium remains there, a straight or curved synovectomy blade is brought in across the intercondylar notch to remove it, as shown in Figure 6.

Creation of a posteromedial surgical portal for synovectomy in the posteromedial compartment is done under direct visualization with a 70-degree arthroscope passed through the lateral surgical portal and into the posteromedial compartment via the intercondylar notch (Fig. 7). Preliminary percutaneous insertion of a spinal needle probe is useful in order to assure that a resector inserted at this point will reach all areas of synovium visualized with the arthroscope. An entry location that is 1 to 2 cm proximal and posterior to the posterior corner joint line is usually

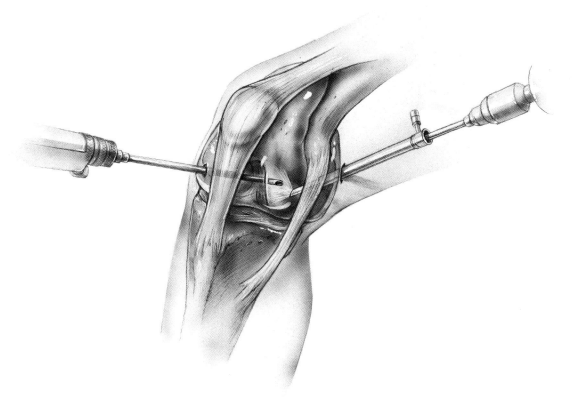

Figure 8. As in Figure 6, switching of the arthroscope and shaver allows completion of synovectomy in the posteromedial compartment.

satisfactory. The knee should be in 70 to 90 degrees of flexion, and the portal should be well anterior to the saphenous nerve. Once the resector removes all visible synovium, the 70-degree arthroscope is withdrawn and the 30-degree arthroscope is inserted into the posteromedial surgical portal. If unresected synovial tissue remains about the posterior cruciate ligament and posterior outlet of the notch, a straight or curved synovectomy blade is passed across the intercondylar notch and into the posteromedial compartment and the tissue is removed, as shown in Figure 8.

Since this posterior-compartment synovectomy technique requires switching of the arthroscope and the resector, it is helpful to establish the initial posterolateral and posteromedial surgical portals with a surgical cannula (shown in Figs. 5 through 8). This facilitates posterior introduction of the 30-degree arthroscope once the resector has been removed, and helps limit saline extravasation into the extracapsular soft tissues.

After completion of the synovectomy procedure, a medium-sized Hemovac drain is placed in the suprapatellar pouch and the portals used in the procedure are closed with Steristrips or stitches, as desired. A sterile muscle-stimulation electrode is applied to the distal thigh (Fig. 9) and a sterile compression dressing is then applied to the limb. The tourniquet is then released. The patient is placed in a CPM machine in the recovery room, with the treated knee moved between zero and 90 degrees of flexion at a slow rate. A cooling cuff or ice is applied to the knee.

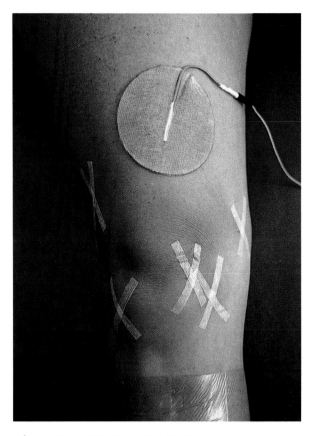

Figure 9. Application of a sterile muscle-stimulation electrode over the distal quadriceps after Steristrip closure of synovectomy portals. A compression dressing is then applied to the knee, leaving the electrode wire exposed for patient access.

POSTOPERATIVE MANAGEMENT

Continuous postoperative epidural analgesia is employed if a concomitant manipulation for capsular contracture has been done with arthroscopic synovectomy. Following synovectomy alone, routine intramuscular analgesia or pain management with aspirin-phenacetin-codeine is generally sufficient. Wound care, pain, and maintenance of joint motion do not pose nearly the same problems as they do after open synovectomy. The patient's Hemovac will usually drain briskly for 5 to 10 minutes only and then slow dramatically. It is usually withdrawn on the morning of the first postoperative day. Between periods of continuous passive motion, the patient is allowed to intermittently get out of bed and ambulate, with partial weight-bearing as tolerated on the surgically treated led and crutches used for assistance. The patient uses the muscle stimulator for four 30-minute periods daily and is taught quadriceps sets and straight leg raising exercises prior to discharge. Physical therapy is usually begun 2 to 3 days after discharge and continued until maximum benefit is achieved.

Continuous passive motion is employed at home for a minimum of 18 hours per day for 1 to 2 weeks or until the patient can freely move the surgically treated limb voluntarily through a normal full range of motion and do stationary cycling both at home and during physical therapy. Aspiration is often performed 1 week postoperatively, at the first postoperative outpatient examination. Intraarticular corticosteroid therapy may or may not be given, depending upon the circumstances of the case. Most patients are fully ambulatory without crutches by 1 to 2 weeks postoperatively and have regained a full range of motion within 2 to 3 weeks postoperatively.

Our expectations after arthroscopic synovectomy depend on the problem for which the procedure is done. For rheumatoid arthritis, the most common indication, the patient will obtain relief of symptoms for from 3 to 6 years. Eventually the synovium regrows and the inflammatory process recurs, but until this happens, patients are comfortable and satisfied with the results of arthroscopic synovectomy. For other diseases, such as PVNS, the results vary with the extent of joint involvement. Although arthroscopic techniques are best for removing the most synovium from the knee with PVNS, it is almost impossible to remove every cell, and recurrences are therefore frequent. Synovectomy associated with degenerative joint disease depends on the extent of arthritic involvement. The more severely damaged the joint, the poorer the result. Therefore, arthroscopic synovectomy offers many advantages in the overall management of patients with synovial disease, but cannot be considered a definitive treatment and varies with the disease process.

COMPLICATIONS

Surgical complications of arthroscopic synovectomy can include neurovascular injury from improperly located portals or overaggressive tissue resection. Proper portal placement is one of the most basic aspects of any arthroscopic technique. Paying attention to anatomic landmarks and using the 70-degree arthroscope when creating access portals to the posterior compartments helps to avoid problems. In my experience, excessive bleeding has never been a problem. Similarly, the continuous use of passive motion postoperatively, along with early and aggressive physical therapy, has kept loss of joint motion from being a problem. Only in those cases in which synovectomy has been combined with joint manipulation for preexisting capsular contracture has subnormal final joint motion been obtained after this procedure. Chronically draining synovial fistulae are a possible complication, although none have occurred in my surgical experience.

ILLUSTRATIVE CASE FOR TECHNIQUE

A 32-year old woman presented with a 2-year history of recurrent right knee effusion, unresponsive both to conservative treatment and to a recent arthroscopic joint lavage and partial synovectomy (done elsewhere, without synovial biopsy). Her past history was significant for an open medial meniscectomy done 5 years earlier. Her joint fluid was sometimes sanguinous, and the diagnosis of PVNS was entertained. A hemosiderin-weighted MRI scan demonstrated large quantities of hemosiderin-laden synovial tissue in her suprapatellar pouch (Fig. 10), as well as what appeared to be similar tissue filling up the entire gastrocnemius–semimembranosus bursa (Fig. 11).

Arthroscopic synovial biopsy under local anesthesia confirmed the preoperative diagnosis of diffuse PVNS. Complete, four-compartment arthroscopic synovectomy was done shortly thereafter, using the technique described in this chapter

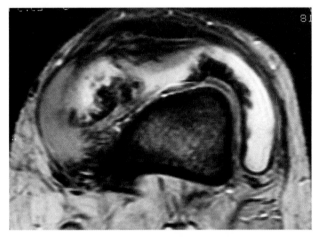

Figure 10. Preoperative, hemosiderin-weighted MRI scan (transverse section) demonstrates a large effusion with proliferative, hemosiderin-laden synovial tissue in the suprapatellar pouch, highly suggestive of PVNS.

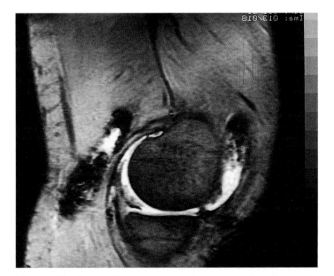

Figure 11. Magnetic resonance image section in medial sagittal plane demonstrates hemosiderin-laden tissue filling the gastrocnemius–semimembranosus bursa extra-articularly.

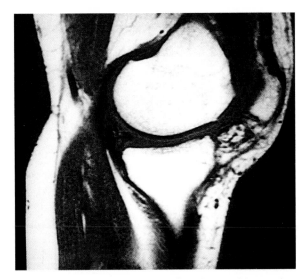

Figure 12. Repeat MRI scan of patient at 18 months postoperatively, shows absence of prior or recurrent PVNS tissue.

along with open posteromedial exploration and excision of the gastrocnemius–semimembranosus bursa, which indeed was distended with rust-colored PVNS tissue. Continuous epidural anesthesia was employed for the first 24 hours postoperatively, along with continuous passive motion. No surgical complications resulted. Continuous passive motion was used at home for 2 weeks, followed by a physical therapy regimen. The patient experienced resolution of her effusions and full knee function was restored. An MRI scan at 18 months postoperatively (Fig. 12) demonstrated no evidence of intraarticular or posteromedial extraarticular PVNS. The patient is now 4½ years past synovectomy with no clinical signs of recurrent disease.

RECOMMENDED READING

1. Rosenberg, T.: *An Illustrated Guide to Arthroscopic Synovectomy of the Knee.* Andover, MA: Smith & Nephew–Dyonics, Inc., 1991.
2. Johnson, L. L.: Arthroscopic synovectomy. In: *Arthroscopic Surgery—Principles and Practice,* 3rd ed. C.V. Mosby, St. Louis, 1986.

Subject Index